A Cancer Survivor's Almanac

Charting Your Journey

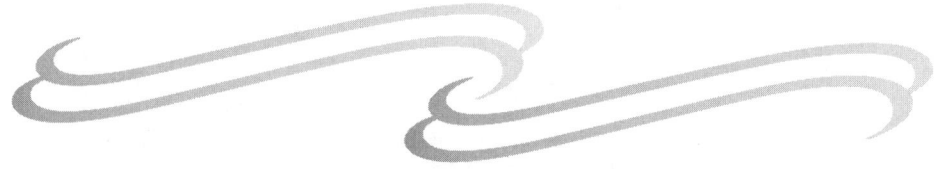

National Coalition for Cancer Survivorship
Edited by Barbara Hoffman, JD

WITH AN INTRODUCTION BY FITZHUGH MULLAN, MD

JOHN WILEY & SONS, INC.

New York • Chichester • Weinheim • Brisbane • Singapore • Toronto

Illustrations are courtesy of Pen & Palette, a not-for-profit corporation which uses art and poetry by cancer survivors to offer emotional support and to benefit cancer research and awareness programs. Pen & Palette, 29 Ver Planck Street, Albany, NY 12206.

This book is printed on acid-free paper. ☉

Copyright © 1996 by National Coalition for Cancer Survivorship. All rights reserved
Published by John Wiley & Sons, Inc.

Published simultaneously in Canada
Previously published by Chronimed Publishing

Illustrations are courtesy of Pen & Palette, a not-for-profit corporation which uses art and poetry by cancer survivors to offer emotional support and to benefit cancer research and awareness programs. Pen & Palette, 29 Ver Planck Street, Albany, NY 12206.

No part of this publication may be reproduced, stored in a retrieval system or transmitted in any form or by any means, electronic, mechanical, photocopying, recording, scanning or otherwise, except as permitted under Sections 107 or 108 of the 1976 United States Copyright Act, without either the prior written permission of the Publisher, or authorization through payment of the appropriate per-copy fee to the Copyright Clearance Center, 222 Rosewood Drive, Danvers, MA 01923, (978) 750-8400, fax (978) 750-4744. Requests to the Publisher for permission should be addressed to the Permissions Department, John Wiley & Sons, Inc., 605 Third Avenue, New York, NY 10158-0012, (212) 850-6011, fax (212) 850-6008, E-Mail: PERMREQ@WILEY.COM.

The information contained in this book is not intended to serve as a replacement for professional medical advice. Any use of the information in this book is at the reader's discretion. The author and the publisher specifically disclaim any and all liability arising directly or indirectly from the use or application of any information contained in this book. A health care professional should be consulted regarding your specific situation.

ISBN 0-471-34669-1

Printed in the United States of America

10 9 8 7 6 5 4 3 2

Table of Contents

ACKNOWLEDGMENTS IX

THE BIRTH OF NCCS XIII

INTRODUCTION – SURVIVORSHIP: A POWERFUL PLACE
by Fitzhugh Mullan, MD XV

PART ONE – TAKING CARE OF YOUR MEDICAL NEEDS

CHAPTER ONE – UNDERSTANDING CANCER, ITS TREATMENT, AND THE SIDE EFFECTS OF TREATMENT
by Patricia Ganz, MD 3

What Is Cancer?	5	Types of Treatment	9
What Is Cancer Treatment?	6	New Approaches	9
Phases of Treatment	7	Clinical Trials	11

SYMPTOMS AND SIDE EFFECTS 12

Pain	12	Skin Changes	19
Fatigue	14	Neurotoxicity	19
Nutrition and		Loss of Concentration	19
Weight Maintenance	15	Respiratory Problems	20
Hair Loss	17	Sexual Functioning	20
Low Blood Counts	18	Contraception and Sterility	21

MEDICAL PROBLEMS OF LONG TERM SURVIVORS 23

Long-Term and Late Effects	23	Other Late Effects	26
Monitoring for			
Recurrence	25		

CANCER PREVENTION AND EARLY DETECTION 27

Eliminating the		Sexually Transmitted	
Use of Tobacco	27	Diseases and Cancer	29
Eating a Well-Balanced		Chemoprevention Trials	29
Diet	28	Reporting Warning Signs	
Avoiding Excessive		to Your Doctor	30
Radiation	28		
Decreasing Alcohol			
Consumption	29		

A CANCER *survivor's* ALMANAC

CHAPTER TWO – WORKING WITH YOUR DOCTOR AND HOSPITAL SYSTEM: BECOMING A WISE CONSUMER
by Natalie Davis Spingarn and Nancy H. Chasen, JD **31**

GATHERING INFORMATION AND CHOOSING A DOCTOR 33
A Historical Perspective	33	The Primary Doctor:	
A Changing Medical Arena	34	Orchestrating Your Care	35
Learning About Your Treatment	34		

COMMUNICATIONS – THE TWO WAY STREET 39
Barriers to Communication	39	
Suggestions for Effective and Meaningful Communication	40	

THE HOSPITAL: A WORLD UNTO ITSELF 43
Evaluating Hospitals	43	Going Home and	
The Hospital Experience	47	Reentering Society	50
Dealing with Hospital Life	49		

KNOWING AND UNDERSTANDING YOUR RIGHTS:
INFORMED CONSENT, CONFIDENTIALITY, PATIENT RECORDS 50
Informed Consent: Your Right to Choose and Refuse Treatment	50	Confidentiality New Challenges to Confidentiality	52 56

CHAPTER THREE – THE HEALTH CARE TEAM: WORKING TOGETHER FOR YOUR BENEFIT
by Diane Blum, ACSW **61**

Social Workers	63	Rehabilitation Specialists	67
Psychologists and Psychiatrists	65	Dietary or Nutritional Services	68
Nurses and Home Health Aides	66	Hospice Care Clergy	69 70

CHAPTER FOUR – UNDERSTANDING THE RISKS AND BENEFITS OF UNCONVENTIONAL TREATMENT
by Natalie Davis Spingarn **73**

CAVEAT EMPTOR: UNCONVENTIONAL TREATMENTS 75
Curious and Willing to Try	75
Categories of Unconventional Treatments	76

MIXING CONVENTIONAL AND UNCONVENTIONAL 78

Out of the Closet	79	Suggestions for Survivors	82
Unconventional Issues	79		

PART TWO– TAKING CARE OF YOUR EMOTIONAL, SPIRITUAL AND SOCIAL NEEDS

CHAPTER FIVE – MIND AND BODY: HARNESSING YOUR INNER RESOURCES
by Neil Fiore, PhD **91**

THE PERSONAL IMPACT OF CANCER 93

Discovering Strategies for Healing	94	Replacing Negative Reactions	97
Diagnosing the Diagnosis – and Your Beliefs	95	Coping with Powerful Emotions	97

THE SOCIAL IMPACT OF CANCER 102

Changes in Self-Perception	102	Gaining Control Over Stress	108
Friends' Reactions	104		
Coworkers' Reactions	104	Transformation – New Potential for the Cancer Survivor	111
Changes in Relationships	105		

CHAPTER SIX – FAMILY CHALLENGES: COMMUNICATION, HOPE, AND LOSS
by Elizabeth Johns Clark, PhD, MSW **115**

CANCER IS A FAMILY CRISIS 118

Family Communication	118	Enhancing Family Communication	123
Barriers to Family Communication	119	Maintaining Family Hope	125
Family Coping Styles	121	Avoiding Family Burnout	127
Multiple Family Problems	122		

LIFE AFTER THE CANCER CRISIS 129

LOSS AND GRIEF 130

Family Tasks During Terminal Illness	130	Recommended Grieving Behaviors	133
Managing Grief	132	Hiding Grief	133

Chapter Seven – Reaching Out: The Power of Peer Support
by Catherine Logan-Carrillo 137

Peer Support in the Cancer Survivorship Movement: A Brief History	139	
The Value of Peer Support	141	
How Peer Support Differs from Professional Counseling	143	
The Role of Health-Care Providers in Peer-Support Organizations	145	
Peer-Led Support Groups vs. Professionally-Led Support Groups	145	
Choosing the Right Peer-Support Program	146	
Have You Found the Right Group?	148	
Guiding Principles of Effective Peer-Support Groups	148	
Rewards of Giving Back to Your Support Group	149	
Creating Your Own Peer-Support Group	149	
Resources to Help You Build and Sustain Your Group	153	
Peer Support with a Multi-cultural Focus	155	
Established Peer-Support Organizations	155	
The Role of Peer-Support Networks in the Culture of Survivorship	161	

PART THREE – TAKING CARE OF BUSINESS: INSURANCE, EMPLOYMENT, LEGAL, AND FINANCIAL MATTERS

Chapter Eight – Straight Talk about Insurance and Health Plans
by Kimberley Calder, MPS and Irene C. Card 167

INTRODUCTION—HEALTH INSURANCE IN TRANSFORMATION 169

TYPES OF HEALTH INSURANCE 170

Fee-for-service (or Indemnity) Policies	170	Managed Care Plans	173	
Catastrophic Insurance and Medical Savings Accounts	170	Hospital Indemnity Policies	175	
Disability Insurance	172	Long-Term Care Insurance	175	
		Medicare	176	
		Medicaid	181	

OBTAINING AND MAINTAINING HEALTH COVERAGE 182

Your Legal Right to Health Insurance	183	
Health Insurance for Individuals and Dependents	189	

GETTING THE MOST OUT OF YOUR HEALTH INSURANCE 191

Collecting Health		Coverage of Investigational or	
Insurance Benefits	192	Experimental Therapies	195

LIFE INSURANCE AND "LIVING BENEFITS" 196

CONCLUSION—WHEN ALL ELSE FAILS 200

GLOSSARY OF INSURANCE TERMS 201

CHAPTER NINE – WORKING IT OUT: YOUR EMPLOYMENT RIGHTS
by Barbara Hoffman, JD **205**

EMPLOYMENT DISCRIMINATION 207

Employment Problems		State Laws	217
Faced by Cancer Survivors	207	How to Avoid Employment	
Reasons for Employment		Discrimination	222
Discrimination	209	How to Enforce Your	
When Cancer-Based		Legal Rights	225
Discrimination Is Illegal	209	Finding a Lawyer	230
Federal Laws	209		

WORKER'S COMPENSATION LAWS 231

UNEMPLOYMENT DISABILITY LAWS 232

VOCATIONAL REHABILITATION 232

CONCLUSION 236

CHAPTER TEN – LEGAL AND FINANCIAL CONCERNS
by Barbara Hoffman, JD **237**

FINANCIAL COSTS AND RESOURCES 239

The Expenses		Public Sources of	
of Cancer Treatment	239	Financial Support	241
Sources of Financial			
Support	240		

PLANNING YOUR PERSONAL AND FINANCIAL FUTURE 244

Personal Planning:		Financial Planning: Planning	
Advance Health Directives	245	for Your Property	248

OTHER LEGAL CONCERNS OF CANCER SURVIVORS 250

Medical Malpractice	250	Adopting a Child	255
Access to Financial Credit	254		

PART FOUR – TAKING CARE OF YOURSELF

CHAPTER ELEVEN – DEFINING OUR DESTINY
by Susan Leigh, RN, BSN..**261**

Cancer Myths	263	Stages of Survivorship	267
Birth of a Movement	265	Seasons of Survival	268
The Semantics of Survivorship	266		

CHAPTER TWELVE – SURVIVORS AS ADVOCATES
by Ellen Stovall and Elizabeth Johns Clark, PhD, MSW **273**

Cancer Survivors Can Advocate for Themselves	276	Cancer Survivors as Advocates for Others	279
Empowered Survivors	277	Conclusion	280
You Can Learn Self-Advocacy	277		

RESOURCES **281**

INDEX **327**

Acknowledgments

This book is the result of the contributions of thousands of cancer survivors, their families and caregivers, as well as health professionals, attorneys, and community leaders who have shared their experiences and knowledge with us.

Barbara Hoffman extends her special appreciation to Elizabeth Johns Clark, PhD and Linda Klein for their invaluable editorial work. She also wishes to thank Fitzhugh Mullan for asking her to coedit the original *Charting the Journey,* Terrence Campbell for laying the initial foundation for the book, and Sally McElroy and Susan Scherr for serving as our unofficial business managers. She is grateful to Jonathan Ebersole, vice president of publications at Chronimed Publishing, and to Philip Spitzer, her literary agent, for their faith in this project.

The authors greatly appreciate the assistance of the many who contributed to individual chapters, including the following persons:

CHAPTER 1: Dr. Ganz's family, professional colleagues and research staff, and patients and friends in the survivorship community who have provided her with the support and encouragement to pursue her interest in improving the quality of life for those affected by cancer.

CHAPTER 3: Myra Glajchen, DWS, who authored the chapter "Helping Therapies and Support Services" in *Charting the Journey: An Almanac of Practical Resources for Cancer Survivors.*

CHAPTER 5: Fran Marcus Lewis, PhD; of the University of Washington at Seattle; Lydia Temoshok, PhD; of Walter Reed Army Hospital; and David Spiegel, MD, of Stanford University School of Medicine for their personal support and excellent research on psychosocial issues.

CHAPTER 6: Ellen Stovall and Karrie Zampini, CSW, for their helpful comments on the manuscript, and Stephenie Jones for her assistance in preparing the manuscript.

CHAPTER 7: Beth Pinkerton and Gena Love of People Living Through Cancer; Anne Shaw Turnage and Martha Maddox, PhD, of CAnCare of Houston; Pat Fobair, LCSW, MPH of *Surviving!;* Linda Williams of Operation Uplift; Edward Madara of the National Self-Help Clearinghouse.

CHAPTERS 9 AND 10: Gail Broder, JD, Daniel Fiduccia, Thelma Hoffman, Frank Hoffman, MD, Ralph Shapiro, PhD, and Samuel Turner, JD, for their invaluable comments on the manuscript; L. Susan Slavin, JD, Theresa Laverhass, JD, and Sonia Ward of the National Cancer Institute for research assistance; and Kristina Thomson, LCSW, for information on adoption services and rights.

CHAPTER 12: Everyone who works to ensure that the voice of cancer survivors is valued across all domains of cancer care: cancer survivors, professional caregivers, and researchers. Their writing, teaching, and advocacy on behalf of cancer survivorship inspired this chapter. Special acknowledgment goes to the founding members of the National Coalition for Cancer Survivorship (NCCS) whose vision provided the leadership for a national survivorship movement and awakened the public to the need for advocacy by and for cancer survivors.

RESOURCES: Carla Sofka, PhD, MSW, for information about online services.

Additionally, the editors and authors express their appreciation to their families and to the staff of the NCCS for their patience, support, energy, and insight.

The Birth of NCCS

The NCCS was founded at a first-of-its-kind national meeting in October 1986. The three-day meeting held in Albuquerque, New Mexico, assembled leaders from across the country who have taken leadership roles in the cancer survivorship movement. Twenty-one participants were chosen from respondents to a national survey taken in the summer of 1986. That survey gathered basic information on organizations and individuals filling two criteria: first, they were addressing the concerns of cancer survivors, and second, they focused on peer support as a fundamental part of addressing those concerns. The survey's respondents expressed a desire to join a national networking organization. To explore the possibility of establishing such an organization, the October national meeting was convened.

The survey and the planning meeting were developed by New Mexico cancer survivors working out of the office of People Living Through Cancer, Inc., New Mexico's cancer survivor organization. Funding was provided by St. Joseph Cancer Center of Albuquerque and St. Vincent Hospital of Santa Fe.

The October meeting, which has been called the "Constitutional Convention" of the cancer survivor movement, provided an opportunity for leaders from across the country to meet, to look at the growing national movement, and to define its needs and potentials. The focus of attention was the strengthening of the national movement.

The meeting began with a sharing of information and an assessment of the then-current state of the movement. That was followed by a lengthy discussion of the needs of individuals and organizations involved with survivorship, and of the potential of the survivorship movement. The participants were then ready to formulate a statement of the goals and objectives of the yet-unborn organization. The primary goal would be to generate a national awareness of cancer survivorship. Specific goals would include developing a communication network and a comprehensive clearinghouse for survivorship materials, advocating the rights of survivors, and promoting the study of survivorship.

During the final day of the meeting, a carefully crafted charter was approved and the structure of the infant organization was established. From among the participants, the founding members (pictured at left), funds were raised to support the organization for its first six months.

The meeting was enormously successful. On October 26, 1986, the new organization was born, and NCCS's work had just begun.

> The primary goal would be to generate a national awareness of cancer survivorship.
>
> Specific goals would include developing a communication network and a comprehensive clearinghouse for survivorship materials, advocating the rights of survivors, and promoting the study of survivorship.

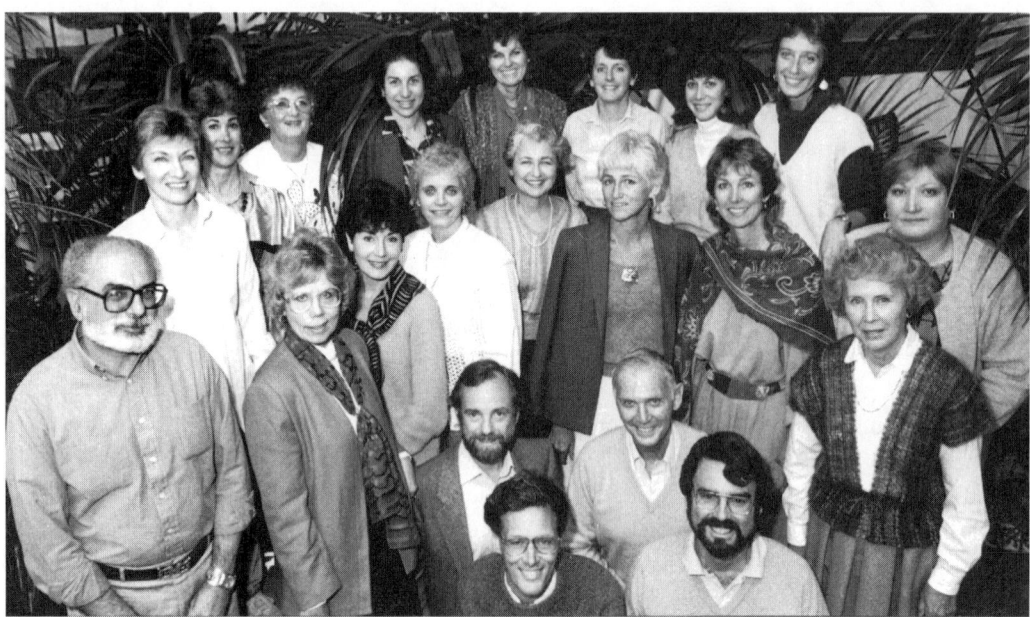

Photo by Michael Rasmussen.

The founding members of the National Coalition for Cancer Survivorship take time for a group photo after the October 24-26, 1986, meeting in Albuquerque. They are (left to right, bottom to top): Michael Lerner, Commonweal, Bolinas, CA; Fitzhugh Mullan, Garrett Park, MD; Neil Fiore, Albany, CA; Harold Benjamin, The Wellness Community, Santa Monica, CA; Pamela La Fayette, Cancer Lifeline, Seattle, WA; Helen Crothers, American Cancer Society, Oakland, CA; Barbara Waligora-Serafin, Harrington Cancer Center, Amarillo, TX; Estelle Weissburg, Cancer Guidance Institute, Pittsburgh, PA; Alice Hiat, Albuquerque, NM; Shannon McGowan. Cancer Support Community, Point Richmond, CA; Peggie Carey, Life After Cancer, Asheville, NC; Al Hiat, Albuquerque, NM; Julie Becker, Cancer Share, Cincinnati, OH; Yvonne Soghamonian, Candlelighters Childhood Cancer Foundation, Washington, DC; Shirley Miller, Cancer Hot Line, Plantation, FL; Patricia Ganz, UCLA Cancer Rehabilitation Project, Los Angeles, CA; Susan Leigh, University of Arizona Cancer Center, Tuscon, AZ; Catherine Logan-Carrillo, People Living Through Cancer, Albuquerque, NM; Barbara Hoffman, Cancer Patients' Employment Rights Project, Philadelphia, PA; Wendy Traber, *Surviving!,* Stanford, CA; Jan Kinzler, Oncology Nursing Society, Pittsburgh, PA.

A CANCER *survivor's* ALMANAC

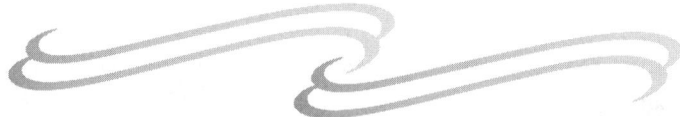

Introduction

Survivorship: A Powerful Place

by Fitzhugh Mullan, MD

"A rocky battle with mediastinal seminoma in the midseventies led me to help found the NCCS in the mid-eighties. Since that time, I have been privileged to serve first as president and now as chair of the Board of Directors of the NCCS. My special interest is developing local cancer support organizations and coalitions."

Fitzhugh Mullan, MD

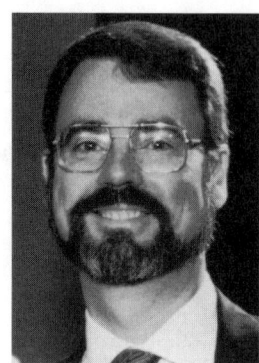

FITZHUGH MULLAN, MD is a cofounder of the National Coalition for Cancer Survivorship (NCCS) and chair of the Board of Directors, serving as its president from 1986 to 1990. Dr. Mullan has written widely about his own cancer experience, including *Vital Signs: A Young Doctor's Struggle with Cancer,* Farrar, Straus and Giroux (1983), and "The Seasons of Survival: Reflections of a Physician with Cancer" in *The New England Journal of Medicine,* (July 25, 1985). Dr. Mullan is currently a professor of pediatrics at the George Washington University School of Medicine and is a contributing editor of the journal *Health Affairs.* Dr. Mullan has recently retired from a 23-year career in the United States Public Health Service, where he rose to the rank of Assistant Surgeon General.

Survivorship is a reason for celebration. It is the act of battling adversity and hanging tough despite bad luck and difficult circumstances. It is living with a constant life challenge that pits the desire to live against the possibility of death. Day-by-day survivorship is a victory because it is the act of living on, no matter what happens.

> No matter how severe the symptoms and the treatments, survival from day to day, week to week, and year to year constitutes an enormous personal and human triumph over what might have been.

Survivorship is not some club you join after several months of treatment—or after five years or ten years. Rather, survivorship is lifelong, beginning with the diagnosis of cancer and continuing for the balance of life—through the medical studies and treatments, the financial and vocational trials, the ups and the downs. Cancer survivorship is the challenge faced daily by millions of Americans who are engaged in defiance of disease and in affirmation of life. The disease-free return to active life and terminal care and palliative treatments are all part of the continuum of survivorship. No matter how severe the symptoms and the treatments, survival from day to day, week to week, and year to year constitutes an enormous personal and human triumph over what might have been.

A cancer diagnosis, however, is always an unwelcome and unexpected intruder in the life of an individual or a family, a one-way ticket across a wide and swift river to a land on the far bank. This becomes the land of cancer survivorship, with its own biology, its own psychology, and its own community. It is a land where family and friends, and doctors and nurses can visit, but where the survivor becomes a permanent resident. It is a land that, until recently, received very little attention and had few maps and no constitution.

That land is changing quickly—and for the better. This book is the product of—and a tribute to—the survivors of today who are bringing a new sense of community and mutual support to this new land. The far bank is now well populated with energetic, gifted, brave people. It always has had ample numbers of new recruits as well as seasoned veterans. What has been missing, though, is recognition, identity, and mission. Too often, cancer has been treated as an embarrassment and a cause for mortal fear, with families and individuals having little awareness that help, information, role models, guidance, and support might be available from others with cancer. This community in the past has tended to live alone, paying little attention to the other inhabitants of that land and taking little strength or sustenance from one another.

Survivorship: A Powerful Place – **INTRODUCTION**

The survivorship movement is changing that by finding ways to map and civilize this new territory. Survivors are talking publicly and writing about their experiences so that others can understand this foreign land. They are meeting together and sharing their experiences, frustrations, and hopes; staffing telephone hot lines; organizing support groups; and publishing newsletters. They are active politically, testifying on Capitol Hill about health insurance reform and research budgets, pressing the National Cancer Institute and the Food and Drug Administration for faster approval for new drugs, and working at the state and local levels for better insurance coverage and fair employment policies. These efforts are making the land on the other side of the river a better place—warmer, more habitable, more informed, and less solitary.

The National Coalition for Cancer Survivorship has led the survivorship movement since its founding in 1986. The NCCS is dedicated to developing a network of people and organizations concerned with all aspects of cancer care—from the personal to the political. In 1990, an NCCS team of survivors and cancer experts working in conjunction with Consumer Reports published the NCCS's first book, *Charting the Journey: An Almanac of Practical Resources for Cancer Survivors*. Rich in poetry, art, and quotations, the *Almanac* addressed all aspects of cancer care—from the basics of oncology to insurance and money matters.

This book carries on the style and tradition of the *Almanac* with the same patient-oriented perspective, but it has been greatly expanded and updated in terms of information and perspective. Both the survivorship movement and the practice of oncology have prospered and changed in the six years since the original volume was published. This book is designed to make the more sophisticated survivorship world of today easily understandable to survivors, their families, and their caregivers.

Neither this book nor the NCCS prescribes a right or wrong way to be a survivor or advocates specific treatments or choices. Every cancer experience is different and what people bring to it varies as much as they do. The authors of this book have recorded their experiences and their advice for you in the spirit of mapping the land and building the community. Their information, counsel, anecdotes, art, poems, charts, humor, sorrow, and wisdom are testimony that no one is alone in the battle against cancer, no matter how newly diagnosed, sick, or discouraged. Survivorship, in fact, has proved revitalizing to many, forging new intellectual, spiritual, and personal connections. Life for these individuals, as the book testifies, is no longer measured in time—but in quality.

Although much has been accomplished in civilizing the land across the river, still more remains to be done. All survivors, as well as their families, friends, and loved ones, have an important role to play in the survivorship movement. We hope that this book will help you and those who care about you in your struggle with cancer and that, in time, you may be able to provide guidance to others.

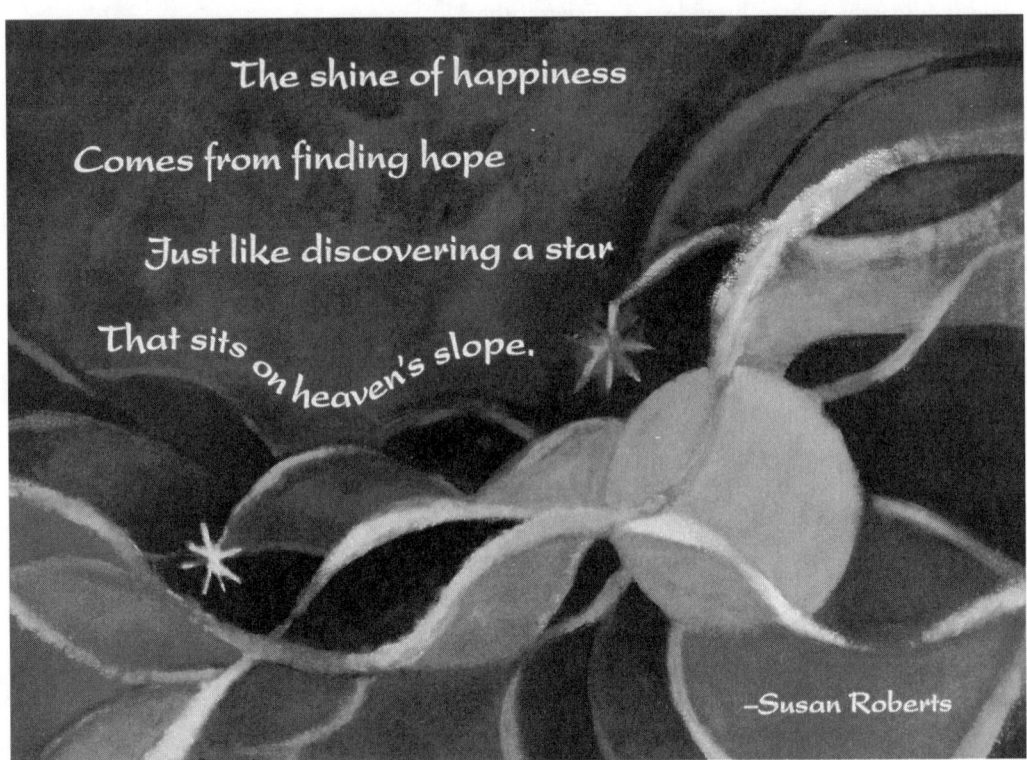

DISCOVERING A STAR

*The shine of happiness
Comes from finding hope
Just like discovering a star
That sits on heaven's slope.
           — Susan Roberts*

Part One

Taking Care of Your Medical Needs

*Understanding Cancer,
Its Treatment, and the
Side Effects of
Treatment* 1

*Working with Your Doctor
and Hospital: Becoming
a Wise Consumer* 31

*The Health Care Team:
Working Together for
Your Benefit*...........61

*Understanding the Risks
and Benefits of
Unconventional
Treatment*..............75

A CANCER *Survivor's* ALMANAC

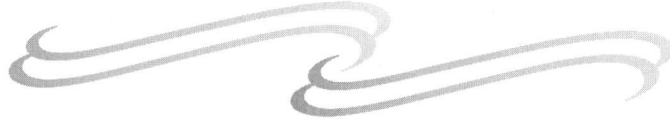

Chapter One

Understanding Cancer, Its Treatment, and the Side Effects of Treatment

by Patricia Ganz, MD

"In my research, I have focused on the long-term, late effects that may occur in individuals with a cancer history. For this reason, it was important to me to be involved in the start-up of an organization like the NCCS, which is primarily interested in cancer survivorship."

Patricia Ganz, MD

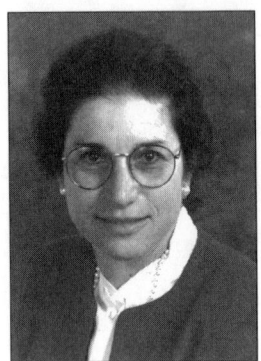

PATRICIA GANZ, MD is a cofounder of the National Coalition for Cancer Survivorship and serves on its Board of Advisors. As a medical oncologist, she has spent the past 15 years doing systematic research on the health-related quality of life of patients with cancer. Dr. Ganz is currently a professor at the Schools of Medicine and Public Health, University of California at Los Angeles, where she also serves as director of the Division of Cancer Prevention and Control Research of the Jonsson Comprehensive Cancer Center. Her research has been sponsored by the National Cancer Institute, the American Cancer Society, California Division, and the Department of Defense. She is the former chair of the Committee on Patient Advocacy of the American Society of Clinical Oncology and is a nationally recognized leader in the field of cancer rehabilitation and quality-of-life assessment in cancer treatment trials.

*A*s YOU BEGIN YOUR JOURNEY — Each of you is part of a growing community of cancer patients who are pioneers experiencing the benefits and difficulties of survivorship. As you journey through the phases of cancer survivorship, you often will be the one to provide information and education to your family, friends, and even physicians about the medical and physical effects of your treatment. Knowing as much as possible about your disease, its treatments, and its potential effects on your body can empower you to take charge of your health and help you make the most of your survivorship experience.

While this chapter could not be comprehensive, it is a starting point for developing your personal educational agenda. Resources referred to throughout this chapter and throughout this book will enable you to familiarize yourself with what you need to know and will assist you in getting the information you require.

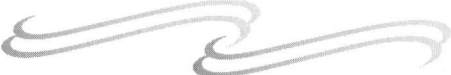

You may find yourself in unfamiliar territory as you begin your journey as a cancer survivor. Part of the challenge is a new vocabulary and a technical environment that a patient cannot avoid. To the extent that you can familiarize yourself with this foreign environment, you will be empowered with greater control over your condition and over your needs for health care.

What Is Cancer?

Cancer is the general term used to describe a large group of diseases whose hallmark is the uncontrolled growth of cells in the tissue in which the cancer arises. Before a single cell commits itself to a malignant and irreversible course, a long precancerous period exists in which cells may appear normal but have already acquired some of the genetic changes that will become cancer. From this single cancer cell, over the course of many years, a malignant tumor will become clinically detectable. The whole process, from the beginning of the earliest changes in the DNA to the detection of a clinically apparent cancer, may take as long as 20 years.

The goals of current cancer screening and prevention efforts are (1) to detect cancers in a premalignant phase—for example, colon polyps—and either to remove them or to prevent the conversion of genetically abnormal cells into malignant cells through the use of medications; and (2) to detect cancers when they are localized and have not spread outside the tissue of origin. Other approaches, such as immunizations against infections that may precede cancer—such as hepatitis B—may in fact reduce the incidence of some cancers—liver cancer, for example.

Cancer cells at first grow locally, but they eventually invade and destroy the surrounding tissues. Cancer cells also have a propensity to spread to other parts of the body through the lymph system or bloodstream. In general, the smaller and more localized the tumor, the better the prognosis. However, some cancers, such as leukemia and lymphoma, are widespread at diagnosis in most cases.

In general, most newly diagnosed cancer patients will go through a series of staging tests, including blood work, x-rays, and scans, to determine the extent of the disease. Your doctor is the best person to consult regarding the details of your illness and treatment; however, it may be useful for you to understand the stage or extensiveness of your disease, as that information will be important to understanding your prognosis—the likely outcome of treatment for your disease.

What Is Cancer Treatment?

After you have been diagnosed with cancer, a treatment plan for your unique medical situation will be developed based on all of the information that has been gathered through blood tests, radiological studies, surgery, and microscopic and biochemical evaluations of your cancer. The treatment plan that your doctors develop will have a specific goal. In general, the possibilities include cure, long-term control of the cancer, or symptomatic relief only.

CURE – Cure is the goal for a wide range of cancers today, and over half of newly diagnosed cancer patients will be cured of their disease. *Cure,* from the medical point of view, means that all of the cancer can be removed successfully by surgery, or completely eliminated from the body through the use of medications or radiation treatments. Cure also implies that the likelihood of the cancer returning at a later date—either in the same local area or in a distant organ—is extremely low. *Curative intent* treatment means that the initial treatment plan is chosen with the expectation that the patient will be cured.

Although some people have focused on five years of disease-free survival as the equivalent of cure, others may have a very high likelihood of long-term cure after as few as two years of treatment. On the other hand, some may be at risk for recurrent cancer for much longer than five years. In terms of treatment, however, the goal is the distinguishing characteristic, not the length of time it takes to attain it. Today, curative intent treatment is a realistic goal for many newly diagnosed cancer patients.

LONG-TERM CONTROL – Long-term control of cancer is the treatment goal for many cancer patients. This means that the aim of the treatment is to modify the course of the disease, usually by temporarily eliminating the cancer, slowing its growth, and controlling its symptoms. In many cases, the cancer becomes resistant to the treatment and returns. Chronic leukemias, myeloma, and some non-Hodgkin's lymphomas are examples of cancers for which treatment provides long-term control.

SYMPTOM RELIEF – Symptom relief only (sometimes called *palliation*) is the treatment goal for most patients with advanced cancers. These cancers, in general, demonstrate only a minor response to chemotherapy or radiation, and are too extensive to be removed with surgery. Chemotherapy and radiation are used frequently with advanced cancers, but primarily for symptom relief rather than elimination of the cancer. In addition to anticancer treatment, measures for pain relief and medication for depression, anxiety, and any other symptoms caused by the cancer will usually be included in the treatment plan.

> When cancer is diagnosed, it has usually existed in a subclinical form for many years. For this reason, you should not be afraid of delaying treatment in order to obtain a second opinion. If metastases have occurred, they have done so during the time before the cancer was detected. Waiting a few weeks to seek appropriate opinions and to define the best treatment plan is an inconsequential amount of time in the life of the cancer.

PHASES OF TREATMENT

INITIAL DIAGNOSTIC AND TREATMENT PHASE – This phase starts with your first encounter with the doctor to report new symptoms or to undergo tests, including a biopsy of the cancer—which is the removal of a small piece of tissue for microscopic examination. Next comes a consultation with a number of experts and consultants to establish the initial treatment plan. For most cancers, a delay of a few weeks to complete various diagnostic tests and consultations should be expected, and this often is the best time to define the treatment plan that will give you the best chance of cure or long-term survival. On rare occasions, treatment will be started immediately.

When cancer is diagnosed, it has usually existed in a subclinical form for many years. For this reason, you should not be afraid of delaying treatment in order to obtain a second opinion. If metastases have occurred, they have done so during the time before the cancer was detected. Waiting a few weeks to seek appropriate opinions and to define the best treatment plan is an inconsequential amount of time in the life of the cancer.

Understanding Cancer, Its Treatment, and the Side Effects of Treatment – **CHAPTER ONE**

MAINTENANCE PHASE – The maintenance phase of treatment is a time when treatment is continued but usually on a less intensive schedule. For example, maintenance therapy is commonly given to children with acute lymphocytic leukemia (ALL). For some kinds of cancer treatment, this may include a consolidation or late-intensification treatment in which high doses of chemotherapy are given as a final booster before discontinuing treatments.

FOLLOW-UP CARE – The follow-up care phase is the time after completion of surgery, radiation therapy, chemotherapy, or a combination of treatments, when it is thought that the cancer has been eradicated completely. During this phase you will be recovering from the short-term effects of treatment and beginning to resume a more normal life, with less frequent visits to the doctor. Initially you may see your doctor every one or two months, and then only three or four times a year. During these visits the doctor will perform a careful interview and physical examination, with emphasis on possible symptoms related to the cancer and any residual side effects from your treatments. You will also have regular blood tests and other studies to monitor your condition. As you get further away from the time of your initial cancer treatment, your visits with the doctor will be less frequent; nevertheless, you will need life-long follow-up because of possible problems which occur secondary to cancer treatment, such as the risk of new cancers or recurrence.

CANCER RECURRENCE – Cancer may recur in the same part of your body where it was found originally (a local recurrence), or it may reappear in a more distant part of your body (a metastasis). In either case, a new treatment plan must be developed. Diagnostic tests will be repeated to determine the extent of the cancer recurrence. The type of treatment that is selected for the recurring cancer will depend on the specific type of cancer, on its extensiveness, and on what previous therapy was given. Some recurrent cancers can still be cured, although the chance for cure is usually lower than it is for the first incidence of cancer.

Advanced and incurable cancer may exist at the time of diagnosis, or it may occur after many years of cancer treatment and follow-up care. In either case, the usual goal of treatment for this phase of cancer is symptom relief. Some patients, however, may want to participate in clinical trials of new experimental treatments (see page 11 for an explanation of *clinical trials*).

TYPES OF TREATMENT

Traditionally, cancer has been treated with surgery, radiation, chemotherapy, or combinations of the three.

SURGERY – Surgery can be performed under local or general anesthesia, and it may be limited to a biopsy or it may be very extensive. A number of cancers—colorectal and lung cancer, for example—are treated with surgery and may be cured by the surgical procedure alone. Other times, surgery will be combined with radiation and/or chemotherapy to limit the extent of the surgery and improve the chance for cure. This approach is called *combined modality therapy*.

RADIATION – Radiation therapy is the treatment of cancer with high-energy radiation. This treatment usually is given to defined or limited areas of the body. Radiation therapy is sometimes used alone to cure certain cancers such as cancer of the cervix and cancer of the larynx, thereby avoiding surgery. More often, radiation is used to reduce the size of a tumor before surgery or to destroy any remaining cancer cells after surgery. Radiation therapy also is used for the treatment of many patients with advanced cancer who require symptom relief; the radiation is used to shrink local areas of the cancer which are causing pain or other symptoms.

CHEMOTHERAPY – Chemotherapy is a general term for treatment with drugs. These medications usually are given by injection or infusion into a vein, but they can also be given by injection into the muscle or skin or be taken orally. Hormone medications are also broadly included in this approach to treatment.

Chemotherapy treatment may be used alone to cure a number of cancers, such as Hodgkin's disease, non-Hodgkin's lymphoma, and testicular cancer; more often it is used in combination with radiation and surgery. The drugs of chemotherapy treatments have the advantage of traveling in the bloodstream to almost all parts of the body and thus are able to destroy cancer cells that are out of the reach of the scalpel or radiation beam. Drugs also are used to provide long-term control for some cancers and to relieve symptoms in patients with advanced cancer.

NEW APPROACHES

Surgery, radiation therapy, and chemotherapy have been the mainstays of cancer treatment for several decades. However, in the past few years, some new approaches to cancer treatment have met with success.

Understanding Cancer, Its Treatment, and the Side Effects of Treatment – **CHAPTER ONE**

ADJUVANT THERAPY is an extra treatment which is added to the primary treatment in order to prevent a recurrence of the cancer and to prolong survival. Distant or local microscopic deposits of cancer may not be detected at the time the original cancer is diagnosed and treated; however, they may show up several years later as recurrent cancer, which is more difficult to eradicate. Therefore, for some cancers, such breast cancer, early treatment with chemotherapy or hormones or both may destroy these microscopic cells and prevent their regrowth. For other cancers, chemotherapy treatments are given before the cancer is surgically removed. This is called *neoadjuvant therapy.*

BONE MARROW TRANSPLANTATION is a treatment in which patients are given extremely high doses of radiation and/or chemotherapy to eliminate the cancer cells which are in the body. The theory behind this treatment is that the higher the dose of chemotherapy or radiation, the more cancer cells will be killed. Unfortunately, these high doses of treatment have serious immediate toxicities on normal tissues in the body such as the cells of the bone marrow—which make white cells, red cells, and platelets—as well as the cells that line the gastrointestinal tract.

The high-dosage treatment ordinarily would cause death because of its effects on blood counts. Through the use of bone marrow transplantation, however, the patient is rescued from the toxic and potentially lethal effects of the treatment on the bone marrow cells. In addition, various growth factors often are used to stimulate the recovery of white cells after the patient receives the high doses of chemotherapy.

Under general anesthesia, about a half-liter of bone marrow is removed from a healthy donor who is genetically identical or extremely well matched to the recipient (an *allogeneic transplantation*). After the chemotherapy and radiation treatments have been given, the cells from the donated marrow are processed and subsequently infused by vein into the recipient. Because this procedure, which includes receiving high-dose chemotherapy and/or radiation, has many side effects, it is performed only at specialized centers. In general, it is not performed on persons over the age of 40 because the side effects increase and the effectiveness of the treatment decreases in this age group. Bone marrow transplantation has become a standard treatment for some cancers, such as acute leukemia.

Recently, more research has been done with very high-dose chemotherapy and with the rescue of patients with their own bone marrow or *autologous transplantation,* a system in which patients have previously donated and stored their bone marrow in the event of a recurrence of cancer, often just prior to the high-dose chemotherapy.

Because there is a risk that the bone marrow may harbor some cancer cells, many centers use a new approach that permits the collection of the bone marrow regenerating stem cells from the peripheral blood. The collection of peripheral stem cells requires high doses of white cell growth factors, which cause the release of the stem cells from the bone marrow into the circulating blood. The blood can be collected and then put through a specialized machine, *pheresis,* which separates out the stem cells from the remaining blood and allows the return of the remaining blood to the patient. High-dose chemotherapy with peripheral stem cell transplantation has become quite common for the treatment of breast cancer, lymphomas, and other solid tumors.

MODIFICATION OF THE IMMUNOLOGIC SYSTEM —This type of treatment uses the body's own regulatory system to resist disease or invasion by foreign substances such as cancer cells. For several decades, researchers have been studying ways to boost the body's own natural defenses against cancer. Until recently, most of these studies have met with limited success. Innovative technologies have permitted the large scale production of new agents, broadly classified as biologic response modifiers, which are derived from the body's own natural products. Interferon, interleukin-2, and tumor necrosis factor are a few substances that are undergoing active study. Some of these agents have already found a place in cancer treatment.

HYPERTHERMIA TREATMENT — This form of treatment uses heat to kill cancer cells. Scientists have known for decades that high temperatures can arrest the growth of cancer cells. Many years ago, patients were given bacterial toxins to induce fever as a means of treating their cancers. We now have more sophisticated ways of applying heat only to the cancer, and we can eliminate exposing the whole body to the side effects of the high temperatures. Hyperthermia treatment still is being studied; it is sometimes integrated into standard cancer treatment.

CLINICAL TRIALS

For most cancers, the majority of physicians and researchers have agreed on a "standard treatment approach"—the way in which cancer should be treated based on years of systematic study and research. However, doctors may have different opinions about how to treat some cancers because several equally effective treatments may be available.

Under these circumstances, seeking a second opinion is helpful in order to learn about all your treatment alternatives. An excellent source of information about the standard treatments for cancer is

for more information
contact

NATIONAL CANCER INSTITUTE'S CANCER INFORMATION SERVICE

800/4-CANCER

PDQ

PDQ, the computerized resource available from the National Cancer Institute. This can be accessed through many public libraries and on-line services, as well as by calling the National Cancer Institute's Cancer Information Service at (800) 4-CANCER.

CLINICAL TRIALS involve research with new experimental treatments and with new ways of using standard treatments. Most trials are conducted at cancer treatment centers affiliated with universities, but many community cancer specialists can participate as well. In general, these trials test the effectiveness of a new treatment, usually in comparison with the best available standard treatment. If a treatment has not been accepted as one of the standard treatments, it is called experimental or investigational. Because of the experimental nature of the treatment, you will be monitored very carefully for side effects as well as for benefits. You must give your informed consent to participate in such research before any treatment is administered (see page 50 for an explanation of informed consent). Unfortunately, very few patients treated in the United States today are given the opportunity to participate in clinical trials, a situation the National Cancer Institute is trying to improve. If you are interested in finding out whether a clinical trial is available for your particular kind of cancer, you should contact the Cancer Information Service at (800) 4-CANCER.

You may want to participate in a clinical trial for several reasons. It may give you the chance to receive treatment that is more effective or less toxic than the standard treatment. You may also be able to get access to a new drug that is not generally available. In addition, your participation in this research effort leads to more rapid accumulation of knowledge that may help others. The clinical trial process is a prerequisite for making progress in cancer treatment.

SYMPTOMS AND SIDE EFFECTS

PAIN

Pain is the most feared aspect of cancer, even though not every cancer patient experiences pain. Most people equate cancer with pain; yet, many are often surprised to find that their cancer was not painful at the time of diagnosis. Pain is, however, commonly associated with advanced cancer and with some treatments. Two types of pain are associated with cancer and its treatment—

- *Acute Pain* – This pain—of sudden onset and relatively short duration—is generally related to the cancer pressing on adjacent tissues or to stretching the organ in which the cancer is located. With successful cancer treatment, usually all of the pain

disappears. If the cancer remains and continues to grow in the same place, the pain often becomes chronic (sustained and permanent).
- *Chronic pain* sometimes develops as a consequence of treatment. This usually occurs in a part of the body where surgery and radiation have been used together, leading to the development of scar tissue which entraps and injures the adjacent nerves.

Although treatment to alleviate pain may be a simple matter, survivors are sometimes reluctant to admit they are experiencing pain because they erroneously believe that—
- pain associated with cancer is to be expected;
- pain is unimportant when life is at stake;
- pain is a sign that the illness is progressing;
- pain medication is addictive;
- people become immune to pain medication if they start taking drugs in early stages of pain.

A reluctance to admit you have pain can result in uncontrolled and unnecessary discomfort that interferes with daily life. You are the best judge of your own pain. You should not hesitate to give your doctor a detailed description of your pain symptoms. If pain becomes an ongoing problem for you, keep a pain diary to chart when the pain began and what helped to relieve it. You need not accept pain as a "necessary evil" in cancer treatment.

The general principle underlying the use of pain relievers is to get the pain under control and prevent it from returning. This can be accomplished by administering scheduled pain treatment whether you are in pain or not, and to give small additional doses of pain medication between the scheduled doses should the pain become worse. Giving pain medication on a regular schedule leads to more effective pain relief and to a lower total dosage of medication than if it is given only when the pain is severe. Ninety percent of all cancer patients can have their pain effectively controlled if they take their medications appropriately. Addiction is extremely rare unless the individual has a history of substance abuse. Efforts to control pain should be made at all phases of the disease, but it is especially important that pain be controlled in the advanced cancer patient. Different treatments are used to control pain from different sources.

Medication is the most common form of pain treatment. Nonprescription analgesics, such as aspirin, acetaminophen and ibuprofen, are effective in relieving mild pain. If your pain is moderate to severe, your doctor may prescribe a narcotic for you to take orally. For extremely intense pain, you may be given narcotics by injection, sometimes continuously using a portable infusion pump.

Radiation or *surgery* to anesthetize pain fibers may be used to control pain that is localized in one area, such as in a bone. Radiation and surgery may also be used to shrink tumors that are causing pain.

Skin stimulation excites nerve endings in the skin and may lessen or block the recognition of pain. Different types of skin stimulation include massage, pressure, vibration, heat, cold, menthol preparations, and transcutaneous electric nerve stimulations (TENS).

The relaxation techniques discussed in Chapter 5 may help eliminate or alleviate pain.

Biofeedback, acupuncture, and *hypnosis* are sometimes used in combination with more traditional pain relief.

Pain clinic – You may find other solutions at a pain clinic.

The Agency for Health Care Policy and Research (AHCPR) recently published a guideline for the management of cancer pain. The guideline recommends that cancer patients should not be denied the opportunity to have their pain controlled. An excellent patient information book associated with the guideline is available by contacting the Cancer Information Service at (800) 4-CANCER or by writing to *Cancer Pain Guideline,* AHCPR Publications Clearinghouse, P.O. Box 8547, Silver Spring, MD 20907.

FATIGUE

Fatigue is one of the most common physical problems reported by cancer patients. Fatigue can occur as a specific symptom of the cancer, especially in persons with advanced cancer. Fatigue, which leaves a patient tired for weeks or months, also results from radiation and chemotherapy. For some patients, energy never returns to pretreatment levels. A few points to consider are:
- Fatigue is a warning sign that the body needs more rest; the best response is to heed the warning.
- Pace your activities according to your energy level, especially during and soon after treatment.
- If possible, exercise routinely to maintain stamina.
- Unless your physician prescribes against it, drink plenty of fluids—at least eight glasses of water per day.

for more information
contact

AHCPR Publications Clearinghouse
P.O. Box 8547
Silver Spring, MD 20907
800/4-CANCER
Cancer Pain Guideline

Nutrition and Weight Maintenance

Cancer survivors experience nutritional and weight problems for a variety of reasons. Cancers occurring in the abdomen can cause problems when they invade or compress digestive organs, such as the stomach. Some patients experience nausea and vomiting, while others feel too bloated to eat. However, most dietary problems experienced by survivors are caused, in part, by cancer treatment.

Although most problems involve weight and appetite loss, some patients, especially those receiving adjuvant therapy for breast cancer, may suffer from too much weight gain, possibly because of decreased physical activity and increased food intake. Because weight gain and a high-fat diet may be risk factors for breast cancer recurrence, these women usually are encouraged to maintain their weight or lose weight if they are overweight.

Below are the seven most common nutritional problems, their causes, and suggestions for relief.

Problems Related to Nutrition and Eating

Problem	Cause	What Will Help
Loss of Appetite	May be caused by illness, anticancer drugs, loss of sleep, depression, or fatigue.	– Light exercise to increase appetite. – A glass of beer or wine before meals (with doctor's OK). – Plan meals with favorite foods; small, appetizing meals in pleasant surroundings. – Speak with a doctor or registered dietitian for suggestions. – Keep nutritious snacks around: offer a snack before bedtime (ice cream with ginger ale, a milk shake, or yogurt). – Use seasonings like basil, oregano, tarragon, and lemon.
Weight Loss	Maintenance of normal weight is indicative of sufficient caloric intake. Weight loss may be part of the disease process, or the result of anorexia.	– Keep a record of foods eaten each day. – Offer between-meal snacks high in calories and protein (for example, add 1/4 cup nonfat dried milk to 8 oz. whole milk; add this milk to sauces, soups, and gravies). – Use cream not milk in cereals. Extra calories may be added with a dietary supplement.
Nausea & Vomiting	May be a result of anticancer drugs or a consequence of the cancer itself.	– Small, frequent meals with no liquid during meals. Drink liquids one hour before meals to prevent large volume of fluid in the stomach.

{Continued on next page}

Understanding Cancer, Its Treatment, and the Side Effects of Treatment – **Chapter One**

Problems Related to Nutrition and Eating (Continued)

Problem	Cause	What Will Help
Nausea & Vomiting (continued)		– Overly sweet foods may cause discomfort. – Greasy, fried foods can cause nausea; try foods like toast and crackers (especially in the morning). – May need to try several antinausea medications to find the one that works. Check with a doctor and keep a record of when symptoms start and how long they last.
Taste	Anticancer drugs may change the way food tastes; for example, sweet foods taste too sweet. Radiation to the head and neck area can cause a metallic taste.	– For overly sweet taste, force fluids. Serve protein at room temperature. Some foods may taste better with salt or sugar. Marinate meats in sweet wine or fruit juices. Salt may need to be restricted if heart disease also exists.
Halitosis	Can occur with anticancer drugs and is caused by breakdown of cells that line the gastro-intestinal tract.	– Use frequent mouthwashes (except when there are sores in mouth) and antacids (check with doctor). Sucking on hard candy can be helpful.
Stomatitis (Inflammation of the mouth)	Both anticancer drugs and sometimes the illness itself can leave a person subject to mouth sores and "furry tongue" indicative of fungal overgrowth.	– A soft, bland diet or favorite foods blenderized. Avoid spicy, hot, or acid foods (orange juice) and coarse vegetables or fruit. Cold drinks are soothing. – Use a straw for easier drinking. – Remove dentures except when needed for chewing. – Mouth care three times a day after meals. – Salt water gargles if mouth sores occur. – Call doctor if sores do not get better after three days. – Soft-bristle brush if mouth sores occur. – Doctor may order topical anesthesia. – Do not use mouthwash that contains alcohol.
Dry Mouth	Radiation to the head and neck area. Pain medication.	– Sips of water frequently. – Lubricate lips. – Artifical saliva may help. – Lemon drops may stimulate saliva.

Note: Each patient is an individual and may or may not have any of these symptoms. No problem is too insignificant to deserve an answer. Call you doctor if you are concerned.

Source: Caring for the Person with Cancer at Home: A Family Caregiver's Manual. *American Cancer Society, 1985.*

Of the seven most common nutritional problems, nausea and vomiting, which are caused by chemotherapy and radiation, can be the most physically exhausting. Chemotherapy-associated nausea and vomiting usually begin about four to six hours after an intravenous injection or within an hour after taking some oral medications. The intensity of these side effects varies with the drug. Many drugs cause no or minimal nausea, while others cause fairly severe nausea followed by frequent vomiting.

To prevent or decrease nausea and vomiting, your doctor may give you several medications, usually by vein. In addition, you may be given pills to take at home, usually for the first 24 to 48 hours after treatment. The preventive medications sometimes cause sedation or drowsiness as a side effect, and you may need someone to drive you home from your treatment. You may be hospitalized because the treatment and preventive medications are so complex that you may need to have more frequent nursing care. If the preventive treatments do not work, tell your doctor or nurse immediately so alternative approaches can be tried.

With effective prevention of post-chemotherapy nausea and vomiting, fewer patients develop "anticipatory nausea and vomiting." This is a problem in which you are conditioned, like the dogs in Pavlov's experiments, to associate many of the aspects of your treatment with the nausea and vomiting that occur after treatment. Patients who have anticipatory nausea and vomiting usually start to feel anxious and nauseated the day before their treatment, with increasing symptoms as they approach the doctor's office. They often will have nausea as they enter the chemotherapy treatment room or have a needle inserted into their vein. These responses are not effectively treated with anti-nausea medications. Instead, behavioral treatments that involve relaxation or self-hypnosis are usually helpful to decondition the response.

HAIR LOSS

Hair loss can result from head and neck radiation and from certain types of chemotherapy. Chemotherapy and radiation result in atrophy of the hair follicle. Your hair becomes weak and brittle, and either breaks off at the surface of the scalp or falls out of the follicle. The amount of hair loss depends on the type, dose, and length of the treatment you receive. Before you begin treatment, ask your doctor whether you are likely to experience some hair loss.

You may lose hair not only from your scalp but also from other parts of your body, such as eyebrows and arms. Most hair loss is temporary. Your hair may return as before or regrow in a different texture and color.

You can take several steps to minimize hair loss:
- Cut your hair in an easy-to-manage style before treatment begins.
- Avoid excessive shampooing, rinse thoroughly, and gently pat your hair dry.
- Avoid heat, such as hair dryers and hot curlers.
- Avoid excess tugging on your hair by brushing only when necessary, by using a wide-tooth comb, and by avoiding hair clips and elastic bands.
- Ask your doctor about scalp cooling. Your doctor may encourage you to wear a cold compress ("ice turban") during chemotherapy. This works by decreasing the metabolic rate of the hair follicles and the uptake of chemotherapy drugs from the blood stream into hair roots. In this way, hair follicles are exposed to a small amount of chemotherapy and have less chance of having their growth disturbed.

You can take several steps to prepare for expected hair loss:
- Choose a wig prior to losing your hair so that you can match it to your natural hair color and texture. Some insurance policies cover the cost of a wig.
- If you do not want to wear a wig, consider a hat, a scarf, or a turban.
- If you do not wish to cover your head, you may want to shave off any remaining hair for a neater appearance. However, keep your head protected from a strong sun to prevent sunburn, and keep it covered in the winter to prevent heat loss.
- At home, consider wearing a hairnet to minimize shedding on your clothes or bedding.

Low Blood Counts

The majority of patients receiving chemotherapy, and some receiving radiation, will experience low blood counts. This is because treatment often slows the growth of cells in the bone marrow, which produces red cells, white cells and platelets. White cells are needed to fight infections. When the white cell count falls below a certain level, it is unsafe to give additional treatments because they would continue to slow the production of white cells. If you are receiving chemotherapy or radiation therapy and develop a fever, you should call your doctor immediately. A fever might be the first sign of a low white blood cell count (also called *neutropenia*) and an associated infection.

If your blood cell counts are too low, your treatments will usually be postponed for several days until the counts improve. If your counts are extremely low, your doctor might prescribe a white cell growth factor (G-CSF or GM-CSF), which is given by injection daily. These growth factors stimulate the bone marrow to make new white cells that will travel into the circulation and prevent an infection. If you develop severe neutropenia with chemotherapy, or if your doctor thinks you will be at high risk for this condition, you may be given the growth factor preventatively to avoid a low white cell count. This preventive approach is particularly common when the doses of chemotherapy are very high, and there is a substantial risk of neutropenia in the majority of patients receiving such treatment. These growth factors now play an important role in preventing life-threatening infections in cancer patients.

Skin Changes

Skin problems in the treatment area can result from both radiation and chemotherapy. Changes can range from a minor reddening to blistering and peeling. Itchy skin, called *pruritus*, is a common side effect of some cancers and treatment.

Your doctor may prescribe antihistamines or cortico-steroid creams for itching. Additionally, you can take several steps to heal dry, itchy, or burned skin.

- Avoid sunlight exposure, which can cause additional burning.
- Lubricate your skin with a water-based, rather than oil-based, moisturizer.
- Drink at least eight glasses of water or other fluids each day.
- Protect your skin from extreme temperatures and wind. Keep indoor temperatures cool.
- Bathe in cool or lukewarm water: cornstarch, baking soda, oatmeal, or soybean powder added to the bath may be soothing.
- Wear loose fitting, lightweight clothing.

Neurotoxicity

Injury to the nerves *(neurotoxicity)* is a side effect of some treatments. Usually this is first noticed as a numbness or tingling in the hands or feet, and rarely as complete weakness in an extremity. Some drugs can cause hearing loss or ringing in the ears. If you are having any of these problems, you should immediately bring them to your doctor's attention so your medications can be altered to modify these side effects.

Loss of Concentration

Many patients report difficulty concentrating, remembering, and thinking clearly while they are receiving cancer treatments. These effects are caused by several factors: direct effects of the chemotherapy and radiation treatments on the brain, side effects from the medications used to prevent nausea and vomiting, and the increased fatigue associated with the disease and its treatment.

It is important to eat and sleep well, to get enough rest, and to do the best you can to maintain your physical condition and stamina. Usually, the greatest loss of concentration will be associated with the treatments themselves (the day of treatment and the first few days thereafter) with return of concentration between treatments. Try to postpone activities that demand your concentration until after treatment.

RESPIRATORY PROBLEMS

Lung cancer patients and other cancer patients may experience shortness of breath which can be caused by the cancer itself, by chemotherapy, anemia, malnutrition, and by other factors. You can improve your breathing in a number of ways.

- Inhale through your nose and exhale slowly through your mouth with your lips pursed as if blowing out a candle. Use your abdominal muscles rather than your chest muscles to pull air in and push it out.
- Rest in a comfortable position when experiencing shortness of breath. For example, you will find it easier to sit up in bed than to lie down.
- Move around as much as possible to help your circulation. Even if you are confined to bed, you may be able to do simple arm or leg exercises. A respiratory therapist can suggest the best exercises for you.
- Aid circulation in your feet by not sitting in one position too long or by crossing your legs.
- Drink at least eight glasses of water a day to help mucous membranes clear your lungs of secretions.
- Cough deeply from within your chest to help clear your lungs.
- Use a humidifier to keep the air in your house from becoming too dry.

SEXUAL FUNCTIONING

A number of sexual problems are associated with cancer and its treatment. Sometimes these are related specifically to the type of cancer (for example, gynecological or urological cancers), but more often they are related to general problems such as fatigue and discomfort. Even in healthy people, fatigue leads to a loss of interest in sexual activity, and this is a very normal response. In addition, certain treatments lead to specific physical problems which affect sexual function (see tables on page 22 for a list of these problems and their causes).

For many women who receive chemotherapy, menstrual periods

may cease and menopause will begin. As a result, a range of symptoms may occur, including hot flashes, vaginal lubrication problems, and lack of sexual desire. Often, hormone replacement alleviates these symptoms; however, for some women hormone replacement may not be advisable. If you have experienced menopause as a result of chemotherapy and have symptoms that are interfering with your sexual functioning, you should talk to your doctor about whether you can receive hormone replacement therapy.

Different sexual problems require different personal responses. Your physician, nurse, social worker, or a sex therapist can offer specific suggestions for coping with the physical and emotional consequences of decreased sexual function. Solutions to some sexual problems include the following:
- reconstructive surgery may help repair a physical loss;
- use of water-based gels may help provide vaginal lubrication;
- hormonal therapy may alleviate symptoms of premature menopause;
- penile prostheses may help provide an erection;
- androgen replacement may be useful in both women and men who have inadequate levels of testosterone as a result of damage to the ovaries or testes by cancer treatments.

CONTRACEPTION AND STERILITY

Cancer and its treatment can affect fertility and fetal development. If you are sexually active during cancer treatment, you should use contraceptives. Both radiation and chemotherapy can lead to malformations or injury to the developing fetus. Conception can occur even if you are receiving treatment. If you wish to have a child, speak with your doctor before trying to conceive. You may be advised to wait several years after your treatments to reduce the risk of a problem pregnancy.

A parallel concern is the risk of permanent sterility from chemotherapy or radiation treatments. Radiation will cause permanent sterility if the testes or ovaries receive direct radiation. For this reason, these organs are usually shielded with lead barriers. Sometimes the ovaries are relocated surgically so that they will not be in a radiation treatment field. When such protective measures are used, subsequent fertility is preserved. It is, however, more difficult to protect these organs from the effects of chemotherapy. Not all chemotherapy treatments cause a decrease in fertility, but some will.

If you have concerns about the effect of cancer treatments on your fertility, you should consider the following:
- Discuss your questions with your doctor before you begin treatment, so that your treatment can be modified, if possible, to min

FEMALE SEXUAL PROBLEMS CAUSED BY CANCER TREATMENT

TREATMENT	LOW SEXUAL DESIRE	LESS VAGINAL MOISTURE	REDUCED VAGINAL SIZE	PAINFUL INTERCOURSE	TROUBLE REACHING ORGASM	INFERTILITY
CHEMOTHERAPY	Sometimes	Often	Sometimes	Often	Rarely	Often
PELVIC RADIATION THERAPY	Rarely	Often	Often	Often	Rarely	Often
RADICAL HYSTERECTOMY	Rarely	Often*	Often	Rarely	Rarely	Always
RADICAL CYSTECTOMY	Rarely	Often*	Always	Sometimes	Rarely	Always
ABDOMINOPERINEAL (A-P) RESECTION	Rarely	Often*	Sometimes	Sometimes	Rarely	Sometimes
TOTAL PELVIC EXTENERATION WITH VAGINAL RECONSTRUCTION	Sometimes	Always	Sometimes	Sometimes	Sometimes	Always
RADICAL VULVECTOMY	Rarely	Never	Sometimes	Often	Sometimes	Never
CONIZATION OF CERVIX	Never	Never	Never	Rarely	Never	Rarely
OOPHORECTOMY (REMOVAL OF ONE TUBE AND OVARY)	Rarely	Never*	Never*	Rarely	Never	Rarely
OOPHORECTOMY (REMOVAL OF TWO TUBES AND OVARIES)	Rarely	Often*	Sometimes*	Sometimes*	Rarely	Always
MASTECTOMY OR RADIATION TO BREAST	Rarely	Never	Never	Never	Rarely	Never
ANTIESTROGEN THERAPY FOR BREAST OR UTERINE CANCER	Sometimes	Often	Sometimes	Sometimes	Rarely	Always
ANDROGEN THERAPY	Never	Never	Never	Never	Never	Uncertain

*Vaginal dryness and size changes should not occur if one ovary is left or if hormone replacement therapy is given.

Source: Schover, Sexuality and Cancer: For the Woman Who Has Cancer and Her Partner, American Cancer Society, 1988.

MALE SEXUAL PROBLEMS CAUSED BY CANCER TREATMENT

TREATMENT	LOW SEXUAL DESIRE	ERECTION PROBLEMS	LACK OF ORGASM	DRY ORGASM	WEAKER ORGASM	INFERTILITY
CHEMOTHERAPY	Sometimes	Rarely	Rarely	Rarely	Rarely	Often
PELVIC RADIATION THERAPY	Rarely	Sometimes	Rarely	Rarely	Sometimes	Often
RETROPERITONEAL LYMPH NODE DISSECTION	Rarely	Rarely	Rarely	Often	Sometimes	Often
ABDOMINOPERINEAL (A-P) RESECTION	Rarely	Often	Rarely	Often	Sometimes	Sometimes*
RADICAL PROSTATECTOMY	Rarely	Often	Rarely	Always	Sometimes	Always
RADICAL CYSTECTOMY	Rarely	Often	Rarely	Always	Sometimes	Always
TOTAL PELVIC EXTENERATION	Rarely	Often	Rarely	Always	Sometimes	Always
PARTIAL PENECTOMY	Rarely	Rarely	Rarely	Never	Rarely	Never
TOTAL PENECTOMY	Rarely	Always	Sometimes	Never	Sometimes	Usually*
ORCHIECTOMY (REMOVAL OF ONE TESTICLE)	Rarely	Rarely	Never	Never	Never	Rarely**
ORCHIECTOMY (REMOVAL OF TWO TESTICLES)	Often	Often	Sometimes	Sometimes	Sometimes	Always
HORMONE THERAPY FOR PROSTATE CANCER	Often	Often	Sometimes	Sometimes	Sometimes	Always

*Artificial insemination of a spouse with the man's own semen may not be possible.
** Infertile only if remaining testicle is not normal.

Source: Schover, Sexuality and Cancer: For the Man Who Has Cancer and His Partner, American Cancer Society, 1988.

imize effects on your fertility. Sometimes you will have a choice between two equally effective treatment programs, one of which has a high rate of infertility and the other which does not.
- Men should consider preserving their sperm in a sperm bank prior to treatment. If your sperm have not been impaired by the cancer itself, sperm banking may increase your chances of having a child after treatment.
- Women cannot preserve their eggs in the same way that men can store sperm. The only way to save a woman's eggs is to fertilize them and store them as embryos. This can be a problem for a woman who does not have a partner or a suitable sperm donor at the time of diagnosis. In addition, the harvesting of eggs may require hormone administration as well as several menstrual cycles (in other words, time) to retrieve eggs for this use. Thus, the opportunities for the preservation of fertility in women are more limited.

MEDICAL PROBLEMS OF LONG-TERM SURVIVORS

Fortunately, an expanding community of long-term cancer survivors have gotten past the early and often complex initial phase of cancer treatment. If you are among them, you will find that as time passes, and you are further removed from the early phase of treatment, you will have a tendency to distance yourself physically and psychologically from the professionals who were involved in your cancer treatment. Although this is natural, you should maintain some form of regular medical follow-up with a physician who knows the details of your previous cancer treatment and its potential long-term side effects.

For example, a patient who has had the spleen removed for staging of Hodgkin's disease is at a life-long risk for serious infections. In these individuals, fever must be treated promptly with antibiotics. Many cancer survivors are at a risk of long-term organ toxicities, infection, and second malignancies as a result of previous treatment. Therefore, it is important for survivors to inform their current physicians about their past treatments so that appropriate monitoring can occur.

LONG-TERM AND LATE EFFECTS

Long-term effects are known or expected problems that may occur with some frequency in individuals who have received certain treatments: for example, the risk of infection after splenectomy or infertility after certain chemotherapy drugs. *Late effects*, in contrast, are secondary conditions that arise as a result of having received certain cancer treatments: for example, leukemia secondary to alkylating agent therapy or congestive heart failure many years after treatment with anthracycline chemotherapy.

Information about the long-term and late effects of treatment on important organs, such as the heart and lungs, is just starting to become available. Chemotherapy and radiation treatments received many years earlier can lead to premature aging of these vital organs. As the number of survivors increases, more information about these problems becomes available, and this information is used to modify the type and intensity of treatment for patients currently receiving treatment. Specific examples of some long-term and late effects of cancer treatment include the following.

HEART MUSCLE INJURY is associated most commonly with high total doses of the anthrocycline drugs (doxorubicin or daunorubicin). In addition, high-dose cyclophosphamide, such as used in transplant regimens, can contribute to chronic heart failure. When chest radiation is combined with these chemotherapeutic agents, the risk of heart failure is possible at lower doses of the chemotherapy drugs. Although heart muscle imaging studies (MUGA scans) are useful for monitoring the acute effects of treatment on how well the heart is pumping, some recent studies have noted the onset of heart failure in cancer survivors many years after their last chemotherapy or radiation treatments. In these individuals, the heart failure was apparently stable and compensated for over many years, until their hearts were stressed by the added physical demands of new situations, such as vigorous exercise or pregnancy.

CORONARY ARTERY DISEASE – Some cancer survivors may experience premature coronary artery disease from past radiation therapy. This may put them at risk for heart attacks at an age much younger than the general population. At Stanford University Medical Center, a detailed study of Hodgkin's disease survivors is underway to examine this problem.

LUNG TISSUE INJURY is an expected long-term problem when the drug bleomycin is used. This drug may lead to lung scarring and to a certain degree of shortness of breath in some individuals, as well as an increased risk of lung failure during anesthesia. Other groups of drugs can also cause this problem (for example, alkylating agents, methotrexate, and nitrosoureas), and these can be a concern in long-term survivors of bone marrow transplantation. Some patients may experience a gradual increase in shortness of breath with exercise, which may be a sign of lung injury from past chemotherapy or radiation therapy.

KIDNEY DAMAGE can occur after treatment with several chemotherapy drugs (for example, cisplatin, methotrexate, and nitrosoureas). These agents can be associated with both acute and chronic toxicities. Rarely, some patients may require hemodialysis as a result of chronic injury to the kidneys.

NERVOUS SYSTEM INJURY, which is commonly associated with the vinca alkaloids and taxol, may cause considerable disability; for example, pain or difficulty walking or using hands. Whole brain radiation, with or without chemotherapy, can be a cause of progressive dementia and cognitive dysfunction in some long-term survivors. This is particularly a problem for brain tumor patients and for patients with small-cell lung cancer who have received prophylactic radiation therapy to the brain. In children with leukemia, a variety of abnormalities (problems with learning and concentration) have been associated with whole brain irradiation.

BLOOD AND IMMUNE SYSTEM PROBLEMS (low blood cell counts, anemia, increased susceptibility to infection) are common during and shortly after receiving chemotherapy and radiation treatments. In some instances, however, some survivors will have persistent abnormalities as a long-term effect of treatment. Immunologic impairment is a long-term problem for patients with Hodgkin's disease, and this may be related to the underlying disease as well as to the treatments that are used. Those patients who have received a splenectomy may also be at risk for serious bacterial infections.

MONITORING FOR RECURRENCE

All survivors should be regularly monitored for recurrence. You should discuss even minor symptoms with your doctor. In order to get the best follow-up care, have the detailed records of your cancer treatment forwarded to your current family physician, internist, or pediatrician. These records should be carefully reviewed by your doctor.

In addition to monitoring you for a recurrence of your initial cancer, your physician should also be aware that some forms of cancer treatment lead to an increased risk of second malignancies. A few specific examples are described below.

ACUTE MYELOGENOUS LEUKEMIA – Acute myelogenous leukemia may occur as a result of intensive therapy with radiation and chemotherapy—initially used to cure cancer—or as a result of prolonged therapy with certain types of chemotherapeutic drugs (alkylating agents or nitrosoureas). In general, this form of treatment-related acute leukemia occurs because of serious damage

CHILDHOOD CANCER SURVIVORS

Childhood cancer survivors are an important and rapidly growing segment of the survivor population. It is estimated that in the 1990s, one in one thousand young adults aged 20 will have been cured of childhood cancer. The special problems of childhood cancer survivors are being actively studied. More information on this special group should be available in the next few years. We do know that some children experience growth retardation secondary to curative treatment (especially radiation to growing bones), and this can lead to some long-term physical limitations and changes in body image. Most survivors of childhood cancer have gone on to have normal fertility and healthy offspring; however, some are unable to have children. Treatment programs are being designed to minimize all of these long-term problems, but currently many survivors of childhood cancer may be experiencing them. Cancer centers that specialize in the treatment of children and the Candlelighters Childhood Cancer Foundation are the best sources for information and guidance about these problems.

Understanding Cancer, Its Treatment, and the Side Effects of Treatment – **CHAPTER ONE**

to the cells in the bone marrow that are responsible for making new blood cells. This type of leukemia is difficult to cure.

The peak time of occurrence of secondary acute leukemia in patients with Hodgkin's disease is five to seven years after initial treatment. Thus, a slowly developing anemia in a Hodgkin's disease survivor should alert the doctor to the possibility of a secondary leukemia. Fortunately, secondary leukemias have not been reported in increased frequencies in women treated with standard adjuvant chemotherapy (for example, CMF—cyclophosphamide, methotrexate and fluorouracil) for breast cancer. Newer investigational adjuvant treatments using high doses of adriamycin have resulted in recent reports of an increased rate of leukemia.

SOLID TUMORS AND OTHER MALIGNANCIES – Cancer survivors who have been treated with chemotherapy or radiation therapy are also at risk for solid tumors and other malignancies. Non-Hodgkin's lymphomas have been reported as a late complication in patients treated for Hodgkin's disease or multiple myeloma. Patients treated with long-term cyclophosphamide are at risk for bladder cancer. Patients who have received radiation therapy for Hodgkin's disease have an increased risk of breast cancer, osteosarcoma, and lung carcinomas.

In these cases, the second cancer usually involves tissues that were heavily radiated as part of the original cancer treatment. In general, the risk of solid tumors begins to increase during the second decade of survival after Hodgkin's disease. As a result, young women who have received radiation to the chest as part of their treatment for Hodgkin's disease should be screened more carefully for breast cancer starting about ten years after treatment. Screening for breast cancer should include a clinical breast examination every six months and a mammogram annually.

OTHER LATE EFFECTS

ENDOCRINE PROBLEMS – A variety of endocrine problems are a result of cancer treatment. Patients receiving radiation therapy to the head and neck region can develop an underactive thyroid gland. This is a particular risk in patients receiving chest and neck radiation therapy for Hodgkin's disease. You should ask your doctor to be sure to monitor your thyroid function if you have had this type of treatment.

MENOPAUSE may start earlier than expected in women who have received certain chemotherapeutic agents (for example, alkylating agents and procarbazine) or abdominal radiation therapy. The risk is age-related, with women older than age 30 at the time of treatment having the greatest risk of treatment-induced menopause. Early hormone replacement therapy should be considered in such women, if not contraindicated, in order to reduce the risk of accelerated osteoporosis and premature heart disease.

TREATMENT-RELATED GONADAL FAILURE OR DYSFUNCTION can lead to infertility in both male and female cancer survivors. Infertility can be temporary, especially in men, and they may recover over time after therapy. Psychological counseling may be helpful to you if you have experienced this long-term consequence of therapy.

Radiation therapy can have effects on the muscles, bones and joints, especially in children and young adults. The radiation can injure the growth plates of long bones and can lead to muscle atrophy. Short stature sometimes occurs as a result of radiation therapy, but it also can be secondary to growth hormone deficiency in some people who have had brain radiation. Finally, abdominal radiation in young girls can change the size and shape of the immature uterus, which may make pregnancy difficult.

CANCER PREVENTION AND EARLY DETECTION

Although cancer survival rates are improving every year, the ideal goal is to decrease the occurrence of cancer through prevention. While screening and early detection of cancer will improve survival once cancer is diagnosed, preventing the development of cancer will provide an even greater impact on mortality rates. Cancer prevention is in its infancy, however, because only some of the causes of cancer are known. In addition, since complex behavioral and lifestyle changes often are required to lower the risk of cancer, prevention of cancer is very challenging. Increasingly, we are seeing the evaluation of medications in clinical trials to prevent the development of cancer in high risk populations, and these may hold some promise as an alternative strategy. What are some of the approaches that can lead to a reduction in cancer incidence and mortality?

ELIMINATING THE USE OF TOBACCO

Tobacco kills approximately 25 percent of those who use it. Approximately 419,000 Americans and three million people worldwide die each year from tobacco induced diseases, including cancer of the lung, head and neck, esophagus, bladder, and pancreas. Roughly half of the cancer deaths each year in the United States are causally related to tobacco use. Many Americans have heeded the warnings of the medical profession and decreased their use of cigarettes, pipes, cigars, and chewing tobacco. Between 1965, when the federal government first required a health warning on packages of cigarettes and 1992, the smoking rate among adults in the United States decreased from 42 percent to 26 percent. In several states, increased tobacco taxes have encouraged further decreases in tobacco use. While adults have decreased their consumption, unfortunately, adolescents are smoking more. Strong antismoking laws also have contributed to making this habit appear less socially acceptable.

Eating a Well-Balanced Diet

During the 1980s and 1990s, Americans began to change their diets significantly to reduce the risk of cancer and heart disease. Morning ham and eggs gave way to oat bran muffins, while fast-food chains promoted salad bars and chicken sandwiches. Although scientists do not agree on the impact that diet has on cancer, they do agree that dietary changes can affect the chances of getting certain types of cancer. For example, high-fat diets increase the risk of colon, breast, and uterine cancer. High-fiber diets decrease the risk of colon cancer. The micronutrients found in many fruits and vegetables have been shown to have anticancer properties. Their high rates of consumption are associated with lower rates of cancer in various populations throughout the world.

A well-balanced diet, low in fat and high in fresh fruits and vegetables, is the most prudent cancer prevention diet. People who do not overeat and who maintain a balanced diet do not need extra vitamins and other supplements, which can be harmful in large quantities. Beware of dietary supplements that claim to prevent cancer. No diet can prevent cancer; it can only affect the risk of some types of cancer. If you need more information on diet and cancer, contact the Cancer Information Service at (800) 4-CANCER for helpful eating hints and information.

Avoiding Excessive Radiation

Cosmetic and pharmaceutical manufacturers are selling a wide variety of sunscreens in response to the evidence that overexposure to the sun is the major cause of skin cancers. During the 1990s, a dark suntan began to lose its value as a status symbol as many Americans avoided the sun during midday and protected their skin with clothing and sunscreen.

Radon is another source of radiation to be avoided. A natural, odorless, radioactive gas, radon in high concentrations increases the risk of lung cancer; radon is found in the ground and can become trapped in buildings with inadequate ventilation. A simple, inexpensive test can measure the amount of radon in a building. Many people in areas with high levels of radon, such as parts of Pennsylvania, New Jersey, and New York, have improved their ventilation systems to decrease the radon levels in their homes and offices.

DECREASING ALCOHOL CONSUMPTION

Alcohol consumption increases the risk of oral cancers, especially when combined with tobacco use. Heavy drinking also increases the risk of liver cancer through the development of cirrhosis. In addition, an overview of several recent studies provides strong evidence for an increased risk of breast cancer with regular daily alcohol consumption.

SEXUALLY TRANSMITTED DISEASES AND CANCER

Cervical cancer and penile cancer are both associated with an infectious agent, the human papilloma virus (HPV). Since the infection is transmitted sexually, men and women can take several steps to prevent the development of these cancers:
- avoid sexual activity as a young adolescent;
- avoid having multiple sexual partners;
- practice good hygiene;
- use barrier contraceptives, such as condoms or diaphragms;
- avoid intercourse with individuals who have numerous sexual partners.

CHEMOPREVENTION TRIALS

Clinical trials are being conducted to test the effectiveness of several medications to prevent the development of cancer. The drug tamoxifen is being evaluated for its ability to prevent breast cancer in women at high risk for this disease. Similarly, the drug finasteride is being tested for its ability to prevent prostate cancer in men 55 years of age and older. While it will be several years before these clinical trials are completed, you should be on the lookout for the results of these important studies. Similarly, a variety of agents (calcium, fiber, aspirin) are being tested for their value in the prevention of colon and rectal cancers. All of these studies are very important, as these diseases are leading forms of cancer.

Reporting Warning Signs to Your Doctor

Although early diagnosis does not decrease the risk of getting cancer, it can dramatically improve the effectiveness of your treatment.
- Report to your doctor any symptoms or warning signals of cancer as defined by the American Cancer Society:
  Change in bowel or bladder habits.
  A sore that does not heal.
  Unusual bleeding or discharge.
  Thickening or lump in breast or elsewhere.
  Indigestion or difficulty in swallowing.
  Obvious change in wart or mole.
  Nagging cough or hoarseness.
- Conduct monthly self-examinations of your skin, breasts (women) and testicles (men). The American Cancer Society and National Cancer Institute have booklets that describe how to perform a self-exam.
- See your doctor for routine physicals which include a screening for breast, cervical, and colon cancer.

Chapter Two

Working with Your Doctor and Hospital System:

Becoming a Wise Consumer

by Natalie Davis Spingarn
and Nancy H. Chasen, JD

"We are all consumers – users of goods and services. Yet, no other area of life exists where we know as little about our choices as we do in the field of health care. And these are choices we must make if we are to work effectively with our doctors toward better health."

Nancy H. Chasen, JD

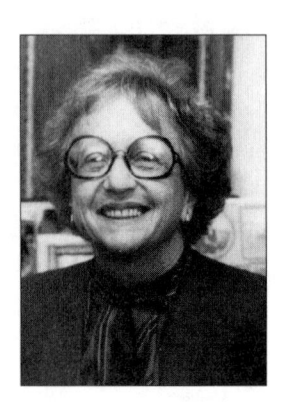

NATALIE DAVIS SPINGARN, a prize-winning writer, advocate, and consultant on health and social policy issues, is vice chair of the Board of Directors of the National Coalition for Cancer Survivorship. Ms. Spingarn founded and served as editor of the NCCS quarterly publication, *The Networker*. Her scores of publications include *Hanging in There: Living Well on Borrowed Time,* which describes her personal experience with metastatic breast cancer and the issues confronting survivors. She won an Oscar at the John Muir Medical Film Festival for her film *Patients and Doctors: Communication is a Two-Way Street*. Based in Washington, DC, Ms. Spingarn has served as an official in the executive and legislative branches of the federal government, as a District of Columbia General Hospital commissioner, and on several advisory committees for George Washington University Medical Center.

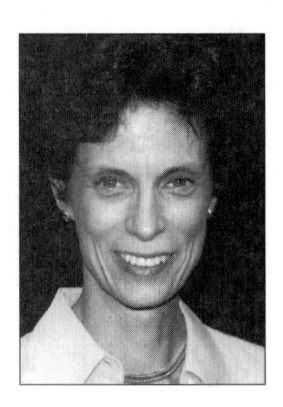

NANCY CHASEN, JD is a consumer advocate and writer in Washington, DC. She was special counsel to President Carter's Consumer Advisor, assistant general counsel for legislation of the Federal Trade Commission, and she has handled consumer issues for Senator Thomas Eagleton (D-Mo.). Ms. Chasen has also worked for several consumer organizations, as staff attorney for the Washington Office of the Consumers Union, and as a lobbyist for Public Citizen's Congress Watch. She served as a producer and consumer reporter for the PBS program, Modern Maturity. Ms. Chasen is the author of *Policy Wise: A Guide to Insurance for Older Consumers,* published by the American Association of Retired Persons and has appeared frequently on panels and before federal agencies to represent consumer interests.

We are all consumers—users of goods and services. Yet, no other area of life exists where we know as little about our choices as we do in the field of health care, and these are choices we must make if we are to work effectively with our doctors toward better health.

It takes a lot of reliable information to make decisions about which physician or which group or which physicians within a group should deliver your medical care. You also need information about your disease, about what each of your potential caregivers can do to help you recover, and about how to live with cancer.

This chapter provides you with a sort of road map to help you find the right doctor and then to communicate with him or her to your best advantage—both in and outside of a managed care setting. The chapter also offers some guides to selecting the most appropriate hospital for your needs.

Gathering Information and Choosing a Doctor

A Historical Perspective

We investigate prospective schools and colleges carefully before enrolling, asking detailed questions about facilities and particularly about the faculty's credentials and record. Whether we buy a big item like a house or car or a smaller one like a refrigerator, we often shop around for weeks, even months, comparing quality and price to see which is the best buy.

Like most cancer survivors of the past decades, you probably did not shop in the same way for the services of someone who profoundly influences your life—your doctor. You came to him or her because of the recommendation of another doctor or friend, or perhaps because of simple convenience or happenstance. You probably did not subject your new doctor—generalist or specialist—to rigorous questioning about credentials or practices.

This behavior is part of a tradition handed down from a simpler time, when patients had one family doctor who took care of them, perhaps for their entire lives. Though these doctors could do little for you if your diagnosis was cancer, you trusted them and were not accustomed to challenging their judgment or that of any other health care specialists they recommended.

But in recent years a revolution in attitudes and a growing candor about medical matters, including preventive health care, have transformed once passive patients, even as health services have burgeoned and changed. Civil rights, women's rights, consumers' rights, and human rights have helped to empower survivors. Now many feel that they can and should have a hand in deciding what part of the highly technical and often remarkable medicine available gives the best chance for more and more "quality" years.

A Changing Medical Arena

When you become a cancer survivor today, you become a consumer in a vast complex marketplace, a never-neverland which you typically enter with little or no experience or training, but where you may want and may be expected to play an active role. Giant strides forward in research and technology confront us with a mind-boggling array of treatment choices and possibilities.

The mushrooming of new systems of medical services has further complicated the survivor's job. More competitive markets require greater sophistication in making choices. Your job as a health care consumer is far more complex and significant than that of consumers looking for the right home appliance or auto repair services. The stakes in choosing medical care can affect your life as well as your pocketbook. Before you select your doctor, you will need to know what options are open to you. For this reason, the material covered in Chapter 8, "Straight Talk About Insurance and Health Plans," is must reading for the wise consumer.

Learning about Your Treatment

Even if you are not the sort of person who is likely to go to the library to study every new "cure," you should read about your diagnosis and the different treatment options available to you. Most survivors feel more secure, more self-assured, and thus more powerful when they understand and participate in crafting a treatment plan. A vast quantity of information is available from government and private organizations and from survivors willing to share their experiences. In "Resources" (starting on page 281), you will find more information on the Cancer Information Service, PDQ, CancerNet, and CancerFax, in addition to other private sector sources of information. All of these resources will provide you with valuable information from which you can make wise decisions regarding your treatment plan.

THE PRIMARY DOCTOR: ORCHESTRATING YOUR CARE

Whether you have been consulting an independent practitioner or a generalist in a managed care plan, you will need a primary care physician to orchestrate your care. For cancer patients, this is usually an oncologist. Your primary care physician will become a significant part of your life, not only during treatment, but perhaps for years of follow-up care.

Keep in mind that the "best doctor" means more than the doctor with the best education, although training is important. It also refers to doctors who practice in fine hospitals; use excellent radiologists and other specialists; tap into such resources as clinical trials; run efficient, patient-centered offices with caring nurses; and communicate in a way that leaves you feeling good about yourself and your treatment.

In a managed care setting, you may be limited to doctors within the network who meet these criteria, or your plan may permit you to look outside the system if you pay a larger share of the cost (the point-of-service option). Older patients may have to face the fact that some doctors they wish to see will not take new Medicare patients.

NO "ONE SIZE FITS ALL" – If you are to be treated successfully, you will need to find a doctor who is sensitive to your needs and your concerns, one who understands you as a person as well as a patient with a disease, and one who has the personality and management skills which enable you to be comfortable in a medical relationship over the long haul.

You should not use a "one size fits all" formula in your search. Patients differ greatly in their preferences and needs. You may not want to conduct in-depth discussions with your doctors about your disease and treatment. You may not want detailed statistics about your chances for long-term survival. Assuming the doctor knows best, you may be more comfortable leaving the tough medical choices and treatment plans to him or her. This is your privilege. Many survivors, particularly older ones, share such views. Others feel better when they are involved actively in gathering information about various approaches to treatment and the decision making process.

IDENTIFYING CANDIDATES – Begin by identifying a few candidates from among your previous doctors, from your health plan, and from the grapevine. You can call the local medical society, the chief resident or experienced nurses at the hospital, or local peer-support groups of seasoned survivors for suggestions. Be cautious: doctors and other medical professionals willingly tell you good news about each other, but they seldom level with you about the bad news.

The National Cancer Institute's (NCI) online service, PDQ (see

"Resources" for a description), includes directories of over twenty-five thousand health care professionals and organizations nationwide, including doctors doing research in specialized areas. You may want to access this list at your public library, since NCI information specialists at (800) 4-CANCER cannot provide the directory information. Your public library may also have the *Official Directory of Medical Specialists* or the *American Medical Directory* (published by the American Medical Association), both of which list doctors and their credentials.

Once you have a shortlist, take the few days required to check out potential doctors' credentials, styles of practice, and hospital affiliations. If possible, check on the experiences of people they have treated. Call the offices of doctors you are considering for any information you still need.

Consider the following in making your choice:

Basic Credentials – Though credentials are not everything, they are still important. Note the doctor's basic credentials, including whether he or she is board-certified in a specialty or subspecialty. Note the quality of the doctor's education, teaching affiliations, if any, and publications and PDQ listing.

Board Certification – Find out whether the doctor is the type of medical specialist you need (for example, medical oncologist, radiation oncologist, general surgeon). Note that some are self-proclaimed specialists, who have not satisfied the requirements for certification established by the professional board that supervises that field.

Certification means that a doctor has passed rigorous peer-administered written and oral examinations in their field and satisfied residency training requirements in the field. Some physicians are *double boarded*, meaning they are certified in more than one field. A few specialty boards require recertification after a certain number of years. Initials starting with an "F" (like F.A.C.P.) after a doctor's name mean that he or she has been honored by election to a specialty college fellowship.

Experience – Length of experience is always important, but medical oncology is a relatively new subspecialty of internal medicine, certified as such only since 1973. So when you consider older doctors who may lack this formal credential, check carefully on other factors, such as reputation among support group members, publications, teaching affiliations, PDQ listing, the study groups to which the doctors belong, and whether they enroll and/or follow patients in clinical trials (or have colleagues who do so).

Hospital Affiliation – Be sure to find out which hospitals the doctor is affiliated with, and which ones he or she prefers and why. Also determine where arrangements will be made for you to have radiation therapy, chemotherapy, or any other such special outpatient treatment.

Style of Practice – How do the doctors you are considering practice? If they practice independently, do they work closely with other physicians? If they are with a group, or in a university setting, do they themselves see you each time you have an appointment, or are you seen by an assortment of associates (and if so, who are these associates and what is the level of their education and training)?

"Chairside Manner" – In the old days, people talked about a physician's "bedside manner." Now, when doctors rarely come to see you in bed, and you are seen in an office chair more often than a hospital bed, it is appropriate to check out the "chairside manner" of a doctor. Do prospective doctors seem warm and concerned with you as a person? Talking with you, do they sit down or glance at a wristwatch while they hover at the door? Do you feel so rushed that your questions have gone unanswered? If called away in an emergency, do they arrange a time to answer your questions?

Office Procedures – When are the doctors usually in the office (days and hours of the day)? Can they be reached evenings or weekends? Who "covers" for them when they are away or not available by phone? How long, on the average, do patients have to wait to see them? Are your prospective caregivers part of that rare breed who still make house calls? How do they want you to proceed in the event of an emergency?

Who manages the office, answers the phones, and deals with the billing? What are the office policies toward the confidentiality of the information you choose to share with them? (see page 54 for a discussion of your right to privacy). Try to find out if the staff tends to be loose lipped about you and your disease, or if they guard your medical information appropriately.

Office Atmosphere – Note the manner in which the doctor's staff conducts business. Are they warm and patient with you and with others—on the phone as well as in person? Do they seem efficient and willing to answer your questions, even if your questions concern such mundane things as your next appointment? Check out the appearance of the office. Is it comfortable and cheerful, or dark, drab, and cluttered? In one major city, patients left a practice because chemotherapy was administered in a small, dark, messy room crowded with black chemotherapy chairs. As one such survivor put it: "That depressing place makes me feel like death warmed over; why make things worse than they have to be?"

Quality of Staff — The nurses and other paraprofessionals who work with a doctor may draw your blood and administer your chemotherapy. Find out how many of them are RNs (registered nurses), and how many have been tested and awarded the OCN (oncology certified nurse) credential. Consider the importance of experience, just as you did in choosing the doctor.

SPECIFIC TIPS — To see if you feel comfortable with a doctor, you will have to visit his or her office. Even then it is sometimes difficult in the first interview to determine whether you have chosen wisely; sometimes it takes months to find out. Here are a few suggestions about what to watch for and how to proceed at the beginning of your professional relationship:

- Some doctors encourage you to take notes during important visits—and even to tape conversations—so you will remember the details of a diagnosis or answers to your questions about treatment. It might be a good idea to inquire about office policy in this regard.
- To test a doctor's ability to relate to you, you might show him the *American Cancer Society's Survivor's Bill of Rights* (reprinted on pages 59 and 60). Ask how he or she feels about statement number one, specifying that those involved in cancer care, for example, should be "sensitive to the cancer survivor's lifestyle choices and need for self-esteem and dignity" and should take symptoms seriously and not dismiss aches and pains. Any marked disagreement about such statements should serve as a warning that you may not have chosen the right doctor.
- If you have other compelling reasons why you want to stay in treatment with a particular doctor—including, for example, the limits placed on your freedom of choice by a managed care plan—you should discuss the matter frankly with him or her. The results of such a conversation can be most positive.
- If your test results, biopsies, and other indicators of the success of your doctor's "recipe" for cancer treatment (including how you feel) do not please you at any time or stage of treatment, get a second or even third opinion (some plans routinely cover and may even require second opinions, while others may ask for your primary care physician's approval of such opinions). Even if you elect to stay with a particular doctor, a second opinion

approving your treatment will make you more comfortable and reinforce your trust.
- If all this does not work, if you feel your doctor does not have the necessary skills, or if you simply cannot feel comfortable with him or her, it makes good sense to start looking for a new doctor. The process will be much the same as the search for your first doctor, except that you have gained experience, know more about what you are looking for, and know what questions to ask.

COMMUNICATIONS—THE TWO-WAY STREET

To work successfully with your doctor, you must be able to talk frankly. As a survivor, you need an anchor, a coordinator, and an interpreter of information with whom you can conduct a comfortable dialogue—a dialogue which may continue for years.

Modern medical care can be highly technical, complex, and difficult to understand. Moreover, it is delivered by a team of specialists, including surgeons, radiologists, and a multitude of nurses and technicians. Psychiatrists, gastroenterologists, gynecologists, neurologists, and others may be consulted. Communicating with these specialists, and getting the benefit of their shared views, is an integral part of survivorship.

BARRIERS TO COMMUNICATION

Communication between the doctor and patient is a two-way street. The responsibility for it rests, in large measure, with the doctor. But, as professional societies are fond of pointing out, it rests with you, as well. In a fine, consumer-friendly 1995 pamphlet, *Making the Most of Your Next Doctor Visit,* the American Academy of Allergy Asthma and Immunology (AAAI) stresses that good communication may be hindered by physician instructions that are misunderstood or not followed by the patient, as well as by time constraints. A decade earlier, in *Communication: It's Good for Your Health,* the American Society of Internal Medicine (ASIM) reported that internists believe that about 70 percent of correct medical diagnoses are made simply through communication between patient and physician, yet patients often hold back crucial information. (To order the AAAI pamphlet, call (800) 456-ASTHMA or write Asthma Monitor, AAAI, 611 E. Wells St., Milwaukee, WI 53202. For the ASIM booklet, primarily intended for bulk mailings to doctors, call (202) 835-2746.)

Why is this so? Conducting a dialogue with a doctor sounds easy, but many survivors report that it is not. They would like to know more about their various therapies. They are not sure just what medicine

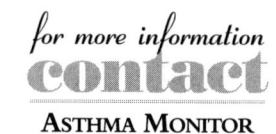

for more information
contact

ASTHMA MONITOR
AAAI
611 E. Wells St.
Milwaukee, WI
53202

202/835-2746

*Communication:
It's Good for Your Health*

they are supposed to take or when or why they are supposed to take it. They may be anxious to learn whether new pains are serious or unimportant side effects of old treatments. Certain attitudes and fears restrain survivors, including the following.

AWE OF THE DOCTOR – Many survivors stand in awe of their doctors, in whose hands their comfort and even their lives rest. They want these doctors to make them better, to like them, and not to consider them pests or hypochondriacs.

LACK OF SELF-CONFIDENCE – Survivors too often fear to ask the questions that lurk in their minds, afraid that the doctor will consider these questions "stupid" or "dumb." They worry: doesn't this busy physician have more important things to do than answer my questions? The answer is "NO!"

DIFFICULTY REMEMBERING – No matter who they are, or how extensive their experience or impressive their education, survivors can grow anxious discussing life-and-death matters with their doctors. Hearing new words and new concepts, they can suffer "information overload." They can have trouble focusing, absorbing abstract ideas and remembering all but certain emotionally charged "buzz words"—like *cure* or *disability*. Survivors commonly return home from an important medical interview and find they are unable to tell family or friends exactly what the doctor said.

"IATROGENIC" BEWILDERMENT – *Iatrogenic*, according to Webster's, means "induced by a physician." Some doctors make it difficult for you to understand them by using complex, technical language instead of plain English (for example, *alopecia* rather than "hair loss"). They may act as though they have no time for you, failing to sit down during your interview, or even hovering near the door. An NCCS survey explains in *Words That Heal, Words That Harm* (available from the National Coalition for Cancer Survivorship) that the doctor who told his patient "You're a walking time bomb," and another who observed that certain treatment was "only palliative," were using negative and harmful words that left patients shaken. Some doctors may simply seem insensitive to hints or cues you give as to how you would like to be treated.

SUGGESTIONS FOR EFFECTIVE AND MEANINGFUL COMMUNICATION

Some survivors argue that medical competence is more important to patients than communication skills. As one lawyer put it, she would rather see a "bleeding bastard" who would cure her, than a less competent, "sweet-talking" physician. Medical competence in today's world, however, requires that your doctor get sufficient information from you and relay important concepts to you.

The following are some practical suggestions, gained from the experiences of many survivors and health caregivers, about how you might communicate effectively with your doctor and other health caregivers.

SPEAK FRANKLY WITH YOUR DOCTOR – Remember, he or she cannot read your mind. Describe your symptoms, not only the obvious aches and pains, but other signs you have observed, such as trouble falling asleep at night, unhealthy eating habits, or overindulgence in alcoholic beverages.

BRING A FAMILY MEMBER OR FRIEND – If you have trouble asserting yourself, bring a family member or friend to speak for you. If several people are involved, be sure you make clear to the doctor to whom and to what extent they have your permission to discuss your case.

JOT DOWN YOUR QUESTIONS IN A NOTEBOOK – Before your visit to the doctor, jot down your questions in a notebook so you do not forget them. With the notebook in hand, you can write down your doctor's instructions.

Be sure these questions cover office procedure and information and confidentiality policies. Ask, for example: "Do you keep copious notes in your patients' medical records? To whom do you send these records? If I want access to my records, how would I get them, and how quickly? I've heard some doctors and hospitals charge an enormous amount to copy records; you won't do that, will you?"

TAPE IMPORTANT CONVERSATIONS – Because most people have trouble absorbing new information when they are upset, some doctors ask patients to tape important conversations so they can listen to the tape again later in the quiet of their homes. That way, they can review medical explanations and instructions in calmer, more rational moments.

INSIST ON PRIVACY DURING IMPORTANT INTERVIEWS – Under no circumstances should such an interview take place in a busy hallway, where anyone passing by can hear it. Preferably, consultations should be conducted with you and your physician seated and facing each other in a private room with the door closed.

GIVE YOUR DOCTOR "CUES" AS TO HOW MUCH INFORMATION YOU WANT AND NEED TO KNOW – Doctors used to tell patients nothing about cancer, not even that they had it. Now they tend to tell everything, including statistical chances for survival. Patients have different "coping styles"; for some it is frightening to know these things, for others it is frightening not to know. If your doctor is overloading you with facts and statistics that you do not want, simply say so; or offer a hint or cue as to how you feel. Try something like, "My father's already gotten the statistics about my tumor from PDQ" or simply "You know best." Sometimes body language—such as turning away and looking down—can help indicate you have had enough. If you want to know more about your disease, its treatment and possible outcome, say so.

ASK FOR INTERPRETATIONS OF LONG, PUZZLING MEDICAL WORDS OR TERMS – Never be embarrassed if you do not understand a word like "metastasis" or "sarcoma." It is reasonable to insist on a translation into plain English. Ask your doctor to show you a diagram or picture of the organs he or she is describing so you can understand where they are in your body and their relation to one another. Your doctor will probably respect your need to have your situation described in a way that makes sense to you.

DO NOT FORGET THAT DOCTORS ARE PEOPLE, TOO – Medical professionals respond to you just as you respond to them: pleasantness is usually met with pleasantness, and courteousness with courteousness. Express your appreciation when your doctor sits down to talk with you—either at the side of your bed in the hospital or on in office chair—and gives you complete attention during your limited time together.

If the doctor is called away from a consultation for an emergency, you should be told when he or she will return. If you are not told, or if the doctor looks at his or her wristwatch in the middle of an important conversation, or takes nonemergency telephone calls, speak up. Say you realize the he or she is a busy person, but you would like to know when you will be able to finish your talk because you still have unanswered questions.

DO NOT PRESENT YOURSELF TO YOUR DOCTOR AS A DISEASE, BUT AS A PERSON LIVING WITH A DISEASE – One survivor reported that she made it a rule to tell her doctor one thing about her life on each visit: that she had been to London, or had seen a ball game, or taken a poetry course. In this way, the doctor learned more about her and could look at her and treat her as a whole person. Another reported that she traveled frequently, but was anxious about going too far from sophisticated medical care. The physician prepared a special medicine kit for her to take along when she went to underdeveloped countries.

BE SURE THAT YOU UNDERSTAND YOUR TREATMENT PLAN BEFORE YOU LEAVE THE DOCTOR – Be sure you understand which tests and medicines have been prescribed, and how long and when you will be taking them. Ask the doctor to repeat whatever you are not sure of, including the benefits and risks involved in your treatment. Find out where you can call him or her and at what time in case a new problem occurs. Do not be embarrassed about taking too much precious medical time. Informed patients are more cooperative patients and doctors report that good communication with patients saves them time in the long run.

IF YOU FIND YOURSELF UNABLE TO COMMUNICATE WITH YOUR DOCTOR, TRY TO FIND ANOTHER ONE – If you feel hurried as you talk, or if you think your questions are not being answered satisfactorily or that you are not being given a fair hearing, try discussing this with your doctor. You may be surprised at the results.

Consider the advice of a support group or a cancer counselor to see how other patients have handled such problems and how you and your doctor might do better. As doctors themselves will tell you, if all this fails, consider changing physicians. Although this may be difficult for some—for patients in managed care situations, for example, or in sparsely populated rural areas, or for older patients who find that some physicians do not accept new Medicare patients—keep trying. With persistence you will probably find new caregivers. (See pages 33-35 for a discussion of how to choose a physician.)

THE HOSPITAL: A WORLD UNTO ITSELF

Cancer survivors do not spend much of their health care time in the hospital, mainly because hospital stays are expensive and outpatient care is used whenever possible. But most survivors do spend some time as inpatients, particularly at the beginning of treatment. This is usually a significant experience which may set the tone for how you view your care in the future.

EVALUATING HOSPITALS

Patients are often unprepared for the hospital experience. You may have been in the hospital briefly to have an appendectomy (a nuisance) or a baby (a joy) or to visit a sick grandmother (a duty). Unless you are an unusually sophisticated consumer of medical services, you probably did not shop carefully for a hospital. In the fee-for-service system, your doctor usually stipulated one of the hospitals where he or she had "privileges." If you were covered by a managed care plan, your choice of hospitals may have been limited.

No matter where physicians and particularly surgeons practice, one of the first questions you should ask them is, "With what hospital, or hospitals are you—or your managed care plans—affiliated." Managed care plans vary widely. Some are restricted to one or two local hospitals; others include services at comprehensive cancer centers in distant cities.

When you have the names of these hospitals, check them out. Again, the public library is a good starting resource. In large cities the main library has the most material. The community relations or public relations office of recommended hospitals should be able to answer your questions. The advice of seasoned survivors, nurses, and other health professionals may be more impartial than that of the local medical society or hospital association.

Gourmet cooking, chintz curtains, or the number of channels on your television set should not be the determining factors in evaluating a hospital. What you are seeking is an excellent workplace for your health team—a humane haven in a difficult period of your life. The following is a check list for you to use as you consider specific hospitals.

TYPE OF HOSPITAL – Today cancer care is offered in many different settings, from major cancer centers to small community hospitals. Find out exactly what sort of hospital you are considering. Is it a comprehensive cancer center—one designated by the National Cancer Institute? If so, it is likely to offer high quality, up-to-date medical care (researchers at these institutions have been involved in many of the most important medical advances).

Comprehensive cancer centers offer a wide variety of services, from counseling and rehabilitation to home-care supervision. If you belong to a managed care plan, find out if it offers a point-of-service option covering the full services of a cancer center. If not, you can still go to one, at least for a consultation, if you are willing to pay for it out of your own pocket.

In addition to these comprehensive centers, clinical cancer centers around the country are funded in part by the National Cancer Institute to carry out research and training programs, as well as patient care. Beware, however that some for-profit hospitals call themselves cancer centers or even comprehensive cancer centers.

But if they are free-standing (not affiliated with medical schools) and do not have research or teaching obligations, they probably are not designated as cancer centers by the federal government. Call

(800) 4-CANCER (the NCI's cancer information service) for a list of NCI-designated comprehensive and clinical cancer centers.

Other important questions to ask when evaluating hospitals include—
- Is this a teaching hospital, and is its cancer program affiliated with a medical school?
- Does a medical school use the hospital for internship and residency programs?

The advantages of medical school affiliation—the availability of doctor-faculty members, round-the-clock medical attention, a broad variety of services, and a greater likelihood of state-of-the-art oncology—usually outweigh the disadvantages (for example, being treated as a teaching case, which means being poked and prodded, especially when the medical team makes its early morning teaching rounds).

ACCREDITATION – If you are considering a community hospital which is not a federally designated cancer center and is not affiliated, either directly or indirectly, with a medical school, be sure the hospital is fully accredited. The Joint Commission on Accreditation of Healthcare Organizations (JCAHO) surveys hospitals carefully before granting them accreditation. A professionally sponsored group employing physicians, nurses, health-care administrators and other experts, the JCAHO holds hospitals to some one thousand staffing, safety, and quality-of-practitioner-care standards. According to the most recent figures available from the American Hospital Association, 1,399 of the nation's 6,467 hospitals were not accredited in 1993.

As an organization maintained by the health care industry, the Illinois-based JCAHO does not offer a consumer-friendly hot line or encourage consumer calls. However, you can ask a hospital's administrative officials about the results of their most recent JCAHO survey. You also can learn about various hospital services from the *American Hospital Association Guide to the Health Care Field,* an annual hospital survey available in most public libraries. Often a hospital's failure to gain accreditation or reaccreditation will be reported in the local press.

Some large-city magazines periodically carry articles rating local hospitals. Such lists include information from various sources, both objective and subjective. *Modern Healthcare,* a magazine for the health care industry, surveyed four thousand hospitals in 1995. The resulting article, "The Best Run Hospitals: For-Profits Spur Efficiency," identified the nation's "best managed" acute-care hospitals (the article may be obtained by calling (800) 678-9595 or by accessing it online at http://www.modernhealthcare.com).

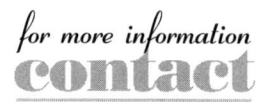

for more information
contact
CRANE COMMUNICATIONS
800/678-9595
http/:www.modernhealthcare.com
"The Best Run Hospitals: For-Profits Spur Efficiency,"
Modern Healthcare

Though articles or consumer books that rate hospitals may be useful, you have to be very careful in reading them to know exactly what they are evaluating. "Best" to one person, for example, may mean "worst" to another—if it means providing the most cost efficient care with the fewest possible resources, instead of the best quality of care for the survivor. Also, highly publicized "best, worst lists" and other information may be oversimplified or skewed in ways only experts can fathom. Hospital mortality rates, for example, can depend on many factors besides the quality of care. A fine cancer center can have high mortality rates because it cares for many patients with advanced cancers, while some public hospitals may have similar rates because they care for a high percentage of very sick patients with a variety of debilitating chronic conditions.

CONVENIENCE – Going to a hospital close to home, where your friends and family can visit you easily, offers many advantages. But if that hospital cannot provide you with the quality of care you need, you should consider another one, even if it is some distance away. A sensible compromise is a consultation at the closest comprehensive cancer center. Often the experts there can make the diagnosis, map out your treatment plan, and consult with your local doctors and hospital as they carry it out. If you cannot travel to a cancer center far from home for family or financial reasons, you may very well find the care you need right in your own community (see Services below).

SIZE AND SOURCE OF FUNDING – Size is a questionable variable when you are selecting a hospital. Some large hospitals (500 or more beds) are very good, some are not so good, and some are poor. The same is true of medium-sized (100-500 beds) and small (less than 100 beds) hospitals. Although bigger hospitals may seem more bureaucratic and impersonal, they may have more cancer treatment resources, such as expensive high-technology equipment. Moreover, staff members often are more experienced, since they see a wide variety of cases.

As for the source of a hospital's funding, public hospitals (like veterans hospitals, county hospitals, and some urban hospitals) may suffer from a poor image, and may not provide certain amenities. But amenities are less important than quality care. If it is affiliated with a good teaching hospital, attracting interns and residents eager to care for a variety of patients, and if it is well organized to deliver care, a public hospital may provide outstanding service.

SERVICES – It is difficult to assess the services of a given hospital until you have experienced them. But you can check on the quality and variety of services a hospital has to offer through your doctor, the hospital's administrative offices, and through other survivors who have used them. If you are going in for surgery, for example, you might ask your surgeon for details regarding the hospital's recovery room or intensive care unit. Ask about the reputation of its pathology laboratory and blood bank.

Some community hospitals do not serve enough cancer patients to have a special cancer unit. They may, however, offer treatment in local alliances, through which you can get CAT scans in one hospital and radiation in another. Such an arrangement may suit your needs. In any case, be sure you have answers to the following questions:
- Where will you be taken care of?
- Will the hospital have the high-tech equipment necessary to treat you after surgery? For example, are radiation therapy and scanning equipment available? If not, where will you receive such therapies when they are necessary?
- What is the reputation of the hospital's low-tech, but all- important services—respiratory and physical therapy, for example, or social work services and post-treatment programs which can give you a head start down the road to recovery?
- Most meaningful perhaps, what is the reputation of the hospital's nursing staff and of the non-RN staff who are performing nursing functions? Whether the people taking hands-on care of you are called "nursing aides" or "patient care associates" or something else, their number and the quality of their work, including their sensitivity to your needs, will affect your health and your well-being.

THE HOSPITAL EXPERIENCE

The hospital scene changes from day to day, but one thing is certain: You will undoubtedly spend less time in a hospital than you would have ten years ago. This is mainly due to insurance strictures.

INSURANCE STRICTURES – Modern hospital practice is governed by insurance strictures as well as by the doctor's orders and administrative wishes. Hospital stays for intensive chemotherapy, for example, are more limited than they used to be, and you will probably stay in a semiprivate room, even if you ask for a single room and are willing to pay the noninsured difference. If you cannot produce evidence of health insurance coverage, you may have trouble getting in at all (see Chapter 7 for more information about insurance coverage).

A preadmission process will save time. A pleasant voice may call from the hospital a few days before you are scheduled for admittance (assuming, of course that you did not enter through the emergency-room door). As an outpatient, you may go through a battery of tests before you are admitted—chest x-ray, EKG, blood tests, and urinalysis—from which you may get your first hints as to the atmosphere of the institution. You can be passed from hand-to-hand efficiently and cheerfully and be made to feel like a human being instead of a diseased body, or you can be worried by a seemingly disorganized bunch of people, jabbing at your veins, or barking orders at you in front of the X-ray machine.

Once admitted, you will become a part of the special hospital culture. You will meet a number of different caregivers who will draw more blood, perform more tests, and care for you in different ways. From them, you should learn about the schedule—visiting hours, lights-out, and meal times. If you have not been told, ask where to store your wallet and other worldly belongings.

A WORLD TO MASTER – The hospital is a world unto itself, a world to experience and to master. This world brings both good and bad news. The good news is that you can feel hopeful, even ennobled, by the marvelous care the modern hospital can offer through many well-trained, devoted, and talented professionals and paraprofessionals. Your caregivers now are more likely to look at you as a whole person, rather than as a lung or breast or set of bones.

The bad news is that a few impersonal staff members wedded to sometimes mindless institutional routines can make you feel dehumanized. For example, they may wake you up to give you a sleeping pill or ask you why you let yourself get cancer. More crucial, even the best hospitals with excellent reputations occasionally make mistakes. Though these mistakes are seldom fatal, survivors should remain alert to the possibilities.

The tragic death in 1994 of Boston Globe health columnist Betsy Lehman made this painfully clear. Though this 39-year old mother of two had chosen one of the country's preeminent cancer centers for bone marrow transplant treatment, and though she repeatedly complained of increasing pain and had a gut feeling that something had gone dreadfully wrong, Ms. Lehman was administered a fourfold chemotherapy dosage, four days in a row. Her resulting death, and the cardiac crippling of a fellow patient in the same hospital program, focused national attention on the issue of hospital errors.

A series of public and private investigations resulted in increased awareness that more hospitals must take steps to oversee quality treatment, including installing computerized techniques for ensuring dosage ceilings, clarifying guidelines for highly toxic drugs, better supervision of junior staff, and the design of unambiguous physician order forms. Essential as such improvements are, they will prove ineffective unless they are supplemented by sensitive professional education and on-the-job training in doctor-patient communication.

Dealing with Hospital Life

Seasoned survivors have found that their attitude—the way they respond to the hospital culture—has a lot to do with their success in taking advantage of the good the hospital offers. Learning to deal competently with the not-so-good is also important. The following are some tips for developing such an attitude and for negotiating with the system.

BE ASSERTIVE – If your common sense tells you something is wrong, learn to act, not aggressively or rudely, but assertively. This means that if someone wakes you up for no good reason or jabs at your veins until your arm is speckled black and blue, ask politely but firmly for an explanation and a remedy. If you cannot speak up for yourself, try to get your spouse, a relative, or a friend to speak up for you.

KNOW YOU CANNOT PERFORM THE IMPOSSIBLE – Be equally assertive in dealing with new and sometimes misguided staff efforts to help you avoid hospital errors. Someone may suggest that you should check your own drug dosages and other aspects of your care. If you wish to do this, and feel well enough to try, fine. If not, and particularly if you are alone with no one to speak up for you, respectfully make clear that you are unable to perform what is really your caregiver's job.

EMPATHIZE WITH OTHERS – Make an effort to treat hospital staff (and your fellow patients) as you would like to be treated, with respect for them and for yourself. Tactfully "stroke" the nurse's aide who forgets to fill your water pitcher or who turns up the television when you are trying to read. This means telling the aide dispassionately that you know how busy the staff is, but that you are not feeling too well and you would appreciate fresh water and a little quiet.

DO NOT TAKE YOURSELF TOO SERIOUSLY – Even as you take your situation seriously, try to keep your sense of humor. When you can laugh and joke and empathize with other people, you will find it easier to stand up for yourself.

STAY ALERT. SPEAK OUT. ASK QUESTIONS – Many people are fearful of hospital authority. An extreme example: the patient who is handed a pill he or she feels sure is wrong but fears to ask questions lest doctors and nurses consider her uncooperative, pushy, or "dumb." You and your caregivers will benefit if you tell them what bothers you and what information you need in order to feel more comfortable (and to be a "better" patient).

IF YOU MUST, COMPLAIN – When you have exhausted your new assertiveness, and things still do not seem to be going your way, by all means complain—to your doctor, to the nursing supervisor on your floor, to the chief nurse, or to the hospital administrator. If your hospital has a patient representative, he or she is a good resource. Present the facts calmly and clearly, asking for attention to your problem.

GOING HOME AND REENTERING SOCIETY

Some patients enjoy the often abbreviated postsurgery part of hospital life. Free of the cares of job and household, they savor their visitors, the plants they bring, the ministrations of the staff, and the companionship of other patients—particularly when the prognosis is good. Others find their hospital stay more stressful than the time spent at home immediately after their release.

Everyone looks forward to going home. Hospitals usually help you plan to assure that your reentry into the real world of self-care and many responsibilities is accomplished smoothly. In the discharge planning process, a nurse, social worker, or some other designated professional works with you to make sure you have the appropriate help and are in other ways prepared to convalesce at home. (See Chapter 3 for a discussion of the roles of these helping professionals.)

KNOWING AND UNDERSTANDING YOUR RIGHTS – INFORMED CONSENT, CONFIDENTIALITY, AND PATIENT RECORDS

INFORMED CONSENT: YOUR RIGHT TO CHOOSE AND REFUSE TREATMENT

Your right to accept or refuse medical treatment is another factor which both complicates good doctor-patient communication and makes it essential. Properly used, informed consent, the process by which patients agree to treatment, is more than a legal exercise. It offers an opportunity to learn about your medical options.

Doctors who take time to explain fully the consent form you must sign before you embark on a specific treatment, are at the same time explaining its benefits, side effects, and possible alternatives. Although state laws vary as to what treatments and procedures require your specific consent, they typically include a course of chemotherapy, surgery, internal examinations such as sigmoidoscopy (examination of the colon), and dye injections for a CAT scan.

RESPONSIBILITIES – *The doctor* – Your doctor has the duty, not to tell you everything about a proposed procedure, but to give you enough information to allow you to make an informed decision about whether you want to undergo it. You must be told the nature and purpose of the procedure; the risk and consequence of the procedure; the medically acceptable alternatives to the procedure; and the risks of not having the procedure. Even if you have given your written consent, it may be invalid if you have not been presented with adequate information.

The patient – If your doctor does not volunteer information about a procedure, ask for it. If you do not understand what you are told, ask for a clear explanation before you sign a form consenting to treatment.

Carefully read the informed consent form itself. When you sign it, you state two important things that help avoid future misunderstandings—that you are an "informed" patient; and that you give your consent to be treated.

THE PATIENT'S RIGHTS – If you do not agree with every statement on the consent form, you can make changes. For example, if the form states that you agree to have your operation videotaped for use by medical schools, and you do not want to be videotaped, just draw a line through that sentence.

By signing a consent form, you are giving your doctor permission to treat you and acknowledging that you understand that a particular result cannot be guaranteed. You do not give up your ability to sue your doctor for malpractice should he or she fail to follow professional standards and cause you harm. Informed consent is not a waiver of the doctor's liability if he or she acts negligently or improperly. (See pages 250-254 for a discussion of medical malpractice.)

WHEN YOUR CONSENT IS NOT NEEDED – Your doctor does not have to obtain your consent if—
- emergency treatment is needed to save your life or to prevent permanent harm;
- you have given your consent to one type of surgery, and during that surgery, a serious unanticipated condition arises (for example, you gave your consent to having cancerous lymph nodes removed, and during surgery, your doctor finds involvement in another organ and therefore removes it, too);

- you waive your right to consent to each treatment and agree to let your doctor make decisions about your care without consulting you;
- you suffer from a progressive illness and, having previously given informed consent to an anticipated course of treatment, are no longer capable of making decisions.

THE RIGHT TO REFUSE TREATMENT – A competent adult has the right to refuse medical treatment, even if the result may be death. Although there are some limits to this right (such as danger to the public if treatment is withheld in the case of AIDS, or the treatment options a pregnant woman with cancer may choose), these limits vary from state to state.

In the case of incompetent patients, states increasingly respect the patient's previously expressed wishes. In the absence of clear direction, credible surrogates may be permitted to refuse treatment on the patient's behalf. (See pages 245-247 for a discussion of your right to refuse treatment and to prepare advance health directives.)

CHILDREN AND INFORMED CONSENT – Under most circumstances, parents have the right to make treatment decisions for their children, although they cannot typically refuse life-saving care for their children. Most states give children the right to choose their own medical treatment at the age of 18. The following are two exceptions to this.
- Minors deemed mature and emancipated (married or self-supporting and living away from home) usually are permitted to make their own medical decisions.
- If a parent's refusal to consent to treatment may cause avoidable harm to the child, a court may decide that the child is suffering from neglect and appoint a guardian to make medical decisions for the child.

CONFIDENTIALITY

We used to take for granted that our doctors, sworn under the Oath of Hippocrates not to "nose abroad" or divulge their patients' "holy secrets," would keep the information we shared to themselves. In those simpler days, medical record keeping was a comparatively simple business, with doctors filing facts about your health on 3x5 cards, and maintaining them—unmolested—from the patients' birth through their death.

You can no longer take the sanctity of your medical records for granted. Even while you, like most survivors, try to talk and deal openly with cancer, you should be aware that some of what you tell your doctors—facts which can include sensitive value judgments about your emotional as well as physical health—may no longer be held in confidence.

Most doctors object as strongly as do survivors to this erosion of doctor-patient confidentiality. But the increasing complexity of the medical marketplace, reliance on third-party insurers to pay medical expenses, and the exploding use of computers speeding information about your health along the information highway, have all but taken the matter out of their hands.

ACCESS OF OTHERS TO YOUR MEDICAL RECORDS – Patients move more, travel more, and take advantage of the skills of more specialists. In an effort to coordinate your care and to treat you successfully and get paid for it, conversations between you and a doctor are likely to be shared with other doctors, nurses, billing staff, and possibly even appointment schedulers.

The Risks – In a managed care setting or in a private physician's office, your medical record may be seen by various caregivers, even though it contains sensitive information such as "patient appears depressed" or "patient reports husband suffers sexual dysfunction." The same is true at hospitals, laboratories, and at the pharmacy that maintains your prescription records.

Your routine signature authorizing your doctor to disclose health information to your insurers triggers a more far-reaching risk. This signature allows access to your entire medical file, including personal information which may not be relevant to a particular claim. But the time-honored bonds of confidentiality that apply to the doctor-patient relationship do not extend to "third party payers" under the law. So insurance companies can, and frequently do, transfer or even sell such information to other data banks.

If you want to be sure your treatment is covered, refusing to authorize your doctor to open your records to insurers is not a realistic option. But keep in mind that you probably can cross out particularly offensive phrases in release forms without dire consequences. One seasoned survivor routinely crosses out "now and forever" from the sentence defining the time frame of her releases, and this practice has never been challenged.

The Benefits – Ready access to your complete medical history can be a lifesaver if you are traveling, relocating, or changing doctors. Well-organized, readily accessible, computerized medical records can eliminate mistakes resulting from a doctor's sloppy handwriting, or they can also avoid the need to retest when x-rays are mislaid or blood counts lost. One metastatic breast cancer survivor reports that she would have preferred submitting her medical data to a host of computers to the experience of searching with hospital authorities one Fourth of July weekend for her spinal x-rays (they had slipped behind a file cabinet).

Still, you should be alert to the fact that your medical records travel routinely along computerized highways at incredible speeds. Your medical information can flow, not only to insurers, but to employers through whom most Americans get their health care paid for (see page 226 for a discussion of what information a doctor can reveal to your employer). In some circumstances, your records flow to data banks maintained by institutions like health maintenance organizations, hospital networks, drug companies, or medical information clearinghouses which collect information from member insurance companies and distribute it to similar companies.

WHAT RIGHTS DO YOU HAVE—CONFIDENTIALITY AND THE LAW – Putting sensitive information in the hands of the wrong person, or even in the hands of the right person who unknowingly misuses it, can stigmatize you. It can result in your losing a job, failing to qualify for insurance, keeping you out of a school or university, or adversely affecting your credit rating.

Yet, our laws fall far short of fully addressing the perils of record-keeping in an age of supercomputers, data banks, and third-party payers. No comprehensive federal law now protects patients from unauthorized or inappropriate disclosure of medical information, although the 1974 Privacy Act does apply some limited standards to records kept by federally funded institutions like the Veterans Administration and military hospitals.

What little protection exists comes from a patchwork of relatively weak, uncoordinated, and sometimes contradictory state laws. Over a dozen states have no protection whatsoever against unauthorized disclosure of medical records. Even in states that do have medical privacy laws, the majority set virtually no limits on what goes into a record, few limits on how long it is kept, and few if any limits on the way in which these records are kept and disclosed.

What rights do you have to the privacy of your medical records? As a practical matter, not very many. Privacy is not mentioned in the United States Constitution but is ambiguously protected as a penumbra (or shadow) of the Bill of Rights. According to Washington attorney and privacy expert Robert Belair, you have a "bundle of rights" to the information in your record (which technically belongs to your health care provider). This permits access to the record, limits dissemination of information in the record, and assures that the information is correct and is used appropriately.

To find out if your state is one of the 35 that currently has a law protecting these rights, and if so, how it protects them and what your remedies might be if they have been abused, call the state attorney general's office or your local Office of Consumer Protection.

Clearly, this is an area where more protection is needed. It is extremely difficult to strike a fair balance between the patient's right to privacy and the public's need to know. While we strive to achieve such a balance, cancer survivors remain at particular risk for loss of privacy.

GETTING YOUR OWN MEDICAL RECORD — You may want to see or obtain your medical records for a number of reasons: to make it easier to seek a second opinion, to change health care providers, to ensure that the records are accurate, or simply to be more informed about your prognosis and health care program. Ready access is particularly important in an emergency or if you or your doctor moves. Given that others may have these records, you also may want to know what they have seen.

If you have been treated in a nonfederal institution (a state, local or private hospital, or a doctor's office), your ability to obtain your records depends on your state law. At present, 25 states now permit access to both hospital and doctor records; six permit access only to hospital records.

Provisions under laws regulating your right to see your medical records vary in several ways, and access to them may depend on—
- the type of records covered (public hospital, private hospital and/or doctor);
- whether any exclusions apply (for example, some statutes permit doctors to withhold records if they believe that reading them would "harm" you);
- who may see your records (you, your family, your lawyer, another doctor);
- the type of access you have (to read or copy in whole or in part);
- when you have access (by request, by court order, by lawsuit, with a doctor's or hospital's consent).

In states without laws providing for access, doctors and hospitals can decide whether to give you your records, but many will do so if you simply ask for them.

However, if you were treated in a federal facility, such as a Veterans Administration or military hospital, you have the right to inspect and copy your medical records—a right established by the Privacy Act of 1974. Under this law, you can ask for your records, and federal agencies are required to respond within strict time limits. If they deny access or fail to meet deadlines, the Freedom of Information Act gives you the right to appeal to the head of the agency with which you are concerned.

When you write to a federal agency, mention that you are seeking your medical records "under both the Freedom of Information Act (5 U.S.C. Section 552) and the Privacy Act (5 U.S.C. Section 552a)," and write "Attention: FOIA/Privacy Act request" on the envelope. That way, the time limits and other benefits of these laws will apply to your request.

Wherever you were cared for, contact the medical records department of the hospital or your physician's office and ask what steps you should follow to obtain a copy of your records. The precise procedures differ from state to state and agency to agency, so you will want to find out what steps you are expected to take. If necessary, make your request in writing and keep a copy. If your request is denied, ask the hospital or doctor to state in writing why they will not let you see your records and how you can appeal their decision.

For further information, consult *Medical Records: Getting Yours* (1995), available for $10 from Public Citizen's Health Research Group, 1600 20th Street, NW, Washington, DC 20009. This helpful and consumer-friendly document describes the laws of each state and provides a step-by-step guide to getting your medical records from federal, state, local, and private institutions.

NEW CHALLENGES TO CONFIDENTIALITY

CONFIDENTIALITY AND GENETIC INFORMATION – One emerging area of concern stems, ironically, from modern genetics, a leading-edge field which holds great promise for cancer survivors and their families. It gives caregivers the exciting potential of improving your lot through more precise diagnostic tools, new medications, screening, and counseling about how to avoid or ease the disease. But at the same time, genetic information poses an ominous threat to privacy.

Calling genetic information your "future diary," one leading medical ethicist, Professor George Annas of Boston University, has warned that access to it "gives others potential power over the personal life of the individual." He warns that when the day comes that a blood test might reveal the extent of your chance of developing an inheritable cancer (some are inheritable, others not)—or your child's risk of getting the cancer you already have—that information will become part of your medical record. These records travel far beyond your doctor's office and open the way to stigmatization and discrimination. Genetic testing expands the scope for invasion of privacy from your definite past to your possible future.

This development is so dramatic, and the prospects for abuse so disturbing, that several states have enacted laws preventing disclosure of genetic information without your permission. If your insurer asks you

for more information
contact

PUBLIC CITIZEN'S HEALTH RESEARCH GROUP

1600 20th St., NW
Washington, D.C.
20009

Medical Records: Getting Yours

for a blood test to conduct DNA-based testing, or if you suspect that you have been discriminated against due to your request for a genetic test or the results of such a test, check with your state insurance department or state attorney general's office to see if your rights have been violated. Some of these laws even bar genetic testing or the use of genetic testing information by employers. (See page 210 for a discussion of how the Americans with Disabilities Act restricts the release of your genetic information in some circumstances.)

CONFIDENTIALITY AND SUPPORT GROUPS – The burgeoning of support groups, important and meaningful as they are, also raises privacy concerns. Whether such groups are professionally or peer-led, participants often grow close and share a great deal of personal information. A 1993 study published in *Hospital and Community Psychiatry,* showed that over half of the group leaders responding to a survey reported experience with group members breaking confidentiality— although almost all of them (87 percent) said they had briefed their groups on confidentiality principles.

But no matter how sensitive group members are to privacy concerns, difficult situations can arise. Consider the dilemmas arising from these examples cited during an expert panel discussion titled "Eavesdropping on Your Cancer" at the National Coalition for Cancer Survivorship's Eighth Annual Assembly in Seattle (1993).

> A survivor absent from a group session called another member to fill her in on what she had missed. When this conversation got back to the group, an active participant felt her confidentiality had been violated.

> A survivor who shared the fact that she had been a long-time member of Alcoholics Anonymous, became very upset months later when a fellow member raised her AA connection in front of new members.

> A couple participating in a group suffered when, at a session which the woman did not attend, her husband asked the group to keep secret the fact that he had sent for a book advising how to end one's life, and that he intended to follow its approach when the time came. The woman later told the group (when her husband was absent) that she knew he had sent for the book but that he would not discuss it. Constrained by his request, the group simply encouraged her to keep trying. When the husband's lung cancer accelerated and he did commit suicide without discussing his decision with his family, the group,

its social work leader, and his physician all agonized as to whether they should have spoken up, even against his wishes.

The doctor-patient privilege is almost always lost when information is discussed in front of other people. That means that each member of the group must trust the others to protect their privacy. While nothing is foolproof, and ambiguous situations may arise, groups should establish an understanding at the outset—perhaps even in writing—that information discussed in the support group is confidential and that no one can discuss what anyone says outside of the room.

The Cancer Survivors' Bill of Rights
WRITTEN FOR THE AMERICAN CANCER SOCIETY BY NATALIE DAVIS SPINGARN

1. Survivors have the right to assurance of lifelong medical care, as needed. The physicians and other professionals involved in their care should continue their constant efforts to be:
   Sensitive to the cancer survivor's lifestyle choices and their need for self-esteem and dignity;
   Careful, no matter how long they have survived, to have symptoms taken seriously, and not have aches and pains dismissed, for fear of recurrence is a normal part of survivorship;
   Informative and open, providing survivors with as much or as little candid medical information as they wish, and encouraging their informed participation in their own care;
   Knowledgeable about counseling resources, and willing to refer survivors and their families as appropriate for emotional support and therapy which will improve the quality of individual lives.

2. In their personal lives, survivors, like other Americans, have the right to the pursuit of happiness. This means they have the right:
   To talk with their families and friends about their cancer experience if they wish, but to refuse to discuss it if that is their choice and not to be expected to be more upbeat or less blue than anyone else;
   To be free of the stigma of cancer as a "dread disease" in all social situations;
   To be free of blame for having gotten the disease and guilt of having survived it.

3. In the workplace, survivors have the right to equal job opportunities. This means they have the right:
   To aspire to jobs worthy of their skills, and for which they are trained and experienced, and thus
   To be hired, promoted, and accepted on return to work, according to their individual abilities and qualifications, and not according to "cancer" or "disability" stereotypes.
   To privacy about their medical histories.

   {Continued on the next page}

Working with Your Doctor and Hospital System: Becoming a Wise Consumer – **CHAPTER TWO**

THE CANCER SURVIVORS' BILL OF RIGHTS (CONTINUED)

4. Since health insurance coverage is an overriding survivors' concern, every effort should be made to assure all survivors adequate health insurance, whether public or private. This means:

> For employers, that survivors have the right to be included in group health coverage, which is usually less expensive, provides better benefits, and covers the employee regardless of health history;
>
> For physicians, counselors, and other professionals concerned, that they keep themselves and their survivor-clients informed and up-to-date on available group or individual health policy options, noting, for example, what major expenses like hospital costs and medical tests outside the hospital are covered and what amount must be paid before coverage (deductibles.)

Chapter Three

The Health-Care Team: Working Together for Your Benefit

by Diane Blum, ACSW

"I have worked as an oncology professional for over twenty years, and I am strongly committed to the concept of survivorship. To me, the survivor is the key person on the health care team, and my work with NCCS is focused on strengthening the survivor's role."

Diane Blum, ACSW

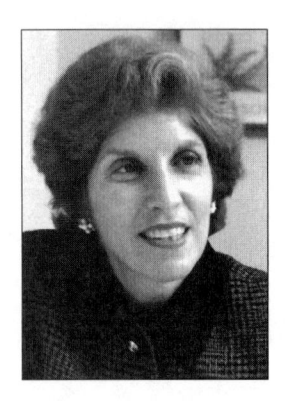

DIANE BLUM, ACSW is executive director of Cancer Care, Inc., co-founded the National Alliance of Breast Cancer Organizations (NABCO), and is a vice president of the National Coalition for Cancer Survivorship. Prior to joining Cancer Care in 1984 as director of social service, she was a social work supervisor at Memorial Sloan-Kettering Cancer Institute and the Dana-Farber Cancer Institute. She serves on advisory committees for the American Association of Retired Persons, the American Society of Clinical Oncology, the Rose Kushner Award for Excellence in Journalism, and the United Way of New York.

Survivorship begins with diagnosis and goes on for the rest of your life. Dealing with each "season of survival" and getting the best possible care is a complicated, demanding process for you and your loved ones. This process can be an overwhelming and lonely experience, and certainly involves much more than medical management. It requires attention to your psychological, social, emotional, and practical needs as well. While medical care is your primary concern, many cancer survivors and their families can benefit from the work of health-care professionals who help them prevent problems from developing and help them resolve problems as they arise.

This chapter describes how social workers, psychologists and psychiatrists, home health and hospice nurses, rehabilitation specialists, nutritionists, and clergy can help you; how you can find them; and how you should expect to pay for their help. All of these professionals are part of your cancer care team who will work together to coordinate your care and help you maintain the quality of your life.

A PERSONAL PERSPECTIVE

When Alan G. was diagnosed with prostate cancer, he was already dealing with the illness of his elderly mother. He felt overwhelmed by the decisions he needed to make about his own treatment and did not know how he could continue to provide the same care for his mother. He joined a hospital-based support group for men with prostate cancer where he got support from sharing his concerns and fears with the other men in the group, and benefited from hearing the monthly medical updates. The social worker who led the group also helped him to arrange for home care for his mother to relieve him of some of his responsibility.

SOCIAL WORKERS

Social workers are professionals who are specially trained to provide counseling and practical assistance to meet your specific needs. Some social workers, called oncology social workers, have chosen to specialize in dealing with the particular issues that arise when a person has cancer. Other social workers may not have specific oncology experience, but have training in working with people who are dealing with medical illness and are knowledgeable about the problems that can arise from a serious health problem. Social workers can provide counseling to help individuals cope with concerns related to diagnosis, treatment, and side effects.

This counseling can be offered to you individually, to your family, or through a support group. The social worker will explain to you what the different types of counseling involve. People frequently express concern about talking in a counseling situation and may feel that they are too shy or just not comfortable talking about themselves or their feelings. The social worker can describe what it is like to be in a support group or to participate in ongoing counseling, and will work with you to determine what is best for you. For many people, talking with a social worker only once or twice is sufficient and meets their needs.

The social worker can help you and your family communicate better, set priorities for the many responsibilities you have, and provide assistance with managing normal feelings of sadness, anger, or worry. Counseling may be particularly important when your treatment is complete and when you may experience anxiety about moving on with your life.

Social workers also have an expertise in helping you find needed community services. They are trained to provide referral to reputable agencies who provide practical assistance with home care, transportation, child care, financial problems, and other concerns that arise frequently during treatment for cancer, including your eligibility for the previously listed services. Social workers can also help when you have concerns about employment or insurance.

The social worker can guide you through the system, including how to apply for Social Security Disability or food stamps, fill out insurance forms, or get information about financial assistance. Social workers help you understand these complex, time-consuming application procedures. They can make telephone calls, write letters, and do follow-up to get you the services you need.

Most hospitals have social workers on their staff who are available to you when you are an inpatient or an outpatient. You can ask your doctor or nurse to arrange for you to meet the social worker or you can call the Social Work Department directly. Most hospitals do not charge for this service, although more hospitals are now billing for counseling sessions.

When you are treated or receive follow-up care in a physician's office, you may have to make more effort to find a social worker. The first step is to inquire in the physician's office about support services in the community, which may include support groups, professionals offering cancer counseling, and local and national organizations that provide information and referral. If you are interested in individual, family, or group counseling, ask about the social worker's experience in working with cancer survivors, what the counseling will cost, and whether the cost is reimbursable.

Social workers are licensed by state agencies. In most states, if a social worker is licensed and has the proper accreditation, health insurance will pay for limited counseling sessions. Do not hesitate to ask questions about experience and licensing and to seek out several social workers if available. Cancer Care, Inc., the National Coalition for Cancer Survivorship(NCCS), the American Cancer Society(ACS), and the Leukemia Society of America are all organizations that can provide you with social work help directly or refer you to community-based social workers and social services. Addresses and telephone numbers for these organizations and many other helpful support and advocacy groups are listed in Resources.

PSYCHOLOGISTS AND PSYCHIATRISTS

Psychiatrists are physicians who are trained to provide psychotherapy and who can prescribe medication. A cancer diagnosis can create feelings of distress or sadness as you try to adjust and incorporate the diagnosis into your life. Chapter 5 goes into more detail on the emotional impact of cancer. Sometimes, the feelings of sadness are more intense when you finish treatment. For most people, sharing their concerns with their family, friends, or someone on the health-care team helps them to feel better.

Other times, however, you may feel sad and discouraged for long periods, and these feelings may affect daily activities. In this situation, the help of a psychiatrist can be crucial. Psychiatrists can prescribe medication for problems such as depression or sleep disturbances. They can provide counseling to help you deal with the emotional impact of your illness and to cope better with your problems. Some psychiatrists also are trained in hypnosis and relaxation techniques that help manage and reduce anxiety.

You may ask your primary physician for a referral to a psychiatrist or call the psychiatry department at your hospital. You also can locate a referral for a psychiatrist by calling a local medical society. The telephone number for the medical society is in the yellow pages under "medical groups." Psychiatric help is covered by most private insurance, but you must determine how many sessions will be covered and at what percentage of cost. In choosing a psychiatrist, you should ask the same questions as in choosing a social worker.

Psychologists are also trained to provide professional counseling, but they are not physicians and do not prescribe medication. In addition to expertise in psychological testing, many psychologists specialize in areas such as marital counseling or behavioral interventions. A few psychologists and psychiatrists specialize in oncology, and many are linked to major cancer centers. Referrals to psychologists are available through your physician. You should determine the individual's credentials, and inquire about cost and the possibility of sliding-scale fees based on your income.

Sometimes people assume that seeing a counselor is a sign of weakness or an indication that they are going "crazy." This is not true; rather it means that you are having difficulty dealing with a very stressful period in your life and need assistance in finding ways to feel better. Being upset by a serious illness is not unusual. Psychiatrists,

A PERSONAL PERSPECTIVE

John R's oncologist suggested that he have a consultation with a psychiatrist when John described his feelings of sadness which made it impossible for him to concentrate on his work, or enjoy his time with his family. Since these symptoms can indicate a serious depression, John met with a psychiatrist several times who evaluated his situation and recommended an antidepressant which began to relieve John's symptoms within several weeks.

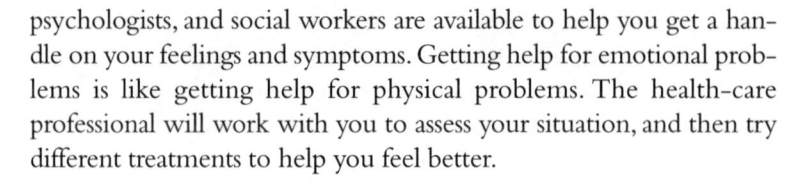

psychologists, and social workers are available to help you get a handle on your feelings and symptoms. Getting help for emotional problems is like getting help for physical problems. The health-care professional will work with you to assess your situation, and then try different treatments to help you feel better.

NURSES AND HOME HEALTH AIDES

Anyone treated for cancer has contact with a nurse, either in a hospital, a clinic, or a physician's office. Many people are not aware of the wide range of skills nurses possess or of their importance in cancer care. Nurses implement the plan of care that is initiated by your physician. They are educated to administer medications and to monitor side effects. Many nurses specialize in oncology, and are very knowledgeable about the symptoms and side effects of cancer treatment. Whether you are receiving treatment as an inpatient or outpatient, you probably will spend long periods of time with your nurse. Look upon him or her as an important resource for tips and advice on how to manage and coordinate your care. Nurses assess your symptoms on a regular basis, administer treatments—often by starting IVs or giving injections—and help you with the side effects of cancer and its treatment. Nurses are also a good source of information about support services in the community and patient education materials and programs.

Many nursing services are available in your home. These services include visits from a registered nurse, a private duty nurse, and a home health aide. Your physician can request that a nurse come to your home to take blood, supervise dressing changes, or monitor IV lines. Nurses may come on a daily basis, or several times a week. They will work with you and your caregivers to deal with problems related to your care. Many people now have chemotherapy administered at home; this works well if you have problems getting to the physician's office. Usually the nurse's visit is brief, less than an hour, and the cost is covered by insurance after approval of the visit is obtained from the physician. Some tasks are not considered skilled nursing tasks, and therefore are not covered by insurance. Be sure to determine the level of insurance coverage available for the services your doctor is ordering.

You and your family also can request a private duty nurse to stay at your home for longer periods of time, such as eight hours of care at night, or during the day when your family members are at work. This care arrangement can provide many advantages by allowing you to stay at home rather than in the hospital. It is very expensive, however, and is not covered by Medicare or Medicaid, and only occasionally by private insurance.

Home health aides also provide care at home for brief visits to help

A PERSONAL PERSPECTIVE

Elsa is a 75-year-old woman who receives chemotherapy for advanced breast cancer. She lives with her husband who has Parkinson's disease. Getting to treatment is very difficult for Elsa. She and her children worked out a plan for her to have chemotherapy administered at home, and she now travels to her doctor's office just once a month.

with bathing and light household chores, such as cooking meals, changing bedsheets, or doing laundry for the patient. This care, which is available during the day and also at night, is less costly than care from a registered nurse. Sometimes it is reimbursed by Medicaid, depending on state rules, and sometimes by Medicare when the care is supervised by a nurse, but rarely by private insurance. Always inquire if there is a sliding scale fee based on your income.

Your physician, nurse, or social worker will know about resources for nursing care and home health care in your community and will be able to refer you to a reputable agency. If you are choosing a home care agency by yourself, you can obtain a helpful booklet called *How to Select a Home Care Agency* available from the National Association for Home Care. The yellow pages also contain home health-care listings. You should check the credentials of the agency, ask about the training of the people providing the care and whether the employee is bonded. Home health-care services can ease the burden of care for you and your family. Sometimes, just a few hours of outside help a week is all that is necessary for family and friends to be able to coordinate their efforts to provide care.

REHABILITATION SPECIALISTS

People who experience physical changes due to cancer and its treatment may be helped greatly by rehabilitation services. These services, which are provided by physiatrists (physicians who specialize in rehabilitation medicine), physical and occupational therapists, rehabilitation counselors, and speech therapists, are offered in hospitals, at outpatient settings, and at your home.

Many people are not familiar with how physical therapy, occupational therapy, speech therapy, enterostomal therapy, or sexual therapy can help them. Physical therapy can strengthen a body part or function weakened by cancer treatment. For example, physical therapy is used after a mastectomy and/or node dissection to reduce swelling of the arm or to regain strength after major surgery. Occupational therapy helps you adjust your routines of getting dressed or moving around the house so that you can continue with your normal activities even when you have a physical disability. Speech therapy helps you learn how to communicate after a laryngectomy or when you have a mouth or facial tumor which interferes with speech.

Enterostomal therapy is provided by nurses who specialize in helping people with ostomies and who give advice and guidance on how to adjust your daily routines to your surgery. Sexual therapists offer help with the problems that may arise in resuming sexual activity following cancer treatment. Managing intercourse after an ostomy, impotence, and loss of sexual interest are all problems that can be

A PERSONAL PERSPECTIVE

Ann, a 45-year-old woman who had a lumpectomy and radiation treatments for early stage breast cancer, utilized physical therapy services which concentrated on arm exercises. She said the four months of weekly therapy plus exercises at home helped strengthen her arm so she could play tennis the way she had prior to surgery. The physical therapy also was a boost to her emotionally, as it helped her feel she was active in her own recovery.

A PERSONAL PERSPECTIVE

Fred's wife, Mary, was upset that he was not able to eat his usual diet because of a bad taste in his mouth. The hospital dietitian made suggestions about sucking on hard candies, drinking ginger ale and mint tea, sprinkling sugar on Fred's food, and using plastic utensils. These tips helped Fred eat with more enthusiasm, and made both him and Mary feel better.

addressed by a professional knowledgeable about sexual functioning.

Hair loss is often considered one of the most devastating side effects of cancer and its treatment. Local organizations can provide help, and social workers or nurses can refer you to providers of wigs and prostheses. It is important that you feel comfortable with your wig or prosthesis, so do not hesitate to ask questions about what to look for and where to purchase them. With the exception of the provision of wigs and prostheses, professionals offering rehabilitation services should be licensed, and rehabilitation physicians should be board certified.

Most physicians will refer you for rehabilitation services. If you are not told about them, ask the physician or nurse about what is available to help you make the adjustment to a physical limitation. Many insurance companies do not pay for rehabilitation, so be sure to check your benefits. If you do not have insurance, or if you want to supplement your professional services, some organizations sponsor rehabilitation programs.

The most well-known agency is the American Cancer Society, which provides programs for women with breast cancer and for people with ostomies and laryngectomies. The YWCA offers its Encore Program for women with breast cancer, and many community based agencies provide wigs, prostheses, and support programs. The American Cancer Society, the National Cancer Institute, the National Coalition for Cancer Survivorship, the Leukemia Society, Y-Me, UsToo, the National Alliance of Breast Cancer Organizations (NABCO), Candlelighters Childhood Cancer Foundation, and Cancer Care, Inc. are all sources of information about rehabilitation programs. Changes in body image or body function can be distressing. Programs that help you adjust to the change and gain strength physically and emotionally are crucial in maintaining your quality of life.

DIETARY OR NUTRITIONAL SERVICES

Many cancer survivors experience weight loss during treatment, usually as a result of a loss of appetite. The most common reason for this is nausea. Other symptoms may be a feeling of fullness, dry mouth, a change in the way food tastes, heartburn, or fatigue, which interferes with meal preparation. You and your caregivers may be upset that you are not able to eat as you did before you had cancer, and that you do not enjoy your food in the same way.

You may be able to minimize weight loss if you follow a diet that meets your needs for calories, vitamins, and protein. Your physician or nurse can refer you to a registered dietitian early in your treatment. The dietitian will suggest food substitutes if your tastes change or if you are able to tolerate some foods better than others. The dietitian will also recommend recipes written specially for people who are undergoing cancer treatment. *Eating Hints for Cancer Patients* is a helpful booklet produced by the National Cancer Institute that provides tips on managing eating problems as well as easy recipes; it is available by calling (800) 4-CANCER.

Most hospitals have a registered dietitian on their staff, and you can request to meet with one. If you are looking on your own, be sure to find someone reliable and not a person or organization that promotes dietary cures for cancer as easy solutions. As with all other professionals, ask about the dietitian's training, experience in working with people with cancer, and fees. You can expect the dietitian to have at least a bachelor's degree and often a master's degree. Anyone can call himself or herself a nutritionist, so be careful in your selection process. Your insurance should cover a consultation with a dietitian in the hospital. Ask your doctor, nurse, or social worker about community-based programs that offer free educational sessions.

Hospice Care

Hospice care, sometimes called *palliative care,* is offered to people with terminal cancer when the focus is on comfort and control of symptoms. Your doctor, nurse, and social worker should work with you to make a decision about hospice care and to coordinate hospice services for you. Most people choose hospice care when they decide that they do not want treatment, such as chemotherapy or radiation therapy, but want to focus on comfort and support. At this time, your doctor will refer you to a hospice in your area. The hospice will evaluate your medical and emotional needs and will work with you and your family to develop a plan of care.

Hospice care usually is provided in the home with backup care in the hospital or in a special unit of a hospital which is called a hospice or palliative care unit. Some hospices which are separate from hospitals and have their own buildings are called freestanding hospices. The most common hospice program is the home hospice program where care is provided in your home.

Hospice care is aimed at physical comfort, especially pain control and emotional support both for the patient and for the family. With hospice care, your health-care team shifts its focus to efforts that provide relief from pain and suffering. A nurse is usually your primary contact with a hospice program, but hospice staff includes physicians, social workers, clergy, and volunteers. All of these people may visit you at home. Someone is always on call to assist you and your caregivers. A hospice also provides bereavement counseling to family and friends after a person dies.

If you are looking for a program on your own, call the National

Hospice Organization (see Resources) or your local Visiting Nurses Association, which you can find in the yellow pages under "nursing care." Hospice programs are available in most communities. If no hospice service is available where you live, your health-care team should coordinate available nursing services as best as possible to insure your comfort.

Many families who have participated in hospice care feel that it offers tremendous comfort and relief to them as they deal with terminal illness. Families report that hospice care helps them provide comfort and a sense of peacefulness in addition to preparing them for the death of a loved one. However, home hospice care is not for everyone, particularly when the family feels it would be too difficult for them to provide care at home to someone who is very sick; when the caregivers are faced with too many other demands; or when it would be too upsetting to have someone die at home.

Sometimes, people want to keep treating the cancer, and they view hospice as a form of giving up. The decision to stop active treatment and focus on comfort is a complicated, emotional one for many families. It is important to gather information about local hospice services, discuss the options with everyone involved, and come to a decision that is shared by the patient and loved ones. The members of your health care team should be involved in this process and should be able to offer you information and support as you deal with this difficult decision.

Clergy

Serious illness frequently leads to questions about the meaning of life, as well as questions such as *why me* and *why now*? You may want to explore these concerns with a member of the clergy in your community. Prayer can be useful as a means of providing hope and comfort. Spiritual counseling can help you find renewed meaning in life during a difficult and stressful time. A compassionate member of the clergy who is trained to provide support can be a valuable asset for you and your caregivers.

Clergy are also important resources for learning about local organizations and agencies that provide other services you may need. Religious agencies such as Catholic Charities, the Council of Churches, the United Jewish Appeal (UJA), the Federation of Jewish Philanthropy, or the Federation of Protestant Welfare Agencies all provide support services that may be helpful to you and your family. Your doctor or nurse can refer you to a hospital chaplain who can, in turn, refer you to community-based clergy or religious organizations.

A PERSONAL PERSPECTIVE

Laura had not gone to church in many years. Her diagnosis of colon cancer created a desire for spiritual guidance, so she sought out the minister in the church she had attended earlier in her life. His recommendation of readings from the Bible as well as books such as *When Bad Things Happen to Good People* by Rabbi Harold Kushner were very helpful to her. Laura met with her minister for guidance and support on a regular basis throughout her course of treatment.

QUALITY OF LIFE CONCERNS

In response to the growing concern about the quality of our health care, the Texas Cancer Council outlined ten "Ethical Principles for Cancer Care" as the moral basis for delivering comprehensive care to people with cancer. Both health-care providers and consumers contributed to this work.

ETHICAL PRINCIPLES FOR CANCER CARE

1. Since cancer affects a person's entire sense of well-being, cancer care cannot be equated with or limited to prevention, early detection, and treatment of bodily disease. To deal with the effects of cancer, this care should address humans as whole persons with biological, emotional, social, economic, informational, moral, and spiritual needs.

2. Benefiting persons with cancer is the highest priority of health-care professionals. Individuals fully benefit when they receive personalized, comprehensive, coordinated, and culturally sensitive care.

3. Patients are to be respected as autonomous, self-governing persons with the right to express their needs and emotions and make informed decisions in their own best interests.

4. To make informed decisions, patients must be provided with information that is understandable, sufficient, and applicable to their circumstances.

5. Effective communication is essential in order to benefit persons with cancer and to respect their autonomy. This communication rests on trust, concern, mutual respect, honesty, and self-awareness.

6. Terminally ill patients are to receive continued health care, support, respect, and assurance.

7. Collegial teamwork is essential for attending to the total human dimensions of cancer care.

8. Teamwork is sustained by caregiver collegiality, which is based on a mutual understanding of and respect for the individual and professional contributions of colleagues.

9. The ability of health-care professionals to care for patients and those close to the patient depends on caregivers attending to their own personal, psychological, social, moral, and spiritual needs.

10. Basic, clinical, and psychosocial research is integral to improving cancer prevention, early detection, diagnosis, treatment, long-term follow-up, and the personal dimensions of cancer care. All research should contribute to, not detract from, beneficial and respectful care of individuals with cancer.

Source: Vanderpool, H, (ed.) The Human Dimensions of Cancer Care: Principles and Guidelines for Action. The Texas Cancer Council and Institute for the Medical Humanities, The University of Texas Medical Branch at Galveston, 1994.

Chapter Four

Understanding the Risks and Benefits of Unconventional Treatment

by Natalie Davis Spingarn

"When I flew to New Mexico in 1987 to keynote the first NCCS assembly… [w]hat I found bowled me over: a sizeable group of feisty, optimistic, knowledgeable, warm, and supportive colleagues.... I was hooked—and I have been active in NCCS and its leadership since."

Natalie Davis Spingarn

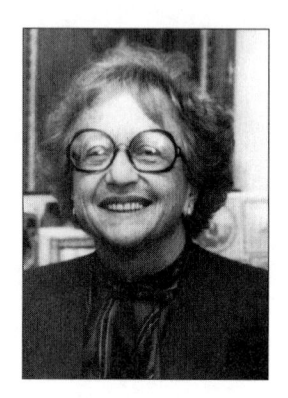

NATALIE DAVIS SPINGARN, a prize-winning writer, advocate, and consultant on health and social policy issues, is vice chair of the Board of Directors of the National Coalition for Cancer Survivorship. Ms. Spingarn founded and served as editor of the NCCS quarterly publication, *The Networker*. Ms. Spingarn won an Oscar at the John Muir Medical Film Festival for her film *Patients and Doctors: Communication is a Two-Way Street*. She is currently on the editorial board of *The Patients Network*, a newly formed international publication committed to patient-centered care. Based in Washington, DC, Ms. Spingarn has served as an official in the executive and legislative branches of the federal government, as a District of Columbia General Hospital commissioner, and on several advisory committees for George Washington University Medical Center.

Caveat Emptor: Unconventional Treatments

One of the most challenging and worrisome questions in your life as a survivor-consumer is whether you should try unconventional (or unproven or questionable) treatments—either in addition to or in place of your conventional medical care as an alternative treatment. Call them what you will, these treatments come to the attention of cancer survivors at every stage of their illness.

Along the clinic grapevine, talking to the retired nurse down the block, at a party of well-wishers, reading newspaper and magazine accounts of holistic or mind-body cures, you sense that something is out there in addition to standard, harsh, "cutting, burning, and poisoning" conventional therapies; that "something" just might ease your pain and might even cure your cancer.

The notion of doing something about your own bodily health is very appealing. Put off by the often impersonal nature of modern high-tech medicine, and depressed by the knowledge that after many years of trying, researchers have still not come up with a sure cure for cancer, you may throw up your hands and ask yourself: Why not try something that won't destroy my body's own defenses, something gentle, easy, nontoxic, and hopeful—like imagining my good cells eating up the bad cancer cells, or eating a restorative grain, or purifying and cleansing my system with coffee enemas?

Many in the medical establishment disapprove of such treatments not only because they are unscientific or even quackery, but also for selfish financial reasons. So, how do you judge the claims made for unconventional treatments, whether they have to do with diet, mind control, detoxification, or some combination thereof? How do you act upon that judgment? How do you separate the good they might offer from the bad? These thorny questions are part of today's survivor culture.

Curious and Willing to Try

Looking around you, you see a do-it-yourself society. Many people are dutifully jogging or at least "eating thin" to fight cholesterol. Personal responsibility, self-help, prevention through sensible nutrition—these are the elements of the health game. Additionally, a good part of the medical leadership seems to encourage a holistic approach

Understanding the Risks and Benefits of Unconventional Treatment – **CHAPTER FOUR**

to prevention and treatment. The National Cancer Institute points to the advantages of eating the right broccoli-like foods, the American Cancer Society talks about "behavioral approaches," and your Harvard-trained physician advises you to take antioxidant vitamins to help prevent recurrence.

In this atmosphere, you, like other survivors, may be at least curious and willing to try one of the currently popular unconventional treatments. Such therapies usually have been developed and offered by practitioners who have chosen to work outside the mainstream. In virtually all cases, this means outside mainstream research, with its animal studies and formal clinical trials. Their practices and interventions generally are not taught in United States medical schools and are not reimbursed by health insurance providers. Unconventional treatments are available throughout the world, but finding them in the United States does not guarantee credibility.

Categories of Unconventional Treatments

The problem for the patient, even if a treatment seems attractive, safe, and effective, is the lack of objective evidence to sort out the potentially helpful remedy from the useless or, worse, harmful ones. To provide a structured way of looking at unconventional treatments, the Office of Alternative Medicine (OAM), created by the United States Congress in 1992, has divided them into seven categories.

DIET AND NUTRITION – Most popular is the macrobiotic diet, consisting primarily of whole grains and vegetables. Based on the Eastern yin-yang philosophy, which aims to "balance" food intake to counteract bodily dysfunction, the diet emphasizes soy beans, seaweed, and soups and avoids meats. Also popular are high doses of different vitamins and minerals intended to strengthen the body's ability to destroy malignant cancer cells, particularly vitamins C and E, beta-carotene, and selenium.

MIND/BODY CONTROL – "Mind over matter" concepts—ranging from prayer and art and music therapy to biofeedback—suggest that you can control stress, and even the course of your illness, if you have the will to do so. Through these techniques, you use your brain to work through your nervous system in an effort to bolster your body's immune defenses. In meditation, for example, the survivor visualizes or imagines the conquest of malignant cells by "good" T cells, and so tries to reverse the malignant process.

PHARMACOLOGIC AND BIOLOGIC TREATMENTS – These treatments use drugs and other preparations made from living organisms and their products. Dr. Stanislaw Burzynski's controversial therapy, Antineoplastons (synthesized urine proteins), remains in demand at his Texas clinic despite its serious legal troubles. The appeal of "Immuno-Augmentative Therapy" (IAT or blood therapy), developed by the late Lawrence Burton, PhD, however,—though still given at his clinic in the Bahamas—seems to have declined with the rise of interest in other pharmacologic and biologic therapies, like shark cartilage pills and suppositories (said to contain a protein inhibiting tumor blood supply). Another treatment is Cancell, a dark brown liquid made up of ordinary chemicals (including nitric acid and sodium sulfite) whose proponents claim they return cancer cells to a harmless "primitive state," but which the Food and Drug Administration (FDA) has found ineffective against cancer.

In and around Tijuana, Mexico, combinations of metabolic treatments using enemas and colonic cleansing, special diets, enzymes, vitamins and minerals, and laetrile are easily available but often very expensive. At the well-known Gerson clinic, patients undergo an elaborate diet and detoxification program to counteract liver damage with a special diet (including veal liver and raw fruit juices) and coffee enemas.

BIOELECTROMAGNETIC APPLICATIONS – These treatments, promoted particularly in Germany, use the low-frequency part of the electromagnetic spectrum to penetrate the body and heal damaged tissues. The OAM has funded a City of Hope (Los Angeles) research project in which electric currents are inserted directly into animal tumors (a technique widely used in China to treat cancer in humans).

ALTERNATIVE SYSTEMS OF MEDICAL PRACTICE – These include folk remedies from Latin American and Native American cultures, as well as ancient healing systems based on Eastern notions about the human body. Chinese medicine, for example, focuses on "chi," the life force. It relies on exercise techniques like Tai Chi to balance the flow of energy and uses acupuncture, acupressure, and herbal remedies. Another popular healing system is India's Ayurveda (LifeKnowledge), popularized by author Dr. Deepak Chopra. Dividing people into three predominant body types, it prescribes specific remedies—including yoga and meditation—to promote health for each type.

MANUAL HEALING – Hands-on techniques to reduce stress and pain have long included the manipulations of osteopathic and chiropractic doctors as well as therapy such as massage, rolfing, and reflexology.

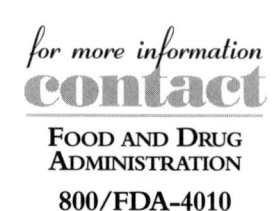

"Therapeutic touch" is a newer version of manual healing in which healers—usually nurses—move their hands a few inches above your body to remove "blockages" to your energy field.

HERBAL MEDICINE – From China to Canada, people have turned to herbal remedies. Many claim they have anticancer effects. One of the few which has gained popularity in North America as an alternative therapy is Essiac (the family name of the Canadian nurse who developed it, spelled backward). Composed of four herbs, including sorrel and slippery elm, it was tested at Memorial Sloan-Cancer Center in New York and found ineffective.

Many other herbs are used, particularly in Chinese medicine, and many have made their way to the United States and enjoyed considerable popularity. Here again, however, it is important to use caution. Even so-called natural substances can have serious consequences. Under the law, the Food and Drug Administration (FDA) cannot apply the same strict regulations to dietary supplements (including herbs used for medicinal purposes) that it applies to drugs. The FDA has been concerned about such supplements containing the "upper" or stimulant ephedrine (like the old Chinese herb *ma huang*) which have caused serious side effects—even occasional deaths. If you have had an adverse effect from any dietary supplement, this government agency would like to hear from you at (800) FDA-4010.

For more information about modern unconventional therapies—their promise and danger, and the subtleties involved in discerning between the two—see "Alternative and Complementary Cancer Therapies," an article by expert Barrie Cassileth, PhD, described at the conclusion of this chapter.

for more information
contact
FOOD AND DRUG ADMINISTRATION
800/FDA-4010
to report adverse effects from dietary supplements

MIXING CONVENTIONAL AND UNCONVENTIONAL

The consensus used to be that survivors turned to unconventional treatments when standard medical treatment had become ineffective in controlling their disease. Medical scientists also felt that people who sought such treatments were rare and somehow marginal—emotionally immature and lacking in courage—or poorly educated and at the end of their ropes.

Today we see a different picture. Many mainstream, educated patients with college degrees are trying unconventional treatments, and if one does not work, they shop around for another. These "new survivors" are as likely to try them at early as at later stages of their illness.

Although exact numbers are unknown, and estimates vary in different parts of the country, between roughly 15 and 50 percent (or more) of cancer patients in the United States currently receive unconventional treatments. The wide range in the estimate probably reflects how treatment is defined, particularly whether it includes the use of complementary therapies with conventional care. In such combinations, mainstream experts agree that some unconventional therapies can be helpful in relieving symptoms and enhancing the quality of life, though no body of scientific evidence supports their effectiveness.

OUT OF THE CLOSET

Unconventional treatment is clearly out of the closet. Developers of certain therapies may still be secretive about the composition of their wares, but general information is available in a wide variety of places, from academic journals to the Internet. Conferences and workshops on alternative and complementary medicine take place at such universities as Harvard and Columbia. Some two dozen medical schools and hospitals have started programs to study the subject. A number of doctors—most often family practitioners, generalists, and psychiatrists—recommend at least some such treatments, usually in combination with mainstream therapies. Treatments once considered "alternative" can become "conventional" when they are proven effective, and vice versa.

Survivors who use unconventional therapies now are usually not engaged in quackery. Laetrile, the famed apricot pit derivative discredited after scientific clinical trials in the 1970s, is no longer popular. Those who turn to unconventional treatment today want to try everything to increase their sense of wellness and to enhance their emotional and physical well-being. Others, discouraged by the oncologist who fails to recognize you on the elevator, by the radiologist who confuses one person's x-rays with someone else's, and by the clinician who coolly states, "I'm afraid there's nothing more we can do for you," turn to what seems to be the warmer, more caring and upbeat world of unconventional treatment.

This is a world of clinics and individual practitioners (and sometimes just homes and health food stores), where herbal teas sit on coffee tables, acupuncture charts adorn the walls, first names and tapes (for relaxation, for sleep, for nervous stomachs) prevail, and the talk is of such remedies as biofeedback, megavitamins, and therapeutic touch.

UNCONVENTIONAL ISSUES

SUPPLEMENT VS. ALTERNATIVE – How are you thinking of using alternative treatments? Some survivors supplement their conventional treatment provided by an oncologist with unconventional treatment. Their chief worry is whether alternative treatments could be harmful or could interfere with their conventional treatment (taken in extremely large doses certain vitamins, for example, could make cells grow). But if you are thinking of quitting your conventional treatment and pursuing the unconventional treatment as an alternative, that is quite a different story.

Michael Lerner, PhD, president of Marin County, California's Commonweal, former MacArthur Prize Fellow and author of *Choices in Healing,* has spent many years studying unconventional cancer treatments, visiting centers in Europe, India, and Japan, as well as North America. A firm advocate of an open mind toward unconventional treatment, he stressed in an interview with the *Living Through Cancer Journal* (Winter 1994), that "conventional scientific medicine has an infinitely better track record for the curative treatment of cancer than any other available system in the world." He recognized that most of today's cancer patients are interested in integrating the best of both worlds.

Like other experts, Lerner is excited about the possibilities of psychological support, citing the watershed studies at Stanford by David Spiegel, MD, and at UCLA by Fawzy I. Fawzy, MD. These studies showed that participation in support groups not only improved the quality of life of patients with metastatic breast cancer, but lengthened their survival time, although replication of this study has been slow in coming. In fact, one recent large study failed to replicate it completely.

Some survivors, however, leave conventional treatment, turn to various unconventional treatments, and suffer setbacks. Indeed, they may suffer not only a progression of their cancer, which might have been checked by traditional treatment, but they suffer outright harm. Such harm ranges from the general weakness—caused by a stringent diet and mild infection resulting from the administration of treatments in unsanitary circumstances—to, in rare cases, outright toxic poisoning.

UNREALISTIC EXPECTATIONS – What are your expectations of the unconventional treatment you are considering? If you are expecting a miracle as a result of the therapy—if you think your tumor will melt away as you take it—you may be in for a disappointment. This is particularly true in the area of mind control, where, at this state of our knowledge the exact connection between cortical function and bodily response in cancer is largely speculative. As Jimmie Holland, MD, Memorial Sloan-Kettering, puts it, only "blips on the screen" reported in the literature indicate psychological interventions might enhance the immune system. Oncologists have no hard knowledge to support any of these findings.

If, on the other hand, you simply expect to at least feel better about yourself and your disease, to relax, and to get rid of some of the pain and stress which can surround cancer treatment, you have a better chance for meeting your goals. Although he found no sure cure for cancer among the treatments he has followed, and little evidence on which to evaluate most of them, Michael Lerner has reported anecdotal evidence that some patients do well while using them. This might be because of the warmth and optimism of the unconventional caregivers, or because people feel better when they are doing everything possible to fight disease. When treatments—particularly mind control treatments—seem to improve your outlook and mood, you are apt to conclude they work for you. You also may come to expect too much of them—that they will affect your tumor as well as your quality of life.

BLAMING YOURSELF – Guilt is a more subtle but equally confusing issue confronting survivors using unconventional treatments. Cancer survivors who already may feel severely punished can feel more so if self-help therapists convince them that their disease is their fault, particularly if the cancer progresses despite their efforts to contain it.

Unconventional mind-control theory is based on the idea that you can influence the course of your disease through psychological means. Advocates claim that long-term unremitting stress can depress the immune system, that positive emotions strengthen it, and that a strengthened immune system makes the possibility of fighting off cancer more likely. So, if you do not succeed at whatever treatment you have chosen, you have not tried hard enough—you are at fault.

Prominent psychoneuroimmunological practitioners insist that they are not pointing the finger at cancer survivors for causing or failing to cure their diseases. For example, former surgeon Bernie Siegel, MD, author of *Love, Medicine and Miracles* and other best sellers, says he is not blaming the patient when he writes, for example, that women who have unhappy love relationships are especially vulnerable to breast or cervical diseases. He claims he is only trying to empower this patient with a will to resist and achieve a more realistic sense of participation in her treatment.

Wellness community leader Harold Benjamin in his book *From Victim to Victor* adds that a woman who died after she refused to give up her "immune-depressive" behavior toward the partner who squeezed her out of her business, should not have blamed herself, as she did. This is because she "can't be to blame for failing to stop something from happening that she didn't know was happening." Nevertheless, the implication of self-blame remains strong in survivors who believe they are responsible for the cause and course of their disease.

COST—A SERIOUS SIDE EFFECT – How much does your unconventional therapy cost? How much does it cost you? The costs of conventional treatment are seldom the main concern of the insured patient. Rather, the main concern is whether it will help you get well or at least help achieve a reasonable quality of life. Unconventional treatment is a different story. Neither managed care nor fee-for-service health insurance plans will likely cover more than an entry office visit and routine blood and similar tests, if that. You will have to pick up the tab even if you are adequately insured.

This may not be true in the case of a once-a-week complementary treatment like guided imagery (which can be practiced at home), which is administered by a qualified health professional. But the bills for unconventional treatment, which may run into many thousands of dollars, usually have to be picked up by survivors themselves. They may be more ominous than anticipated, because practitioners reluctant to disclose details of their treatment are often specific about the manner in which you will have to pay, including the amount you have to pay up front.

As far as costs to the whole community are concerned, the estimates have risen dramatically. In 1987, a Louis Harris and Associates study for the Food and Drug Administration estimated the cost of "questionable" cancer treatments at $141 million a year. In 1990, a Harvard study published in The *New England Journal of Medicine* reported that Americans spent over $10 billion (and that did not include insurance coverage for treatments such as acupuncture).

SUGGESTIONS FOR SURVIVORS

Until sure cures for cancer preclude such issues, how do you approach unconventional treatment? People do not seek out "alternative" treatments for diseases with proven cures, like tuberculosis. At this point, when the medical community still lacks conclusive answers regarding the validity of unconventional therapies, it is no wonder that survivors continue to use them, particularly for hard-to-cure cancers. Even renowned experts can be forced to clarify and explain themselves. For example, psychologist Barrie Cassileth and the late, famed author Norman Cousins called a press conference in the 1980s to bemoan the fact that the public had placed them on opposite sides of the mind-body controversy. A highly respected researcher, Stanford's David Spiegel, MD, reported in 1989 that metastatic breast cancer patients in a support group lived longer than patients not in a support group. In 1996, a large, impressive study of similar patients published in the *Journal of the National Cancer Institute* (with an accompanying laudatory editorial by Dr. Speigel) failed to prove this to be true.

"[F]or cancer patients, it is not simply mind over matter, but instead [experts] point the way toward how in future research it may be possible to determine how mind does matter."

David Spiegel, MD, "Psychological Distress and Disease Course for Women with Breast Cancer: One Answer, Many Questions," Editorial, Journal of the National Cancer Institute, *Vol. 88, No. 10, May 15, 1996*

When such experts disagree, what are you, as a survivor, to think and do? The following list of practical suggestions may help.

UNDERSTAND YOUR CONVENTIONAL TREATMENT – Take time to gather as much information as you want and need about what your doctors expect surgery, radiation, chemotherapy and/or hormone therapy to do for you. Understand your options. Weigh the costs and the benefits—the utility of each conventional treatment for the kind of person you are and for your lifestyle. For example, are you the sort of person who would choose a more radical treatment, getting it over with as fast as possible? Or would you prefer longer-term, more cautious treatment?

TELL YOUR DOCTOR WHAT YOU ARE THINKING – Reportedly, many survivors do not even tell their doctors of their interest in unconventional treatment. This is a mistake. Doctors experienced with cancer patients are most qualified not only to help you figure out risk-benefit questions—whether or not a coffee enema, for example, will adversely affect the electrolytes in your body—but to monitor their effects if you do decide to try them. Knowing why you wanted to try an unconventional therapy—that you were dissatisfied with your pain management, for example—can help your doctor take better care of you.

CONSIDER COMBINING CONVENTIONAL AND UNCONVENTIONAL TREATMENTS – If the prospective practitioner will give you unconventional therapy only if you leave conventional treatment, reconsider. If you are still determined to have the treatment, try to find another practitioner who will cooperate with your primary physician.

CAREFULLY CHECK CREDENTIALS AND UNDER WHAT CONDITIONS HE OR SHE PRACTICES – Some well-trained nurses, psychologists, and even physicians may give the kind of treatment for which you are looking. They may offer it under optimum professional conditions.

Try to be hard-nosed when you investigate, taking off any blinders you may be wearing in your search for help. Avoid the double standard. If either conventional or unconventional practitioners are unlicensed, without a degree, or occupy dirty office space, your antennae should go up.

HOLD UNCONVENTIONAL PRACTITIONERS ACCOUNTABLE FOR THEIR TREATMENTS – Find out everything you can about their track record—if one exists. Normally you would look at the literature published about treatment efficacy. Have patients taking it participated in controlled studies? What effect has the treatment had on them? Have they lived longer or at least enjoyed a better quality of life?

When it comes to unconventional treatments, however, such literature may be nonexistent. What little is available may be full of unsubstantiated testimonials claiming that it is safe or effective. But unlike "experimental" therapies undergoing clinical trials, these advocates will not be able to prove that experiments are being conducted on unconventional treatments.

Nonetheless, call the clinic or practitioner and ask for all the available literature about the treatment you are considering. Look at the medical literature for anything written about its efficacy by experts not personally involved. Ask the clinic or practitioner directly what the treatment consists of and what its claims are for your particular cancer. Demand supporting evidence. Ask about both positive and negative effects.

Be cautious: You might believe a treatment is effective if you are told it is being used in a Food and Drug Administration (FDA)-approved clinical trial under an Investigational Drug Application. The agency has studied some unconventional treatments, but that does not mean it has endorsed them. Indeed, one small trial of a controversial treatment, limited to patients with advancing disease and no other options, resulted in litigation.

CONSULT SOURCES IN A POSITION TO HELP YOU – These include:

- "Alternative and Complementary Cancer Therapies," an excellent survey of the field, published in the March 15, 1996 issue of *Cancer* (Volume 77, Number 6) by a preeminent expert, Barrie R. Cassileth, PhD, and Christopher C. Chapman. This dispassionate article will bring you up-to-date on subjects ranging from the stalling of an OAM shark cartilage study (because the cartilage received was found to be contaminated), to the severe liver and kidney damage caused by a limited number of herbal remedies, to the soothing effect of such therapies as relaxation techniques for patients who use them to complement medical regimes. You can get copies of this article for a small handling fee of three dollars by writing to Dr. Cassileth at 8033 Old NC 86, Chapel Hill, NC 27516.

- The Food and Drug Administration Cancer Liaison Office, opened in 1994 "to serve as a resource on cancer issues from the patient's perspective," is located at 5600 Fishers Lane, Room 9-49, HF 12, Rockville, MD 20857; tel: (301) 443-0104. This office will try to answer consumer questions about

for more information
contact

DR. BARRIE CASSILETH
8033 Old NC 86
Chapel Hill, NC 27516

"Alternative and Complementary Cancer Therapies"

FOOD AND DRUG ADMINISTRATION
5600 Fishers Lane
Room 9-49 HF 12
Rockville, MD 20857

301/443-0104

questions about the FDA drug approval process

the FDA drug approval process and specific treatments—conventional, unconventional, and those under investigation.

- *Unconventional Cancer Treatments,* is a 300-page report commissioned by the U.S. Congress, and published by the now defunct Office of Technology Assessment in 1990. Based on a four-year study, it covers the laws and regulations affecting unconventional treatments, as well as the treatments themselves, and the patients and practitioners who used them at the beginning of this decade. This report (No. 91-104893) is still available through the National Technical Information Service for $56.50 plus $6.00 for shipping and handling. To order the book, you may call (703) 487-4650, or you may fax your order and credit card information to (703) 321-8547. A 38-page summary of the report (No. 91-142273) is available for $22 plus $4.00 shipping and handling.

- Your local American Cancer Society (ACS) office or the ACS hot line (800) ACS-2345 can send you the free ACS pamphlet *Questionable Methods of Cancer Treatment Management* (1993) which includes a list of information resources on this subject. In addition, if you call the hot line to request information on a particular therapy, the ACS will send you information from its database.

- The National Institutes of Health's Office of Alternative Medicine (OAM), set up by the U.S. Congress in 1992 to further research on alternative medicine, can supply you with a variety of informational material including a list of the research projects and university-based research centers it has funded. As a research group, the OAM does not answer individual queries. The OAM Information Center, 5120 Executive Boulevard, EPS Suite 450, Rockville, MD 20892; tel: (301) 402-2466, fax: (301) 402-4741.

for more information
contact

NATIONAL TECHNICAL INFORMATION SERVICE
703/487-4650
Unconventional Cancer Treatments

AMERICAN CANCER SOCIETY HOT LINE
800/ACS-2345
Questionable Methods of Cancer Treatment Management
or to request information on a particular therapy

NIH OFFICE OF ALTERNATIVE MEDICINE
OAM Information Center
5120 Executive Blvd.
Suite 450
Rockville, MD 20892
301/402-2466
informational material, including a list of the research projects it has funded

FINALLY, ARE YOU COMFORTABLE WITH THE PROPOSED TREATMENT? – Do not try something that does not seem to fit in with your style and values.

What can you do if you have tried zealously to find out about a treatment and have not been successful? if you have found conflicting information about it? or if you have found information about the risks it entails, but do not know how to evaluate the risks?

Here, good rapport with your doctor is like money in the bank. If you are able to talk openly with him or her, you will get valuable help in weighing the possible risks and benefits of prospective treatments. Other people you trust in your medical setting, the chief nurse at the clinic, for example, or a very experienced survivor, may be able to give you good advice.

TO CARE

To many people, the C-word is cancer. The C-words in this poster, however, express positive aspects of caring. Words such as compassion, commitment, and cooperation reflect the dedication of health-care professionals and other caregivers in their mission "to care" for those touched by cancer.

To Care was the signature poster for the First National Congress on Cancer Survivorship in Washington, DC, in November 1995. It was presented to Hillary Rodham Clinton, honorary chairperson of the conference.

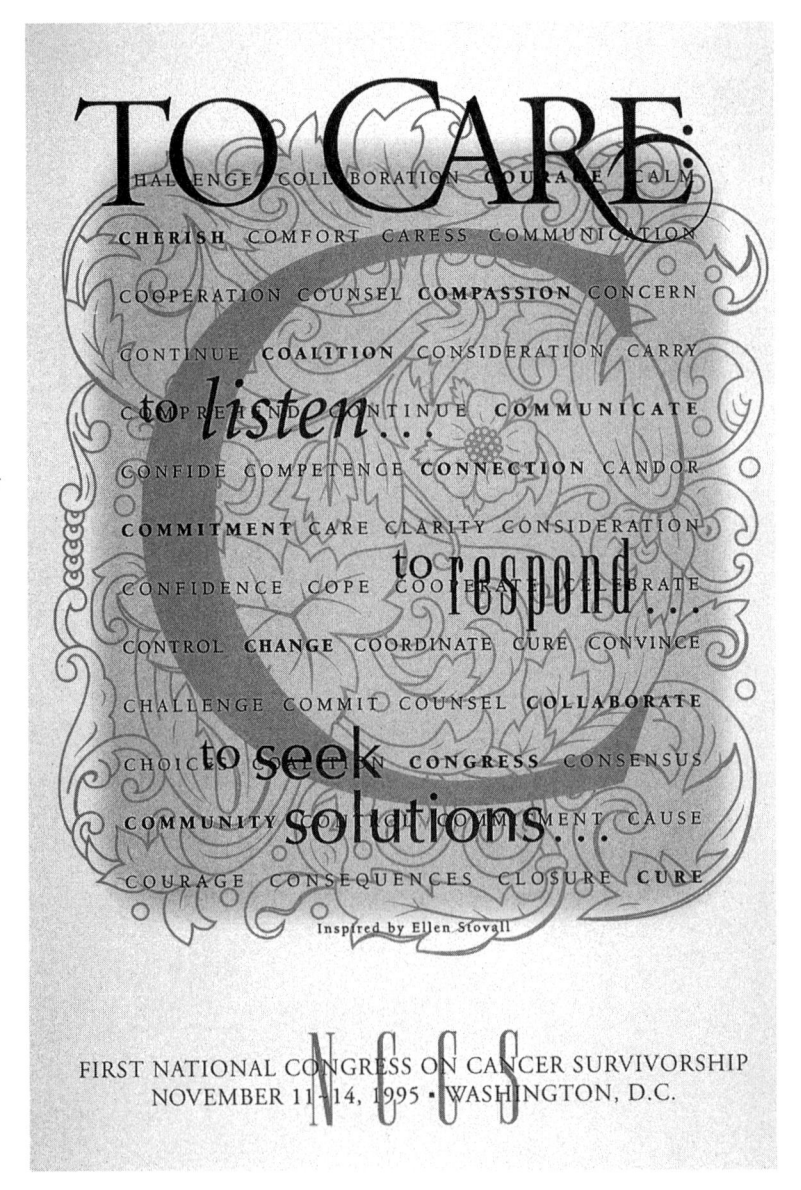

A CANCER *survivor's* ALMANAC

Part Two

Taking Care of Your Emotional, Spiritual, and Social Needs

*Mind and Body:
Harnessing Your Inner
Resources 91*

*Family Challenges:
Communication,
Hope, and Loss 117*

*Reaching Out: The Power
of Peer Support 139*

Chapter Five

Mind and Body: Harnessing Your Inner Resources

by Neil Fiore, PhD

"As a founding member of NCCS, I was honored to participate in one of the most satisfying organizational events I have ever witnessed. Ten years ago, 25 extremely strong individuals buried their egos and gathered together to create an organization that would bear witness to the unmet needs, the rights, and the responsibilities of the majority of individuals who have cancer."

Neil Fiore, PhD

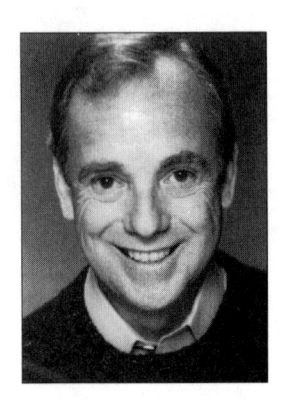

NEIL FIORE, PHD is a founding member of the National Coalition for Cancer Survivorship and serves on its Board of Advisors. Dr. Fiore is a cancer survivor and a licensed psychologist practicing in Berkeley, California, as well as a former paratrooper in Vietnam. He specializes in the areas of health psychology, optimal performance, stress management, and clinical hypnosis. Dr. Fiore is the former president of the Northern California Society of Clinical Hypnosis, a nationally known speaker, and the author of three books. His latest book, *Fully Alive: Learning from Those Transformed by Crisis,* will be released in the spring of 1997.

The Inner Journey

...seeing illness as an occasion to make positive changes in your life beyond the disease itself is a creative adaptation to a major life threat.... Your illness is an occasion to reevaluate life—a wake-up call, not a death knell. When your life is threatened, take hold and make the most of it; don't give up on it.

—David Spiegel, MD,

Living Beyond Limits: New Hope and
Help for Facing Life-Threatening Illness

The Personal Impact of Cancer

A personal battle against cancer is, in many ways, like any other fight for survival—it requires a toughness of mind, an intense focus on the task; and a refusal to be deterred by the enemy, self-doubts or seemingly rational fears. More than toughness, however, it requires resilience, patience, humility, and flexibility. Surviving cancer and surviving with cancer is not a street fight that is over in a few seconds. Surviving is more like a spiritual journey that teaches you how to change your life and your relationships.

Too readily survivors identify with their diagnosis and forget that they are more than the host of a serious illness. Even with advanced cancer, the healthy portion of the body continues to fight. Less than one percent of you has cancer. The rest of you—your inner mental and emotional resources, your immune system, and your very life force—cooperates with your medical treatment to combat cancer.

In the course of coping with cancer, survivors learn to respect their own emotions and to distinguish them from irrational and unhelpful worries. Survivors learn different ways to express emotions—sometimes verbally, sometimes in writing, and sometimes with those fellow survivors who will understand.

Caregivers have understandable fears of cancer and death that survivors should not take personally. Survivors need to remind themselves: "I am more than my cancer. A healthy part of me is fighting for my life; I want to live my life—not someone else's image of who I should be and how I should feel. I intend to be fully alive in my life until the last moment."

In charting the journey of survivorship, survivors can learn to protect their precious, limited energy in order to make it available for healing. As one colon cancer survivor said: "If I want to go to a party the day after my chemotherapy treatment, I make sure not to squander my energy on getting myself upset the way I used to. It is as if the elastic band of my emotions has been stretched. I can handle a lot more without snapping."

DISCOVERING STRATEGIES FOR HEALING

Managing energy, time, and relationships is part of the empowerment that can come from surviving a crisis. Studies of survivors show that several activities appear to contribute to a healing of the spirit and often to a healing of the body including—

- *practicing hypnotic or meditative relaxation* for stress and pain reduction;
- *expressing honest emotions*—especially the more difficult emotions of anger and sadness, rather than stoic denial or false cheerfulness;
- *accepting the reality about one's medical condition* and facing the possibility of death;
- *mourning our losses*, then moving on and adapting to the present condition, rather than struggling to hold onto the past;
- *maintaining a sense of wonder* about how your body will cooperate with medical treatment and how your emotional strength will see you through difficult times, rather than insisting on knowing the future; for example, "I wonder how I'll get through this one? This is going to be interesting. I wonder what unknown resources my body and mind will muster to cope with this?";
- *participating actively in your health care*—maintaining some control over medical decisions, asking the doctor questions, knowing whether diet and exercise could enhance the effects of medical treatment.

The current mystery about what causes cancer leaves us vulnerable to potentially harmful speculation about a connection between our health habits—specifically our mental activity (thoughts, beliefs, and images)—and cancer. Sandra Levy, MD, former chief of behavioral medicine at the National Cancer Institute, states that "the most important determinant of cancer outcome is the biology of the tumor and the medical treatment." If the cause of cancer has a psychological component, it is most likely minimal. Yet we can do things, mostly behavioral (such as stopping smoking, eating more fruit and vegetables, and reducing fat in our diet) and some psychological, that

---

Research conducted at the University of California, San Francisco, found improved survival rates among patients who expressed their emotions, were realistic about their disease, and actively participated in their health care. These patients had significantly more healthy white cells at the site of their tumors, slower growing tumors, and a better prognosis than those patients who did not exhibit emotional expression, realism, and active participation.

can improve our chances of surviving cancer.

Research conducted at the University of California, San Francisco, found improved survival rates among patients who expressed their emotions, were realistic about their disease, and actively participated in their health care. These patients had significantly more healthy white cells at the site of their tumors, slower growing tumors, and a better prognosis than those patients who did not exhibit emotional expression, realism, and active participation.

While researchers in medicine and psychology continue to debate the physical and emotional factors that contribute to illness and health, almost all serious professionals agree that—

- *you cannot wish away cancer* nor can you get cancer by having negative thoughts or painful emotions;
- *many factors and events beyond your control* determine if and when you will get cancer;
- *supportive therapies*—such as groups, counseling, and meditation or prayer—can contribute to your peace of mind, emotional well-being, immune system strength, and improved survival time; and
- *unproven treatments* often put patients through unnecessary expense and discomfort and can be dangerous if they keep you from receiving prompt medical care.

Diagnosing the Diagnosis—and Your Beliefs

Many diseases are more severe, traumatic, and fatal than cancer. Yet the stigma attached to this disease makes the diagnosis of cancer disproportionately terrifying. The meaning of the word "cancer" is very different for the doctor who deals with it every day, for the person who has survived "terminal cancer" for eleven years, and for the patient hearing the diagnosis for the first time.

SELF-BLAME AND GUILT – When the diagnosis is first presented, the emotional shock can be so great that survivors tend to look for an understandable cause in order to make some sense of what is unimaginable. Some people might even prefer self-blame and guilt to the greater discomfort of loss of control, unknown causes, and the feeling of being a random victim.

Everyone has remnants of a child's pattern of taking on inappropriate levels of responsibility for things beyond our control. For young children, the thought that their parents might be imperfect, unstable, or mortal is unthinkable. Since they must depend on adults for shelter, protection and food, children frequently blame themselves for problems that occur in their families rather than imagine that parents and God may not be powerful enough to always keep them from harm.

In 1989, a study led by Dr. David Spiegel of Stanford University demonstrated that women with advanced breast cancer who participated in a support group survived eighteen months longer than those who did not. This research offers evidence that psychosocial treatments not only can make you feel better, they may affect the length of survival with cancer. In his book, *Living Beyond Limits: New Hope and Help for Facing Life-Threatening Illness,* Dr. Spiegel summarizes much of the psychosocial research:

"All of the studies… point in the same direction: You do better when you learn to take charge of the course of your illness realistically. You cannot control everything, you cannot undo what has been done (like getting the disease), but you will benefit by taking hold of your current situation in whatever way is possible.… When your life is threatened, take hold and make the most of it; don't give up on it."

These findings encourage survivors to focus on what they can do after a cancer diagnosis to cope realistically with the situation and actively participate in their health care.

> Many diseases are more severe, traumatic, and fatal than cancer. Yet the stigma attached to this disease makes the diagnosis of cancer disproportionately terrifying.

In a time of crisis, adults may revert to this childlike illusion of control to explain how bad things can happen to good people. This protective device temporarily keeps adults from facing a chaotic world in which cancer and accidents can randomly touch anyone's life, regardless of how well we live, how we handle our emotions, or how positive or negative our outlook. Similar to children, adults feel safer blaming themselves rather than accepting vulnerability to a world that is not under their control.

Unfortunately, denying human limits leaves survivors feeling guilty about lack of control over uncontrollable events. Certain phrases in your internal dialogue may reflect a "refusal to mourn" the loss of the illusion of control. It is not unusual for survivors to say to themselves: "You should have known better. If only you had done things differently this wouldn't have happened. I don't believe it. I can't stand it." Statements such as these are symptoms of being stuck in a fantasy about how life should be and of finding it difficult to accept life on its terms.

Overall, self-blame as a means to explain uncontrollable events is damaging to your ability to cope with cancer. It can result in feelings of depression that contribute to a delay in seeking medical treatment, a reluctance to discuss worries and fear, and a diminished ability to form helpful relationships with doctors, social workers, and family members. Realistic information about cancer and its causes, however, can help you adjust to the unpleasant realities of a tough situation and can help you find support in doing something about it.

TESTING YOUR FAITH – The strength and compassion of religious and spiritual beliefs are tested by the psychological and emotional stress of cancer. Some survivors may need to reexamine the source of their beliefs if they contribute to feelings of guilt rather than serve to comfort. In *When Bad Things Happen to Good People,* Rabbi Harold Kushner writes of his message to a young man in his community who was dying of a degenerative disease:

> I don't know why my friend and neighbor is sick and dying and in constant pain. From my religious perspective, I cannot tell him that God has His reasons for sending him this terrible fate, or that God must specially love him or admire his bravery to test him in this way. I can only tell him that the God I believe in did not send the disease and does not have a miraculous cure that He is withholding.

In his attempt to understand how bad things can happen to good people, Rabbi Kushner concludes that the laws of nature affect all alike and that not even God interferes with these laws.

Any beliefs that lead you to think of cancer as punishment from God should be examined carefully with the help of clergy or counselors. Personal and spiritual beliefs that accept human suffering as a natural part of life and facilitate forgiveness for being vulnerable human beings, are more likely to assist rapid adaptation to illness and even lead to spiritual transformation.

REPLACING NEGATIVE REACTIONS

Examining your initial reactions to a cancer diagnosis and the beliefs that underlie them is the first crucial step toward developing alternative attitudes toward cancer and discovering alternative ways of coping. Here are some common negative reactions to cancer and some suggestions for useful responses to them.

Negative Reaction: Why me? Why now? Life is unfair. I feel pitiful.
Response: Now that it has happened and it is me, what can I do about it? As awful as this situation is, what can I do to improve my chances of beating cancer?

Negative Reaction: Cancer is powerful and my body is weak. Cancer means death.
Response: Cancer cells are, in fact, abnormal cells that are weak. These confused cells cannot reproduce when exposed to chemotherapy or radiation. My immune system routinely identifies and destroys malformed cells and removes them from my body. My body can cooperate with medical treatment in destroying cancer.

Negative Reaction: If I had lived life differently I wouldn't have cancer. If only I knew then what I know now. I wish I could do it over again.
Response: The past is over and I cannot control it or change it. It did happen! It does hurt. But brooding about what is beyond my current control only weakens my ability to deal with what I can do now. I do have control over how I make myself feel in this present moment and over my attitude in the future. I will focus on what I can do now!

COPING WITH POWERFUL EMOTIONS

If you have ever felt the ground shake beneath your feet from an earthquake or have lived through a war or a near-fatal accident, you know how quickly feelings of tranquility can change to overwhelming anxiety. The emotional response of cancer survivors to their diagnosis is just as legitimate as the shock, anger, and depression expected in those who survive accidents and wars, and recovery involves similar steps of emotional and physical rehabilitation.

Worry about recurrence and wonder about changes in the rules of life make the task of "getting back to normal" a complex one for any cancer survivor. One survivor said, "Sometimes it feels like I'm living

> Similar to children, adults feel safer blaming themselves rather than accepting vulnerability to a world that is not under their control.

under a centipede, waiting for the other 99 shoes to drop." It takes the experience of many calm days before we can relax and stop bracing for another catastrophe.

Over time, it is not so much the strong emotions themselves that cause difficulties as it is the fear of expressing them. With understanding and patience, physicians, family members, and survivors themselves can find helpful avenues for the release of legitimate feelings.

ANXIETY – Feelings of anxiety are to be expected during any part of the cancer experience, but survivors have ranked the time of diagnosis as the most upsetting. During this time, thoughts about life and death predominate and survivors are most vulnerable to psychosocial problems. This is a period of monumental adjustment to—
- the shocking news that your life is in danger;
- the consideration of treatments that may be more severe than any of your cancer symptoms;

AN EXERCISE TO HELP IDENTIFY UNDERLYING BELIEFS

This exercise can help you identify troublesome beliefs that persist from your initial diagnosis, and which unnecessarily tax your energy and cloud your thoughts. Developed at the University of California Medical Center, San Francisco, the exercise may be useful to sharpen your awareness of initial reactions to cancer and give you an opportunity to share these reactions, often for the first time, with those close to you.

In preparation for this exercise, read through it, setting aside 15 to 30 minutes to experience the exercise and talk about it with your family. You may want to tape record the instructions and play them back so that you can be completely relaxed.

START READING THE EXERCISE HERE: Begin by settling into a comfortable position, perhaps sitting in a chair with your feet flat on the floor. Take three slow, deep breaths, holding your breath briefly, and then exhaling slowly and completely.

Give yourself time to take three slow, deep breaths, and, with each exhalation, float more deeply into the chair. Let the chair support you; you can let go of holding with your muscles. Just allow the relaxation to flow down over your body. There is no need for you to hold those muscles. Just allow the chair to support your body and the floor to support your feet and legs. With your conscious exhaling you are letting your body know that there is no place to go for the next few minutes; that the strong part of you is choosing to face a fear and to resolve any blocks to living fully.

Now, simply drift back to that time and place when you first were told

- the loss of your physical integrity;
- rapid changes in your work and relationships;
- the possibility of a long period of rehabilitation.

During this initial period, especially, the expression of anxiety, sadness, and anger are quite natural and potentially healing. Some studies suggest that survivors who were more expressive of their anger and sadness fared better than those who were less so. This does not mean that survivors should force themselves to be emotional, but that it may be better if they do not repress their natural feelings. After all, attempting to remain stoical during times of great trauma takes energy—energy that might better be used by the body for recuperation.

Other studies indicate that survivors who maintain a support network of friends and family are more likely to weather this difficult time without major psychological problems. The first months of cancer therapy are intense but some comfort can be gathered from

---

of the diagnosis. Imagine being in that place: Recreate for yourself that room, the furniture, the colors and lighting, and the sounds and the voices. Just be there and allow your mind to present what it will. Just let it happen.

Once you are there, back in that place, at that time, focus your attention on three areas within you:

- *Become aware of what you are feeling physically*—your muscles, your breathing, your pulse and heartbeat, and anything that makes itself physically evident.
- *Become aware of the thoughts* and images that are going through your mind and of what you are saying to yourself—what your attitude is and how you are coaching yourself.
- *Become aware of what you are feeling emotionally.* Just notice fear, anger, frustration, and wonder. Also, notice that you can shift your focus from one area to another, indicating that you are taking control over your attention and feelings.

All your reactions are legitimate and, whatever your reactions are, simply note them. You coped as well as you could under the circumstances given your former beliefs, your needs, your history, and the information you had at the time.

Now your job is to reexamine those beliefs and attitudes to see which ones still serve you. Identify and replace any beliefs that only cause you stress. Acknowledge that these old beliefs helped you to adapt to your former environment. Now, equipped with "new ways of thinking," you are choosing to adjust to your illness and make positive changes in your life.

knowing that the second 100 days probably will be less stressful, as you adjust to your medical treatment and the process of healing.

Once the initial shock of the diagnosis is past, the next task will be to become familiar with the treatment steps and options—what can be done medically and what survivors can do for themselves. At that time, the disbelief and anxiety about having cancer generally will give way to the tasks of living and adapting to life after cancer.

DEPRESSION − Depression, a common reaction among cancer survivors and their supporters, is often regarded as a negative emotion. In fact, depression may be a natural way to cope with shock by conserving energy and providing a time to think about ways of adjusting to change. Cancer survivors, says Jimmie Holland, MD, chief of New York's Memorial Sloan-Kettering's Psychiatry Service, are no more depressed than people with other severe medical conditions. The type of depression experienced by cancer survivors, reactive depression, differs from that of patients suffering from chronic mental depression. The Psychiatry Service of Memorial Sloan-Kettering reports that half of the cancer patients they see have suffered from acute stress and reactive (as opposed to "chronic") depression.

The relatively short-term, reactive depression that often accompanies the stress of a cancer diagnosis and treatment can be handled more easily if it is accepted as natural and if a "mourning" process is allowed. Recovery from the depression of cancer is helped by acknowledging the loss—loss of control, loss of a body part, and loss of self-image.

Another contributor to depression is the passivity that is required of patients as they follow orders and fall into the "sick role." Hospital regimes encourage dependence, adding to the sense of helplessness, and reinforcing the negative image of "cancer victim."

Hospital employees who demand extreme compliance by patients and offer little opportunity for patient participation in their own health care can contribute to patient depression and rebellion. Studies have shown that many patients stop taking their chemotherapy, not simply because of treatment side effects, but because they never had a chance to consider alternatives before they chose their treatment.

A National Cancer Institute study demonstrated that the majority of those patients who turned to unconventional therapies had been told by their physicians that they had a "terminal disease" and that nothing else could be done. (See Chapter 4 for a discussion of unconventional treatments.) These patients—who felt abandoned and unable to participate in conventional medicine—turned to treatments that required them to take an active role in getting involved and changing their lifestyles.

Recovery from the depression of cancer is helped by acknowledging the loss—loss of control, loss of a body part, and loss of self-image.

Affirmations for a Positive Self-Image

Cancer survivors often find personal affirmations helpful in making the transition to a new, robust self-image and greater strength to cope with changing relationships. These affirmations are a way of being there for yourself despite the events in your life. Affirmations can be like Ivan's credo in Dostoyevsky's *The Brothers Karamazov*: "…[i]f I lost faith in the order of things, if I were convinced that everything is a disorderly, damnable, devil-ridden chaos, if I were struck by every horror of man's disillusion—still I should want to live…." *The part of us that still wants to live, even after so many losses, is the part that speaks the affirmations to the part of us that is understandably afraid and discouraged.* The following are suggested affirmations that cancer survivors can give to themselves, thereby providing compassion and creating an internal safe and comforting place.

Regardless of what happens in life, you are worthwhile.

Regardless of how your body is scarred by the experiences of life and survival, I accept you.

Regardless of whether you win or lose, you deserve love, pleasure, and freedom from self-criticism.

Regardless of what you can or cannot do, you always have worth to me. Your worth is not based on what you do, but on who you are.

Regardless of what happens to you, you deserve to be treated with human dignity and respect. I will always respect you.

Regardless of who stays or who goes, I am on your side, always in your corner. I will never abandon you.

Regardless of how healthy or ill I become, I appreciate the effort, wisdom, and protection of my body. I am committed to protecting you.

Regardless of how negative or intense your emotions become, I acknowledge their validity for you. All your emotions and thoughts are understandable.

Regardless of how uncomfortable others are with you, your feelings, body, or illness, I always remain at peace with you.

Regardless of what happens out there, you always have a home in here. You are always welcome and safe in my home.

Even if you cannot heal your body, you can always heal your spirit. You are safe with me. I will be with you all the way through to the last moments of life.

In order to lessen depression and hopelessness, you can accept some level of depression as normal, let go of trying to control everything, mourn your losses and avoid assuming a passive role in your treatment. You also can talk to your doctor and health-care team about what can be done to reduce treatment side effects that might be contributing to depression. Ask about counselors and support groups to help with the emotional components of surviving cancer. (See Chapter 2 on how to communicate with your doctor and hospital staff. See Chapter 7 for information about support groups.)

Once you have acknowledged that you are in a distressing situation and must face many hard choices, you can direct your thoughts toward the future by asking yourself, "Where do I go from here?" You do not have to be thrilled with where you are today, but to improve your situation, you do need to recognize the appropriate paths that are available to you. By coping realistically with the emotional impact of cancer, you have prepared yourself to move beyond the initial reactions of *if only*, *what if*, and *why me* to a more productive question: "What small steps can I take today to improve the quality and length of my life?"

The initial shock of the cancer diagnosis will soften as you become more familiar with the steps of your treatment—with what can be done for you and what you can do to improve your health. Most likely, you will find that your actual experience of cancer will be very different from your initial beliefs and fears.

By understanding how cancer affects your emotions and relationships, you prepare yourself to master the skills of coping with trauma, transition, and survival. Concerns about life-and-death issues, while never totally dismissed from the thoughts of any cancer survivor, can give way to the challenges and joys of daily life.

> I feel as if my life has belonged to someone else. What bothers me is not that I might die, but that I never really got to live. Much of my life I lacked confidence and was depressed. But having cancer has taught me to take charge of my decisions and to feel powerful. How can I use this in my daily life? ... I want so much to live my life even if that is only for a few months or years.
>
> Jean, thirty-eight year old mother diagnosed with ovarian cancer, in Neil Fiore's Fully Alive

THE SOCIAL IMPACT OF CANCER

Even though the shock of a cancer diagnosis appears to be mostly physical, a major portion of the impact is emotional and social. Consequently, it can affect how you perceive yourself and how others react to you.

CHANGES IN SELF-PERCEPTION

If a cancer diagnosis is your first experience of being vulnerable to serious illness, its influence on your self image can be especially traumatic. You may feel betrayed by your body, as if your cells have turned against you. In a very concrete way you realize that you are human and mortal, that life does end, and that your time is limited.

A dramatic change in self-image is most evident in teenagers and young adults with cancer. It makes them different from their carefree friends who seldom believe that the threat of death or even serious illness applies to them. They have not had to face the body's gradual decline that adults begin to experience in their forties. Usually they have not seen illness and death strike their peers, so they are unprepared for a life-threatening illness. It shocks them and makes them doubt their underlying assumptions about how the world is supposed to work.

But this rapid change in perception can take place in people in their 60s as well—people who are accustomed to good health and energy. These individuals seem to maintain a teenager's sense of invulnerability and immortality well beyond the age of 60. For people whose self-image has remained stable for decades, a diagnosis of cancer can be dramatically inconsistent with their view of life.

The experience of facing a life-threatening event unites survivors around a new view of the world and human courage. It also separates survivors from those who cannot appreciate the cancer experience. Cancer changes not only the self-perception of survivors, but how others perceive survivors.

Physicians will treat your physical losses, but you, your family and friends, and your psychosocial counselors must deal with the emotional and psychological changes. You can improve your self-image by accepting mortality and vulnerability to disease as reality for all human beings rather than as signs of personal weakness or failure. A more hardy and realistic self-image will enhance your ability to fight for your life. It will equip you with a better understanding of the social impact of cancer and will prepare you to cope in ways that contribute to your mental and physical well-being.

As a cancer survivor you may feel quite isolated at times, as if no one could possibly understand your shock and agony. In *Live the Pain, Learn the Hope,* Wayne Keeling expressed his reactions to his cancer diagnosis as follows:

> Self-doubts begin to play tricks with your head, and you might ask yourself, "Does anybody give a damn whether I live or die?" You begin to see and hear evidence that nobody does. No one else seems panicky, just you. The doctor seems cool, scientific. Your spouse and parents are cool, sad-looking. Your boss is cool and has a few sad, sympathetic words that sound like "have a good trip" (to wherever).

This young man felt that everyone was indifferent toward him, but some survivors feel they must be strong and repress their own needs because no one else seems capable of coping. They may even think that their doctor or spouse is too emotional about the diagnosis to consider the feelings and needs of the patient. Sometimes survivors find themselves comforting distraught family members, while wondering: "Who's going to listen to my feelings? I'm the one with cancer!"

Mind and Body: Harnessing Your Inner Resources – **CHAPTER FIVE**

Friends' Reactions

Others in the survivor's community may attempt to help by offering a new "miracle cure" they have read about, or by giving unsolicited religious advice. Some may need to avoid the cancer survivor, because cancer for them is an uncomfortable reminder of their own mortality. Even doctors and nurses, at times, may have difficulty visiting patients whom they cannot help without showing their emotions.

Although a social stigma is still attached to having cancer, cancer is discussed more openly now than ever before. Some people may shy away during times of crisis, but you may also be pleasantly surprised by offers of help from unexpected sources. Survivors can lessen their own hurt and disappointment by appreciating the good intentions of others and by letting them help in whatever way they can.

During the course of your cancer treatment, you may need someone to give you rides, buy groceries, clean the house, and listen to your concerns. Accepting this type of help from people can ease your own burdens and reduce the feelings of inadequacy others may have concerning their inability to help. Prepare yourself for a variety of social reactions to cancer, and try to accept the humanity and good intentions behind most people's actions.

Coworker's Reactions

A job or some form of work, paid or volunteer, can be a stabilizing influence for cancer survivors. It gives you the opportunity to focus your attention on something other than cancer and to experience yourself as more than someone with a disease. When work expands the roles you play in life, it can have a healthy effect on your self-image.

With some cancer treatments the disruption of the work schedule and the impact on coworkers is minimal. Many cancer treatments, however, do require lengthy periods of recuperation and rehabilitation. Survivors sometimes encounter prejudice on returning to work, with reactions ranging from avoidance to curiosity. When you are prepared for a variety of reactions, you have more understanding and are less apt to be overly shocked and hurt.

The fear of cancer among colleagues and coworkers can result in additional feelings of isolation for the cancer survivor. When coworkers deny their vulnerability to the caprice of fate—and the same laws of nature that affect us all—they often attempt to support their erroneous view with attitudes such as:

- He's different from us. He's no longer healthy; he's going to die.
- We who have lived life correctly don't have to worry about death.

Conventional misconceptions about the severity of the various types of cancer and their cure rates lead some people to wonder if and when you are going to die, or they may be shocked that you look so well. Insensitive statements such as "You don't look like you're dying" and "Just my luck—I finally get some help in this department and he gets cancer" are not uncommon. Most people will not be that blunt or insensitive, but colleagues and employers may—even with good intentions—treat you as if you are preparing to die rather than fighting to stay alive.

Others may simply wonder about your ability to pull your share of the load, whether they will need to hire someone new, and whether you will be a financial burden on the company. Such concerns can lead to overt and covert job discrimination and isolation from fellow workers who fear cancer. Prepare yourself to cope with the emotional, as well as the financial and legal consequences, of being a cancer survivor at work. (See Chapter 9 for information about your employment rights.)

Changes in Relationships

Throughout the course of your treatment you will probably experience significant changes in your relationships. Some may become deeper, some more superficial, and some may end. When your treatment causes you to appear weak or sick, even some old friends may avoid you, resuming their friendship when you appear healthier. Whatever relationships remain will be intensified and strengthened during this challenging period of your life.

A healthy relationship should be a major source of support, not something that drains you emotionally. During the early stages of combating cancer, you will need to reduce the stress of your attitude, your diet, your job, and your relationships, making more energy available for coping with cancer and healing. This is a time when your first priority must be to yourself and your health. Loving friends and family will do what they can to be supportive of the way you want to fight cancer and of how you want to maintain the quality of your life. You may need to change those relationships which do not support your commitment to survival.

Changes in relationships need not be painful or negative. In fact, honest confrontation about your changing roles can heighten the quality of healthy relationships. A supportive family and understanding friends can lessen the devastation of cancer and clarify the importance of relationships in your life. The next chapter provides more information regarding the family's role in cancer survivorship.

Mind and Body: Harnessing Your Inner Resources – **CHAPTER FIVE**

SEXUAL RELATIONSHIPS – Sex generally becomes a low priority during times of stress and preoccupation with survival. This is normal with any serious illness or medical treatment. For most survivors, as physical energy and feelings of vitality return, so will the sense of attractiveness and an interest in sex. The psychological component of sexuality is strongly influenced, however, by a person's feelings of self-worth and security. This adjustment may require more than just the return of physical energy and health. Counseling may be required to restore self-esteem and to provide training to overcome sexual dysfunction when illness or medical treatment have affected interest, ability, and comfort.

AUTOGENIC EXERCISE

Autogenics means self-control of your body, and this particular exercise is directed toward warming your hands and relaxing your entire body. You can achieve this only by letting go of conscious attempts at control, and by allowing the automatic part of your nervous system to do its job.

In doing this exercise, you will be performing the amazing feat of dilating the blood vessels and capillaries in your hands and fingers. You cannot achieve this by commanding it to happen, the way you might if you wanted to open your hand. It is only possible when you speak in a language that your unconscious mind understands, and when you trust your inner wisdom to bring you deep relaxation and rapid recuperation for your own health and benefit.

Start by sitting erect with your feet flat on the floor and with your hands on your thighs. Breathe deeply; hold your breath for a moment, and then exhale slowly and completely. Do this three times, counting each time you exhale. Let each exhalation be a signal that you are letting go of any remaining tension. Now allow your eyelids to close softly. You can try to keep them open, and then find that it is much more comfortable to allow them to float down over your eyes. And now, allow that relaxation to flow down over your entire body.

Now you can focus your attention on the chair. Let yourself float down into the chair, and let it support you. Let go of any unnecessary holding in those muscles. Shift your attention to the floor, and let it support your feet. Now you can let go of those muscles. As you let go, continue to exhale away any remaining tension.

During these next few minutes, there is nothing much for you to do except to allow your conscious mind to be curious as your body and unconscious mind cooperate with the process of providing you deeper and deeper relaxation with each of the phrases you will say.

As you repeat each phrase, just imagine, visualize, and feel the change happening. By imagining, visualizing, and feeling the direction given in each phrase, you are stating your will in a language your body can under

{*Continued on next page, 107*}

Counseling is available to help survivors feel comfortable with the many ways of experiencing physical pleasure and of being sexual after the trauma of cancer. But one of the most prevalent reasons for a loss of interest in intimate contact among cancer survivors is a feeling of being defective or "damaged goods." Certainly, your medical condition and physical health should be checked if you have any sexual dysfunction. You also can address, however, the psychosocial component of sexual problems. Concern about how your mate will react to the loss of a breast, to a colostomy, to changed sexual functioning, or to fatigue, can have a profound effect on your ability to relax and

---

Autogenic exercise (continued)

stand. You are letting the will give direction in a passive way, without using force and without trying to make anything happen.

Quietly let the change happen, using your body's natural tendency to cooperate. Now you can be comfortable. Continue to breathe deeply and slowly and repeat quietly to yourself the following:

> I feel quiet. I am beginning to feel quite relaxed—my feet feel quiet and relaxed. My ankles, my knees, and my hips feel light, calm, and comfortable. My stomach and the entire center of my body feel light, calm, and comfortable.

> My entire body feels quiet, calm, and comfortable. My arms and my hands feel quiet and warm. My entire body feels quiet and warm. I feel calm and relaxed. My hands feel calm, relaxed, and warm. My hands are relaxed. My hands are warm. My hands are slowly becoming warmer and warmer as I continue to breathe deeply and slowly.

> My entire body is quiet, calm, and comfortable. My mind is quiet. I withdraw myself from my surroundings and feel serene and still. My thoughts are turning inward. I feel at ease. Within myself I can visualize and experience myself as quiet, calm, and comfortable. In an easy, quiet, inward-turned way, I am quietly alert. My mind is calm and quiet. I feel an inward quietness.

> I will continue with these thoughts for two minutes and then softly open my eyes feeling fine, relaxed, quietly alert, and better than before. It will be interesting to discover how deeply relaxed I can become in a time that normally would seem so short. But even a few minutes of clock time can be all the time in the world for the unconscious mind to dream, to problem-solve, and to achieve deep relaxation and recuperation.

You can now open your eyes and feel adequately alert and completely relaxed, comfortable, and better than before.

experience pleasure. You and your mate may need help promoting self-acceptance, adjusting to a new body image, and removing any sense of defect. A personal sense of attractiveness, desirability, and well-being are the best insurance against sexual problems.

Although reassurance from one's mate is a great asset for self-confidence, self-esteem, and the return of sexual desire, ultimately it is up to the survivor to accept himself or herself as lovable and capable of loving. As one survivor, after months of adjusting to a new sense of self, put it: "I want to grasp every moment as it presents itself to me as I am now, without fretting over how I should be, should feel, or should think."

Gaining Control Over Stress

The stress caused by cancer and cancer treatment is psychological and emotional as well as physical. Your usual strategies for coping with events that are not life threatening may prove inadequate for coping with the stress of cancer. (See the next chapter for a discussion of how families cope with stress.) The ability to manage stress, however, can be learned.

Stress management techniques can be used in the following ways: (1) for physical control over a body whose very cells seem to have gone awry; (2) for cognitive control over the flood of distressing and counterproductive thoughts and images; and (3) for assertiveness to maintain personal control and worth in an environment of strong social pressures.

Because people often experience illness as a loss of control over their bodies, gaining the ability to calm anxiety and to manage pain can restore a sense of connection that is revitalizing. The ability to relax deeply, to experience the release of tension, and to feel that your body can still provide pleasure is a powerful sign of hope when facing a life-threatening illness. Learning that you can achieve a state of relaxation at will brings a feeling of confidence that you are once again in touch with your body. In addition, relaxation itself is recuperative and can lead to a decrease in the need for some types of medication.

Different methods for relaxing provide varying degrees of comfort: listening to music, warm baths, massage, exercise, yoga, meditation, autogenic training, self-hypnosis, and biofeedback. Your personal comfort with and preference for an activity that involves physical movement and contact or mental stillness will determine which method is best for you.

Thoughts, beliefs, and attitudes can lead to either calm or panicky feelings. Just as you can scare yourself by viewing horror films, you can soothe yourself by watching scenes of nature. You can, therefore, gain some control over your feelings by choosing the movies you permit to run in the theater of your mind. With some practice, you can learn to focus your attention on those thoughts, feelings, and behaviors that are the most beneficial, pushing aside—or considering later, when you have more information—those thoughts and beliefs that are disturbing.

You can learn mastery over your internal physical, mental, and emotional states. However, to be effective in controlling external pressures, you will need to communicate your wishes in a forthright, assertive manner. Being assertive does not guarantee that you will always get what you want, but you will at least receive the satisfaction that comes from standing up for yourself. Moreover, communicating to your doctor and family your fears and preferences regarding your medical care may well lead to changes that reduce stress and worry.

COPING THROUGH IMAGERY – Most cancer survivors are exposed to negative images of their bodies as helpless victims of a virulent disease. Some survivors are given negative images imbedded in diagnoses such as: "the cancer has spread to your lymph nodes" or "chemotherapy is highly toxic and will cause your hair to fall out."

Healthy imagery combats these negative images and provides a way of reducing stress, enhancing well-being, and promoting cooperation with medical therapies that may save your life. Many survivors find comfort in actively replacing negative images with ones that promote realistic hope rather than distress.

The negative images of the "spread of cancer" or the side effects of chemotherapy and radiation for example, can be supplanted by more balanced images and thoughts, such as

> My body is trapping the malformed cancer cells in the lymph nodes and the lungs' filtering mechanisms where healthy immune system cells cooperate with chemotherapy or radiation to destroy and remove them. The weak cancer cells, with their confused nuclei, cannot recover from the chemotherapy or radiation the way my healthy cells can. My healthy hair and skin cells are only temporarily affected by cancer treatments which seek out and destroy rapidly dividing cells. Hair loss and nausea—which may be side effects of my treatment— are, therefore, signs that this powerful ally is destroying cancer cells.

Once you do your part by seeking medical treatment and reducing the tumor with surgery and chemotherapy or radiation, you can begin to trust your body to use its white cells ("killer T-cells") to destroy any remaining cancer cells while your macrophages ("scavenger cells") remove them.

Healthy imagery encourages survivors to allow the body to work naturally without conscious direction. Instead of worrying about doing the "right kind" of imaging, you can delegate responsibility for maintaining the proper functioning of your immune system to the "wise, inner healer" (or "inner physician") of your body. You thereby reduce stress and make more energy available to your body to continue its fight against cancer. For example, during stressful medical treatment, a survivor might say to himself or herself:

> I can relax my efforts and allow the superior wisdom of my body do what it knows best. There's nothing much for the conscious me to do, except to allow the flow of relaxation, recuperation, and remission. I am letting go of tension as I exhale, and I'm turning that energy over to a part of me that knows more than I know about washing away the cancer cells while protecting my healthy cells.

By delegating the task of fighting cancer to the superior wisdom of the body and its immune system, you can avoid concern about the correctness of the image, of sufficient "will to live" and "right-thinking."

Three types of imagery are particularly useful for cancer survivors—autogenics, centering, and healthy imagining.

Autogenics influences bodily functions, such as blood flow to warm your hands, by using a language your body and mind can cooperate with. Through autogenics you learn to use "passive volition" to communicate words and images that produce relaxation, recovery from fatigue, and improved circulation. In this first stage of gaining physical control through relaxation, you can achieve satisfactory levels of relaxation with increasingly improved results within a week or two of

---

CENTERING EXERCISE

Begin by taking three slow breaths, and then just float down into your chair or bed. Let go of any unnecessary muscle tension. With your next three breaths exhale away all thoughts and images of work from the past. Clear your mind and your body of all concerns about what "should have" or "shouldn't have" happened in the past. Just let them go.

With your next three breaths let go of all images and thoughts about what you think may happen in the future—all the *what ifs*. Clear your mind and body of all concern about what you expect to happen.

With your next three breaths, choose to be in the present where there is nothing much for you to do now. Just allow the natural processes of your body to provide you with deep relaxation, recuperation, and remission. Let go of trying to be in any particular time or striving to be any particular way—just be here in this moment, where it does not take much effort to breath comfortably and to make more energy available for healing and recuperation.

daily practice of 10 to 15 minutes. Resist the urge to test out your new skills against the most stressful events in your life until you have practiced and achieved a satisfactory level of relaxation.

Centering is a rapid, two-minute procedure which brings your mind back from fretting about the past and future into the present, where your body must be. This helps you clear your mind of past or future problems that cannot be addressed now. As you withdraw your thoughts from these problems, you also release their accompanying guilt and stress, and experience a stress-free moment in the present. You already are practicing centering your attention in the present whenever you experience moments of joyful abandonment or intense concentration. With the centering exercise you can learn to bring about these relaxing and recuperative moments at will.

Healthy Imagining centers around the concept of the "inner healer." The inner healer is that wise part of you that knows more than all of modern science about cellular biology and the strength of your immune system. Use healthy imagining when you are ready to replace negative images about cancer and treatment with more relaxing, robust images. If you are new to imagery, you might first start with the autogenic exercise, the centering exercise, or your own form of meditation or prayer. Use any of these methods to just become relaxed and to experience the way your body responds to your words and images.

As you practice these relaxation and imagery exercises, your ability to control stressful images will improve. You will find that you have more effective communications between your mind and body. With mind and body working together, your imagery exercises become a mental shield, giving you time to push aside negative images, to let go of tension, and to make decisions about medical treatment.

TRANSFORMATION—NEW POTENTIAL FOR THE CANCER SURVIVOR

During the process of coping with the cancer diagnosis, treatment decisions, and adjustments to side effects, it is difficult to imagine any benefit coming from the experience of cancer. Yet those who have written and spoken of their survival experience often tell of the positive changes that have taken place in their outlook and character as a result of facing the challenges of cancer.

For many survivors, cancer calls forth a transformation in attitude, health habits, and self-image. They learn to replace ineffective and limited ways of coping with healthier methods of dealing with work and social challenges. In this sense, any crisis offers an opportunity for positive change. Facing a life-threatening experience stretches your abilities beyond previous limits and gives you a chance to achieve your greatest potential.

Most cancer survivors are forced to develop their latent skills, to refine their strengths, and to drop negative habits. Some survivors stop worrying about money and begin traveling around the world. Others leave destructive relationships and unsatisfying jobs. Some just take life a little less seriously.

The experience of cancer will not make you more powerful over nature, the economy, world events, or other people. But it can show you the power you have over your thoughts and attitudes, and that—regardless of the events in your life—you can be in charge of how you make yourself feel.

Life-threatening experiences remind us that life is a precious, limited resource to be experienced fully each moment. For many survivors, discovering the ability to live fully in the present can bring about unexpected feelings of calm and power. For some, the possibility of death can bring freedom from worry about the future and about defending a former identity. Others may find that the power to change their lives comes more from a new appreciation of life once

> Cancer… gives you an experience so intense, so frightening, and so energy-creating, that it's almost like being launched from a pad. You must, must change. …life is finite and can't be predicted. It could be cancer or it could be the truck coming around the bend, and so some effort has to be made to wake up and live a day, every day, as if it matters.… It just isn't the same anymore. Because of that, all kinds of things become possible.
>
> *Valerie, a thirty-year old breast cancer survivor, in Deborah Hobler Kahane's* No Less a Woman

HEALTHY IMAGINING EXERCISE

Focus your attention on any part of your body about which you are concerned. Take a deep breath and exhale through that area, releasing any tension you may be holding there. As you let go, allow your muscles to relax, permitting your blood vessels to dilate, and your circulation to improve the flow of oxygen and potentially healing elements to that area. By exhaling and relaxing your conscious efforts and concerns, you are assisting your body in healing itself. Continue to breathe slowly and deeply and—changing my words to fit your own style—say to yourself:

> Ninety-nine percent of me is healthy and working for the removal of the weak, confused cancer cells. Even now, as I am sitting here, breathing easily, I am making millions and millions of healthy, new blood cells every minute—and I don't even know how I do it; but my mind and body do know how, and they do it for my protection and for my healing and recuperation, even while I sleep.
>
> I imagine my body bathed in sunlight and clear water, washing and dissolving cancer cells out of my body while coating and protecting the healthy cells. I see and feel my chemotherapy as a powerful cleanser, and radiation as bullets of light removing cancer cells from my body while doing little harm to my healthy cells. My body is strong and can rapidly heal and recover from surgery, chemotherapy, or radiation. My body welcomes the help of my medical treatment and works with it to free me of cancer.

health and energy return after prolonged illness.

Some survivors have noted that they never had such an opportunity to change their roles with their families as when they had cancer. Even those who are shy find it easier to express their wishes, feeling: "Since I have nothing to lose, I have nothing to fear." The impact of cancer can shatter old roles and senses of identity and leave survivors without a set of rules on which to fall back. Many survivors must mourn the loss of the old securities and fashion new rules of life based on personal values and priorities. This focus turns survivors inward toward previously untapped reserves and resources. It gives survivors a second chance to discover and shape their "true self," apart from the family's and society's pressures.

In short, the cancer experience holds the possibility of making one's life more meaningful. Learning to control stress, worry, and social pressures can prepare survivors for the burdens imposed by cancer as well as energize them for a fuller life after cancer.

Chapter Six

Family Challenges: Communication, Hope, and Loss

by Elizabeth Johns Clark, PhD MSW

"Social oncology, the study of personal and social problems caused by illness, has been my professional area of interest for 20 years. But equally as significant is the fact that a close family member lives with cancer on a daily basis. It is my hope that this chapter will provide some assistance to other families who are just learning to navigate the cancer survivorship journey."

Elizabeth Johns Clark

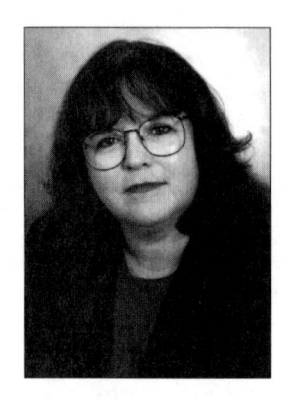

ELIZABETH JOHNS CLARK, PHD is the president of the National Coalition for Cancer Survivorship and was cochair of the First National Congress on Cancer Survivorship, which was held in November 1995 in Washington, DC. She currently serves as director of Diagnostic and Therapeutic Services at Albany Medical Center Hospital and as an associate professor of medicine in the Division of Medical Oncology at Albany Medical College. She holds a doctorate in medical sociology and master's degrees in both medical social work and public health. Dr. Clark has lectured and published extensively in the areas of social oncology, loss and grief, hope and burnout.

After the usual biopsies and other tests, I was told that I had a potentially fatal disease. Now that gets your attention. The Big C. The word "cancer": it overwhelms the psyche—just the word. I couldn't believe it. I was unprepared for the enormous emotional jolt that I received from the diagnosis.

—Sandra Day O'Connor
Associate Justice, United States Supreme Court

As Justice Sandra Day O'Connor so eloquently said, a cancer diagnosis causes an intense emotional jolt. Usually, you are not prepared for such a crisis and are not equipped with adequate problem-solving strategies. As a result, you face a normless situation where you may not know how to think or talk about the problem, how to evaluate reality, or how to take action. You need information, but due to the shock and unfamiliarity of the situation, you may be unable to understand the information you do receive. As Dr. Fiore pointed out in the previous chapter, you probably will be thrown into a state of panic.

The research literature on crisis theory emphasizes that all crises are time-limited, and that the crisis period usually lasts from one to six weeks. After that time, the individual has found a way to deal with the problem or has become more used to it so that it no longer fits the definition of a crisis. One of the difficulties of living with cancer, however, is that the disease creates a series or sequence of crisis situations. The first crisis may result from the diagnosis and the initial treatment. A new crisis may be caused later by treatment failures, protocol changes, or recurrence of disease. The end of intensive treatment and the beginning of the waiting period to see if the treatment was successful may trigger yet another crisis.

Eventually, you become an expert about your own illness and treatment. You know more or less what to expect medically, and you learn how to navigate the health care system. You develop the needed language and coping skills to manage the crisis periods. In short, you learn how to live with cancer. You may face recurrent crisis situations, both physical and psychosocial, but gradually the panic and lack of coping skills you first experienced after your diagnosis subside.

CANCER IS A FAMILY CRISIS

Due to your cancer, your family will have a similar crisis experience. A family is a social system. Change in one part of the system causes change in the other parts of that system. Therefore, a diagnosis of cancer for one family member significantly alters the pattern of the family system and affects all other family members. Many researchers have found that some of the most difficult problems faced by cancer survivors are the reactions of their family members, friends, and coworkers.

In times of individual crisis, families are often viewed as a refuge, a place of support when trouble occurs. Even the word "home" has special significance for most people in times of stress. Stress is an expected part of family life, but cancer is an extraordinary stressor. By virtue of its ability to threaten the continuity of family life, cancer results in a family crisis. The magnitude of the cancer crisis is such that the family system is thrown into distress and family functioning and quality of family life can be compromised.

A diagnosis of cancer in one family member will have an impact on each member of the family. The intensity of that impact will vary depending on individual factors such as closeness to the cancer survivor, developmental level, and personal strengths and coping abilities. Serious illness generally intensifies relationship patterns that already exist within the family, but excessive and prolonged stress can have a negative impact on even the strongest and closest family. Cancer can also offer the chance for personal growth and can bring about a stronger family unit.

During the initial cancer crisis, the family unit faces many tasks and challenges. Family members need to obtain adequate information so that treatment decisions can be made. They need to decide who to tell and what to tell them. They may need to reassign role responsibilities, at least on a temporary basis. They may have to make financial decisions. They have to find ways to support one another emotionally. As individuals and as a unit, they need to manage fear and uncertainty, and they need to maintain hope. Each of these tasks requires family communication.

FAMILY COMMUNICATION

The communication patterns of most families are well established; they may be either functional or dysfunctional. If communication within the family is open and honest, it should serve a positive function in times of crisis. Some families, however, have less than optimal communication patterns, and serious illness may make communication even harder.

Your family may have difficulty talking about subjects that have an emotional component. For example, crying in front of others may

> Stress is an expected part of family life, but cancer is an extraordinary stressor. By virtue of its ability to threaten the continuity of family life, cancer results in a family crisis.

not be acceptable in your family; yet, a diagnosis of cancer for yourself or for a loved one causes sadness. As a result, family members may be forced to cry alone in their cars, their offices or in the shower. A lack of communication and the inability to express emotion in front of others can cause increased isolation and anxiety.

Open communication and the expression of feelings within the family are crucial to creating a healing environment and for helping one another gain the strength necessary to deal with the crises of cancer. Remember that while each cancer crisis is time-limited, cancer is a chronic illness. You will need to maintain or develop good family communication skills so your family can adapt over the long haul.

Good family communication skills can be learned, but you may need to get some specific training for dealing with cancer-related communication issues. This training often is available in your hospital or community through patient education programs or through mutual self-help and support groups. In order to improve family communication, you first need an understanding of what kinds of factors create communication barriers.

Barriers to Family Communication

Fear – Fear is a major barrier to communication. When someone is first diagnosed with cancer, the major fear for the cancer survivor and the family is that cancer will lead to death. Even with unrealistic myths about cancer dispelled, and even when the prognosis and statistics are favorable, the fear of death requires some management. If not managed adequately, fear and sadness can drive a wedge between helpful family communications.

Refusal to Discuss 'Sad' Topics – An additional burden is an almost instinctual need for family members to protect the cancer survivor from the realities of the cancer. This protection may extend to other family members who seem vulnerable and overburdened. The problem can be compounded by some therapies that encourage positive thinking as part of the treatment for cancer. Due to these theories, some family members do not want to hear sad or scared talk for fear of jeopardizing their loved one's recovery. This means the cancer survivor, as well as other family members, is cut off and isolated from talking about cancer-related fear and sadness. This isolation may increase the burden of the illness.

Anger – Anger is inevitable during the cancer experience. Angry outbreaks on the part of the cancer survivor and family members are to be expected. Try to look beyond the anger to its source. It usually is not a result of something someone has done; rather, it is a way of responding to the accumulated high stress and helplessness that the cancer survivor or angry family member feels.

Guilt – Guilt, over real or imaginary events, can be another communication barrier. Family members may blame themselves for not insisting that the patient see a doctor sooner, or for various other illness-related concerns. Family members may feel guilty that they are well and that it is another person in the family who has the illness. This may especially be the case among siblings when the cancer survivor is a child.

Guilt is often related to feelings of inadequacy. Perhaps a family member feels guilty because he or she is embarrassed by the way the cancer survivor looks during the treatment process. Hair loss, disfiguring surgery, or other changes in appearance take time to get used to. Questions and comments from friends or strangers may be difficult to handle.

> Small children can also have guilt related to the cancer diagnosis. Perhaps they did something that they should not have done, or when angry at the family member, wished that he or she would die. Children need reassurance that nothing they said or did caused the cancer.

Gender Differences – Family members often deal with problems differently, and they usually rely on coping behaviors that they have found useful in the past. Men and women sometimes respond differently to fear and anxiety-producing situations. Men may present a brave front, denying the seriousness of the illness, especially when it is the female partner who is the cancer survivor. This denial sometimes helps men cope with feelings of powerlessness and anxiety.

Some women also use a form of denial, but it generally relates to their own illness, not to that of their partner or child. They may find themselves trying so hard to calm the fears of their immediate family members and their relatives, that they have little time to acknowledge the concerns and fears they have for themselves. They repress their own fears in order to help family members cope. Their responses to their own illness seem stoical, and others may comment about "how strong you seem," or that they "don't know how you do it." This "strong" behavior on the part of a woman with cancer eventually has a negative effect. In the face of personal threat or poor physical health, it becomes more and more difficult to be the person providing the majority of the family support.

Conspiracy of Silence – Both men and women with cancer may need help in voicing their fears and anger and in accepting emotional support and assistance. When communication is not possible among family members, confusion can result. The cancer survivor may feel resentful that no one really understands the difficulty he or she faces. Family members feel they cannot let their guard down or discuss their real feelings. Sometimes this leads to what is termed a conspiracy of silence, a situation in which information is withheld from either the cancer survivor or a family member for fear that they will not be able to deal with it.

FAMILY COPING STYLES

It is important to realize that family members respond to high stress differently. One person may resort to anger as a response to feelings of helplessness. Another may withdraw emotionally or try to be out of the house as much as possible. Still another may appear not to care, or to act as if nothing has changed. These various coping styles may be misconstrued by other family members and may lead to conflict within the family system.

Whatever their level of knowledge or understanding about cancer, children are aware that a tremendous change has occurred in the household. Changes in daily routine, long absences of one or both parents, preoccupation of parents or siblings, and feelings of tension are all obvious signals that something is wrong. Young children need to know that they will continue to be cared for and supported. In addition, they need to make sense out of the sadness, anxiety, and despair of the adults around them. If they are given inadequate information, they will make their own assumptions. They need to know what is happening or they will fill in the gaps with their own interpretations, and what they imagine is often worse than the reality.

Teenagers in the family also need reassurances. Sometimes their needs are overlooked during family crises. Since they are approaching adulthood, their needs may be grouped with those of other adults. They may be expected to act like adults and take on adult responsibilities. This is not always possible for teenagers and may lead to increased stress and result in further family conflict.

A family crisis such as cancer disrupts normal adolescent processes. Just as the young person is beginning a gradual emotional withdrawal from the family and is starting to establish an individual identity, the illness of a parent forces them to have intensified family contact. They may be willing to accept increased household and babysitting responsibilities, but they also may act out their resentment in various ways. Teenagers need support and an opportunity to ventilate and talk about their mixed feelings. Perhaps a relative or close family friend could serve this support function for the adolescent.

Sometimes grown-up children are initially left out of the family communication loop; this may be purposeful or accidental. While these children generally live outside the parents' home, they still remain a part of the extended family system and should know about a family problem as soon as it occurs. Not telling them about your illness isolates them and does not afford them the opportunity of receiving or providing family support. You may think you have very good reasons for not informing your grown-up children about your diagnosis or for putting off telling them. Perhaps they are struggling with a crisis of their own, or are overwhelmed at work or school or with parenting issues. Regardless, they will be hurt if they find out about your diagnosis from a sibling or relative or an acquaintance. They may feel guilty that they were not able to be supportive of you sooner.

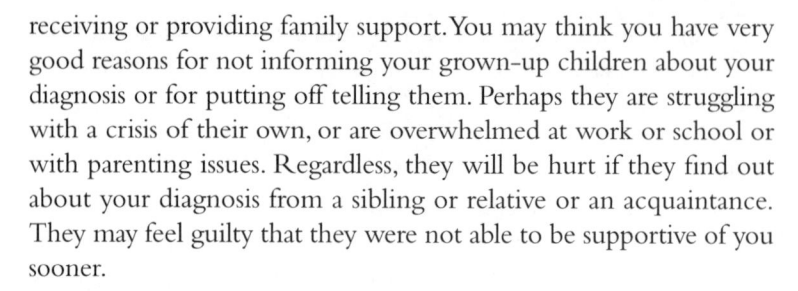

MULTIPLE FAMILY PROBLEMS

The crisis of serious illness seems to intensify the family relationship patterns that already are in place. It also may intensify existing family problems. For example, if a child is not doing well in school, his or her grades will not likely improve when an additional family problem is introduced. Likewise, marital discord or financial problems may be made worse when a serious illness is identified. Alcoholism, drug abuse, and eating disorders may also become more severe for a family member when new problems are introduced.

Sometimes, existing problems do seem to "self-correct" for a short

> Getting teenagers to talk about feelings can be the most frustrating effort a parent faces. So don't. But make time to just be together. Don't set it up as "our time to talk." If your teenagers are taking a stab at expressing themselves, just try to reflect back what you hear. "I hear a lot of anger and that's okay. I am angry, too."
> *Kathy LaTour, breast cancer survivor, author, and mother. From* The Breast Cancer Companion, *1993:298.*

TIPS FOR CHILDREN TO COPE WITH CANCER IN THE FAMILY

- Don't be ashamed or afraid of the way you feel. Others in your situation have felt the same way.
- Sometimes things get better if you talk about them. Share your feelings with your parents or another adult or a friend you can trust.
- Learn about cancer and the way it is treated. What we first imagine about cancer is often far worse than what is really happening.
- Try to find other people your age who have a person in their family with cancer or other serious illness. You may be able to share your feelings with them.
- If you overhear someone talking and what you hear scares you, ask them to explain what they said. Don't assume that you heard everything and understood what it meant; ask about it.
- Don't forget the adults other than your parents who can help you.

Abstracted from the booklet When Someone in Your Family Has Cancer. *Available from the National Cancer Institute (Publication No. 90-2685).*

time as everyone focuses on the immediate family crisis. Eventually, however, the increased stress will probably take its toll. If someone in your family has a personal problem or is engaging in destructive behavior, do all you can to get them to seek counseling or go together to see a family therapist so that your family energies are not fragmented and dispersed. If your loved one will not seek help, seek counseling without them so you can gain assistance in managing your own responses to the ongoing family problem and to the new crisis.

Enhancing Family Communication

The following are suggestions for avoiding some of the barriers to family communication:

TRY TO PUT CANCER IN PERSPECTIVE — Family members need to recognize that cancer is a disease like any other disease. It can be cured, it can be treated, it can be controlled, and it can be managed. Do not let the negative myths and fears about cancer impede communication.

Both the cancer survivor and family members need accurate and honest information about the illness and the treatment course. Knowledge can increase personal control and can help minimize a sense of helplessness on the part of all family members. Family discussions about the type and extent of treatments and about expected side effects and changes in appearance are useful. Family members should discuss openly within the family worrisome things that they hear from their friends or colleagues. Troublesome comments and questions about suggested miracle therapies, for example, can be brought to your health-care team for clarification.

Educational materials to help your family understand cancer and its treatment are available from your hospital, your physician, your oncology nurse, or your social worker. Booklets related to specific types of cancer can be obtained free of charge from the local unit of your American Cancer Society at (800) 227-2345 and from the National Cancer Institute at (800) 4-CANCER. Excellent educational resources have been written for younger age groups. Two recommended resources for children include *It Helps to Have Friends When Mom or Dad Has Cancer* from the American Cancer Society; and *When Someone in Your Family Has Cancer,* available from the National Cancer Institute (NIH Publication No. 94-2685).

DISCUSS NEEDED CHANGES IN FAMILY ROLES AND ACTIVITIES — Will a vacation or family event need to be delayed or canceled? Will the cancer survivor need to be absent from work for a period of time, and if so, will this have an impact on family finances? What will

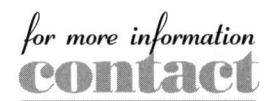

for more information
contact

AMERICAN CANCER SOCIETY
800/227-2345
It Helps to Have Friends When Mom or Dad Has Cancer

NATIONAL CANCER INSTITUTE
800/4-CANCER
When Someone in Your Family Has Cancer
(No. 94-2685)

Family Challenges: Communications, Hope, and Loss — **CHAPTER SIX** remain the same—for example, your love for one another, honesty with each other, valuing family time, and continuing special activities? How will family chores and responsibilities be distributed during the treatment process? Who will be available to help with transportation, shopping, meal preparation, and homework?

The shifting of responsibilities for household tasks, managing family finances, and providing care for the cancer survivor or for children creates stress. Family members can feel overworked, unappreciated, or left out. Discussing these changes and related feelings in an open manner, and being accepting of anger, disappointment, and differences can go a long way toward stabilizing the situation and helping the family system to adapt to the crisis.

Even if a loved one is extremely ill, try not to exclude him or her from the family decision-making process. While some role shifting may need to occur due to the illness, all family members, including the cancer survivor, need to feel that they are a respected and valued part of the family system.

DETERMINE WHAT IS ACCEPTABLE TO DISCUSS WITH FRIENDS AND EXTENDED FAMILY MEMBERS ABOUT THE CANCER SURVIVOR AND THE ILLNESS – Many friends and neighbors will be curious about the illness and prognosis. Most will ask questions because they want to offer assis-

---

CHECKLIST FOR THE FAMILY

Are you pressuring the person with cancer to—
- stop talking about his health because it is morbid?
- stop feeling sorry for himself?
- prove that he is feeling great even when he is not?

Instead, help by—
- letting him talk about his problems and finding positive topics to talk about;
- keeping his interest up about home, work, and world affairs;
- being sympathetic but emphasizing the good things about life;
- not pressuring him to be a cheerleader for you to keep up your spirits;
- letting him level with you about his feelings.

Morra and Potts, Triumph: Getting Back to Normal When You Have Cancer, *1990:211.*

tance and support. Some people, however, are simply interested in gossip. Keep in mind that the cancer survivor has a right to privacy and that you are not obligated to discuss the situation. It is useful to go over some of the myths about cancer and to help family members form responses to difficult questions that might be posed by others.

SEEK OUT ADDITIONAL EDUCATIONAL RESOURCES FOR THE FAMILY – Classes like the American Cancer Society's "I Can Cope" and group meetings can provide education and support to meet the challenges of cancer. Mutual support and self-help groups and special programs designed to help individuals and families cope with family changes and problem solving are readily available in most communities (see Chapter 7). Let the cancer survivor and other family members know if you are planning to attend a support group or a cancer-related education program. Keeping attendance a secret will not foster family communication.

> Hope does not equate with denial; in fact, true hope always is based in reality.

MAINTAINING FAMILY HOPE

Hope is a way of thinking, feeling, and acting. It functions as a protective mechanism and is essential for managing and adapting to an illness as serious as cancer. Maintaining hope is not always easy. At times of crisis you may need additional support and assistance from your family, your health-care team, and other cancer survivors.

Many people have never thought much about what role hope plays in their lives, or about how they hope, or even how they learned to hope. Yet research tells us that people hope very differently and that our personal hope is affected by various social factors. One of these is the way your family hopes.

Families have well-established ways of hoping. These patterns are called family hope constellations. They contain your family's values and norms regarding hope, and the strategies used to maintain hope. For example, some families use a religious or spiritual basis for their hope. As a result, statistics and medical facts may not be as important to this family because they believe God will determine the outcome. These family members may draw great strength from attending religious services, from prayer, and from interaction with clergy.

Another family may use an educational or information basis for their hope. Their hoping strategies lean more toward fact gathering. They read about cancer and its treatment. They seek second, third, and fourth opinions. They use cancer information lines and medical libraries. For them, information equates with control and hope.

No one family hope constellation is the best or most functional. What is important is that you recognize how your family thinks about hope and what strategies they use to maintain it. You should

How People Hope

People hope differently. While hope is individualistic, your own hope strategies are influenced by how your family of origin and your present family use and maintain hope.

Families tend to have similarities in the ways they hope, but family hope constellations are not mutually exclusive.

Different types of hope constellations may lead to conflict between the cancer survivor and family members or friends. They also can lead to conflict between the cancer survivor and family and the health care professionals who care for them because health care professionals also hope in individual ways.

Most people have never thought about "how" they hope. They just assume everyone hopes in the same manner that they themselves do. This does not refer simply to optimism or pessimism, but to the strategies people use to look forward and for maintaining a positive outlook on the future.

Most health-care professionals are not trained to do "hope assessments" or to recognize different hoping styles. They often think only in terms of "therapeutic" hope, and equate other hope with denial. This can have a negative impact on your interactions with them and can make you vulnerable to broken hope.

It is important to think about your own hoping strategies and to be direct with family, friends, and professional caregivers about what is most helpful to you with regard to using and maintaining hope. Never let anyone tell you that there is nothing further to hope for or that there is no hope. There is always something to hope for, and you and your family have the right to determine for what, when, and how you hope.

Abstracted from the booklet You Have the Right to be Hopeful, *by Elizabeth Clark. Available from the National Coalition for Cancer Survivorship at (301)650-8868.*

recognize that individuals within your family may hope differently, particularly if they are part of your family through marriage and were raised in a different family.

You also need to recognize that hope is broader than just the therapeutic aspect of treatment and control of disease. Hope has many dimensions. It changes over time as situations and reality change. For example, when first diagnosed with cancer, you may have hoped for a cure. If you have a type of cancer that cannot yet be totally cured, you may shift your hope to control—long-term control. Even if hope for survival dims, individuals and families can find something else to maintain hope. Perhaps you are hoping to have a family reunion, or hoping to see a child graduate from college, or hoping to welcome the birth of a new grandchild. It is important to always choose hope because hopelessness leads to despair and helplessness.

> Burnout is defined as a syndrome of emotional exhaustion that frequently occurs among individuals who do "people work," which means they spend considerable time in close encounters with others under conditions of chronic tension and stress. Two major clues to burnout are increased cynicism and feelings of being indispensable.

AVOIDING FAMILY BURNOUT

The concept of burnout has generally been applied to individuals. Only recently have the concept and consequences of institutional burnout been explored. By definition, burnout is applicable to families, too.

Burnout is defined as a syndrome of emotional exhaustion that frequently occurs among individuals who do "people work," which means they spend considerable time in close encounters with others under conditions of chronic tension and stress. Two major clues to burnout are increased cynicism and feelings of being indispensable. This definition can easily fit family members during the initial cancer crisis and over the duration of a treatment regimen that may extend for many months or even years.

The signs and symptoms of burnout range from physical symptoms such as fatigue and exhaustion, frequent headaches, or sleeplessness, to behavioral and psychological symptoms, such as being quick to anger, feelings of being unappreciated, and being unable to make decisions. Sometimes they result in escapist behavior and an individual may begin using alcohol or drugs to avoid the overwhelming feelings of stress. You may become cynical about the treatment regimen or about the health-care team or despair that the situation will ever get better. This cynicism may be linked to anger, and those angry feelings about the situation or your sense of hopelessness may be displaced onto others such as a physician, a family member, or even the patient.

Feeling indispensable can be equally dysfunctional. Family members who believe they have to be present constantly and in a caregiving role will delay any personal gratification or plans so that they can be readily available to the cancer survivor and other family members. All family members must take care of their own health. This means eating right, exercising, and getting enough rest and relaxation. You do not need a family martyr—one person who sacrifices personal well-being for the family's sake.

A side effect of having one "indispensable" family member is that other family members may take advantage of the person and after a while, they stop asking to share the burden and are relieved that they do not have to be so constantly involved. Eventually, the constant caregiver will burn out, and the family will be unprepared for the consequences; or, the stress for the individual will be so great that he or she will become sick. A new illness will further compound the family crisis.

If you or a family member are feeling indispensable, have a family conversation about the situation. To avoid burnout, you must know your own strengths and weaknesses and freely admit these to others. When everyone is together, do an assessment of family skills and see how each person can contribute. Perhaps you will find that one person becomes panicky about being present at treatment procedures or simply can not tolerate needles. Yet, that person's strength may be in planning family activities or managing finances or preparing tax returns.

As time goes on, give individuals the opportunity to change "assignments" so that they do not become too burdened by any one task or responsibility. Avoid having all of the personal care tasks fall on only one person. Plan routine breaks for each family member. Let teenagers and close family friends share the burden. For example, a teenager who drives could take the cancer survivor for radiation treatments or to a doctors appointment. This will enable him to learn something about the treatment process, will make him feel like a fully functioning member of the family, and will provide an opportunity for private and meaningful conversation between the teenager and the cancer survivor.

If you are feeling burned out, you may want to attend some educational programs or join a support group (see Chapter 7). Maintain a personal support network that includes people outside of the family circle. When two people are involved in the same crisis, it becomes almost impossible for them to support one another equally because their emotional energy is going into managing the crisis. As needed, you should be able to draw emotional support from a friendship and coworker network. Take routine breaks from discussing and living the cancer crisis.

As much as possible, the family, including the cancer survivor, should try to maintain usual activities and routines. Continue outside interests, hobbies, sports, and exercise programs. If needed, recruit assistance from your extended family and friends for carpooling and other services. They will be glad they can be useful.

TAKE TIME OUT – Vacations, even if only for a day or two, are essential so that you can maintain perspective. Guilt because you take a day or two off from the family crisis is an indication of feelings of indispensability and may be a strong warning signal for burnout. It also is important to encourage the cancer survivor to divest of the patient role as soon as possible. Too often families become overly protective during the treatment phase. They continue to limit or discourage individual and family activities even when no physical limitations warrant doing so.

ASK FOR WHAT YOU NEED – Another task for family members is asking assertively for what they need. At times of serious illness and tension, many persons put their own needs on hold and feel that it would be selfish to ask for something they personally want or require. After a while, this denial of personal needs can become the family norm, and resentment builds up. Do not assume that other family members know what you think, feel, or need. Remember that they are as involved in the crisis as you are and have probably not taken your needs into account. Similarly, you may have overlooked their needs and concerns.

While acute crises are time-limited, the burden of caregiving for family members can extend over long periods. The family, as a whole, may become worn down, depressed, or less functional than they were at the beginning of the illness. If this is the case, you may need some professional advice or counseling to help you move beyond family burnout. You may also need additional tangible support from home health aides or community agencies.

> Asking for help is a sign of courage and control. Asking for help provides others the opportunity to feel fulfilled. Asking for help promotes everyone's recovery.
>
> *Wendy Schlessel Harpham, physician, author, and cancer survivor.* In After Cancer: A Guide to Your New Life. *1994:237.*

LIFE AFTER THE CANCER CRISIS

Cancer in the family permanently changes that family. Although everyone longs to "get back to normal," a "new normal" must evolve in order to move forward. The new normal includes elements of the cancer crisis, such as increased medical checkups, living with uncertainty, and fear of a cancer recurrence or the end of a remission. Some experts liken the aftermath of an acute cancer experience to a post-traumatic stress reaction. It may take years for the cancer survivor and the family to feel safe again. Periodic episodes of flashbacks and heightened anxiety that are unrelated to cancer often arise around periodic checkups or minor illness episodes.

Uncertainty may result in a hesitation to give up your patient identity and your dependency on the health care team. You may be frightened to start over and to trust the future again. Resuming life-oriented thought processes after living with an acute fear of death is a difficult transition. The ability to make long-range plans can take

> Cancer in the family permanently changes that family. Although everyone longs to "get back to normal," a "new normal" must evolve in order to move forward.

months or even years to acquire. To move forward, you will need to take the experiences and the related skills and strengths you have acquired and integrate these into your "new normal" life.

Managing a crisis frequently leads to a higher level of functioning on the part of both the cancer survivor and the family. Families may have drawn closer together and can now handle minor problems and stressors more easily. They may be able to communicate more directly. They may know one another better and be able to recognize and acknowledge one another's strengths and weaknesses and provide support as needed. In some cases, though, the stress of the illness is too great and family members become alienated and more distanced than before the crisis. If the family infrastructure was weak before the illness, it may not be strengthened by adversity. Again, family or individual counseling may be desirable to deal with the aftermath of a cancer crisis.

As a family, you probably will retain an interest in cancer related topics for a long time. You may follow developments in cancer research and may serve as a resource for other individuals and families who are in the midst of a cancer crisis. Frequently, cancer survivors and their family members want to give something back and turn to personal and community advocacy on behalf of persons with cancer. (For a discussion on how to become an advocate, see Chapter 12.)

Loss and Grief

Some cancer survivors and their families live with a chronic state of illness for many years; other cancer survivors never achieve remission of their cancer. Still others, despite excellent care and initial responses, experience one or more recurrences or even the development of a second, unrelated cancer diagnosis. These situations sometimes become life-threatening, and approximately half of all persons diagnosed with cancer eventually do die from their disease.

Loss is a recurrent theme in cancer. While undergoing cancer treatment, you may experience physical and psychological losses such as hair loss and loss of autonomy. Families also experience losses such as the loss of feelings of security, financial losses, and loss of dreams. Nothing, though, ever prepares us for the really bad things in life, such as the death of a loved one.

Family Tasks During Terminal Illness

During the terminal phase, numerous family tasks must be accomplished in preparation for your loved one's death. It is important to know preferences. What kind of medical care does your loved one want? Is the family in agreement about the death taking place at home? Can family members handle the caregiving and be available around the clock? Should you ask for a referral to a freestanding hospice or to a home-care hospice program (see Chapter 3 for an overview of hospice services)? Even with home-care hospice services, if your loved one dies at home, how will death be pronounced and by whom?

Legal considerations need attention. Has an advance directive been completed? Has a durable power of attorney been selected and finalized? Has a will been made or updated? Does your loved one want to donate any organs?

Chapter Ten discusses many of the legal decisions that need to be made. Another excellent resource is the book *Ready to Live, Prepared to Die,* written by Amy Harwell and published by Joshua's Tent, (available at (800) JHS-TENT). Getting any necessary paperwork done and collecting needed documents in advance can help the tasks that are required immediately after the death go more smoothly.

Perhaps the most difficult tasks facing the family are making preparations for the final weeks of life and planning the funeral. If your loved one is staying at home, will you need to make changes in sleeping arrangements or other home accommodations? How will caregiving duties be shared? How will you know when death is near? How and when will you notify family and close friends about impending death? Who will notify the funeral home?

Your local hospice or health-care team can help you with many of these questions. They can also tell you what to expect during the final hours and how to deal with the physiological changes as death occurs. An excellent resource that helps families prepare for a loved one's death at home is called *Dying at Home.* Written by professionals at the Massey Cancer Center in Virginia, a copy may be obtained by calling (804) 828-0450.

Desired funeral arrangements may have been expressed previously by your loved one. Decisions must be made about burial or cremation. If burial is chosen, a cemetery must be selected and a plot must be purchased. Will there be a tombstone or a grave marker, and how should it be engraved? Will there be a wake or viewing? Will you have a religious ceremony or a memorial service? Will the burial be private or open to the public? Does your loved one want flowers or prefer that memorial contributions be made to a favorite charity or community agency? Will the death be announced in the newspaper and what information will be included in the obituary?

Reading the above paragraphs may make you think that you cannot handle the death-related tasks. You may even think that you cannot broach the subject of death with your loved one, but you can. Almost all patients in the terminal phase of life realize that they are going to die.

for more information
contact

JOSHUA'S TENT
800/JHS-TENT
Ready to Live, Prepared to Die
by Amy Harwell

MASSEY CANCER CENTER
804/848-0450
Dying at Home

Family Challenges: Communications, Hope, and Loss – **CHAPTER SIX**

They can feel themselves getting weaker. They may have asked a member of their health-care team if they are dying. You do not want to waste the time you have left together trying to keep the truth from one another. Instead, use this time to say all of the important things you want to say—how much you have loved the person and how wonderful it has been to have him or her in your life. Express how much you will miss him or her. If possible, resolve past issues and make peace with the things that were not always right with your relationship.

Having said all of the above, it is important to note that people generally do not make many changes during their final weeks or days of life. A person who has a lot of anger will probably die angry. Persons who have had a difficult time expressing personal feelings may still be unable to say all of the things they would like to say. Approaching the final hours with as much openness as is possible for you and your loved one is the best that you can do. Sometimes touching takes the place of talking and touching can be a very important form of communication.

Managing Grief

When your loved one dies, family members will need to grieve. Perhaps anticipatory grief began while you were making preparations for the death and the funeral. Even if it did, the actual death, the reality of it, is still overwhelming. For the first two weeks or so, you may feel numb. You cannot accept the reality of the loss and you move through the days following the death and funeral as if you are in a fog.

After the numbness wears off, you begin to acknowledge the finality of the loss and a period of despair ensues. While people vary in how they deal with grief, the syndrome of acute grief is remarkably uniform. Most people have periods of crying and sadness. Expect physiological disturbances like being unable to eat or sleep or restlessly pacing and sighing. You probably will engage in what is termed searching behavior where you search for your loved one's face on passing buses and cars. You also may have auditory and visual hallucinations in which you are certain you briefly see your loved one or are convinced you hear his or her voice or hear the car pull in the garage at the usual time. These thoughts are caused by psychological cues and will decrease in time. They do not mean that you are going crazy; they are a normal part of the grieving process.

You also may find comfort in an object that links you to your loved one. You may wear a piece of his or her clothing or sleep in your loved one's bathrobe. This, too, is normal grieving behavior, and the need for the linking object will lessen over time.

Recommended Grieving Behaviors

The four major tasks of mourning were identified over 50 years ago. They are (1) to accept the reality of the loss; (2) to experience the pain of the grief; (3) to adjust to a changed environment in which your loved one is missing; and (4) to emotionally relocate the loss in your life and move forward.

Grief counselors recommend certain behaviors for the period immediately following the death of a loved one.

BE GENTLE WITH YOURSELF – The experience of caring for a loved one over an extended period of time and witnessing their suffering and death is extremely difficult and draining. It will take time for you to recover physically and even longer for you to recover emotionally.

DO NOT EXPECT TOO MUCH OF YOURSELF or of other family members who are grieving. Defer making important family and personal decisions, such as moving to a different location or making major purchases for several months or even a year or more.

RECOGNIZE THAT GRIEF CANNOT BE POSTPONED – It has to reach expression in some way. If you cannot express your grief openly, it will be transformed to another emotion such as displaced anger, guilt, anxiety, or physiological symptoms.

ALLOW VARIATION IN GRIEVING PATTERNS among family members. Grief, like hope, is individualistic, and each person has to do it in his or her own way.

Hiding Grief

American society is uncomfortable with grief. We prefer that individuals hide their feelings and emotions. Many persons reach adulthood without having experienced a loss by death. As a result, most people do not know what to say when someone dies, and they are unfamiliar with the normal grieving process. Added to this is the organizational approach to grief which often allows an employee less than a week to bury a loved one and mourn the loss.

Denial of the significance of the loss makes grief harder. Bereaved persons are forced to hide their grief in public and act as though they have completed their grieving process and are "back to normal." This inability to be open about grief may extend the grief process.

Many people ask how long grief lasts. Others ask if it ever ends. The answer is somewhere in between. Death ends a life; it does not end a relationship. However, after the death that relationship must change. Researchers estimate that it takes at least one year to work through the grief process (note they do not use terms like "finish grieving" or "resolve the grief" or "get over the loss"). Two to three years may be a more realistic estimate. A full year is considered a minimum because it takes a year to experience all of the anniversary dates with the loved one missing for the first time. These dates include holidays, birthdays, wedding, and other anniversaries, and finally, the anniversary of the date of the death. You probably will have more difficulty during these periods, and you should recognize that this is normal.

You will be able to tell that your acute grieving is coming to an end when you can think about your loved one without feelings of intense pain. One woman was able to describe eloquently the pain she felt when her daughter died. She said that at first it felt like total body pain. Everything about her hurt. Eventually, it did not hurt quite so much, and after a longer time, she could think about her daughter without being consumed by painful feelings. She said that now (several years after the loss) she keeps the pain in a special place in her heart. It is always with her; it just does not hurt so much anymore.

Some people who lose loved ones will benefit from grief counseling. Ask your doctor or other members of the health-care team if they can recommend a counselor who specializes in helping people deal with grief; or call your local hospice and see what services they have to offer. Almost all hospices provide mutual support groups for persons who have lost loved ones, and you may find that a support group is right for you.

Perhaps the most important thing others can do to help friends or loved ones who are experiencing grief is to recognize their right to express their grief and to encourage them to verbalize their feelings and sadness. Through expression comes healing.

Cancer is a family matter. When a loved one has cancer, the entire family is affected, and the family should be viewed by health-care professionals as the unit of care. Cancer causes a sequence of crisis situations for the cancer survivor and the family during the illness experience, and each crisis must be managed. However, as you learn more about the disease process and cancer treatments, and as you gain familiarity with the health-care team and the treatment setting, the impact of subsequent cancer-related crises should decrease. Armed with experience and information, you and your family will be more equipped to handle subsequent problems and to limit the impact of the crisis.

If your family has inadequate communication, seek assistance from

RIGHTS OF THE BEREAVED

The bereaved have a right to expect optimal and considerate care for their dying loved one.

The bereaved have the right to a compassionate pronouncement of the death and to respectful and professional care of the body of their loved one.

The bereaved have the right to view the body and to grieve at the bedside immediately following the death, if this is their wish.

The bereaved have the right to expect adequate and respectful professional care (both physical and emotional) for themselves at the time of their loved one's death.

The bereaved have a right (except when contraindicated legally) not to consent to an autopsy and not to be coerced into consenting to an autopsy, regardless of how interesting or baffling the patient's disease.

The bereaved have the right to an adequate explanation of the cause of their loved one's death and to answers regarding the illness, treatment procedures, and treatment failures.

The bereaved have the right to choose the type of funeral service most consistent with their wishes and financial means and not to be coerced into those of which they are not supportive.

The bereaved have the right not to be exploited for financial gain or for education or research purposes.

The bereaved have a right to observe religious and social mourning ritual according to their wishes and customs.

The bereaved have a right to express openly their grief regardless of the cause of the loved one's death, suicide and violent death included.

The bereaved have a right to expect health professionals to understand the process and characteristics of grief.

The bereaved have a right to education regarding coping with the process of grief.

The bereaved have a right to professional and lay bereavement support including assistance with insurance, medical bills, and legal concerns.

Elizabeth J. Clark. "Bereaved Persons Have Rights That Should be Respected." In A. Kutscher, et al., (eds.), Principles of Thanatology. *New York: NY: Columbia University Press (1987).*

your health-care team, attend mutual support groups or community programs specific to cancer-related problem-solving, or seek individual or family counseling. It is important for your family to maintain a future positive outlook. To do so, you will need to understand how your family hopes and then maximize that hope.

Individuals who are under constant and chronic stress can experience burnout. So, too, can families reach a stage of emotional and physical exhaustion. You need to share the burden of caregiving and be alert to signs and symptoms that signal family burnout. With adequate support, family burnout is usually temporary and reversible.

While we now have excellent treatments for most cancers, and over fifty percent of persons with cancer will be cured, others will die from their disease. Terminal illness is one of the most difficult crises faced by the family system. Yet, with open communication and through caring and support, even this crisis can be dealt with in a positive way. Family members can acquire a new perception and appreciation of each other. They can be enriched by the gifts of love they give and receive during their final days together.

Chapter Seven

Reaching Out: The Power of Peer Support

by Catherine Logan-Carrillo

"NCCS is where I meet my peers–those who are struggling to sustain local grassroots programs. And it is those peers who remind me how vital my community-based work really is."

Catherine Logan-Carrillo

A CANCER *survivor's* ALMANAC

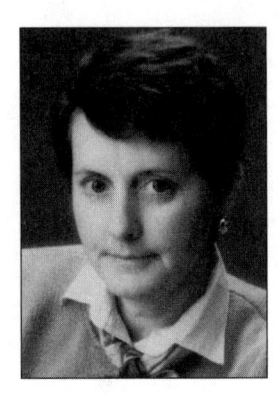

CATHERINE LOGAN-CARRILLO, a 17-year cancer survivor, was one of the initial organizers and a cofounder of the National Coalition for Cancer Survivorship. She served as its first executive director from 1986 to 1991, managing the organization through its formative years as it became a leader in the national cancer survivorship movement.

Ms. Logan-Carrillo is also the founder of People Living Through Cancer, Inc. in Albuquerque, New Mexico. She has facilitated thousands of support group sessions, written for and edited the *Living Through Cancer Journal,* and has been instrumental in the development of all of the organization's programs.

Something very special happens when people facing cancer turn to one another for help. The resulting peer support can have a profound impact on how they feel about themselves and on how well they manage their lives after cancer.

Peer support can take many forms: support groups, one-to-one consultations, telephone hot lines, newsletters, and even Internet exchanges by computer. It also can be found at week-long retreats with intimate groups and in larger groups, such as annual survivors' day celebrations, educational workshops, and conferences.

Whatever its form, whether used by cancer survivors or their loved ones, peer support is empowering. Reaching out for help from your peers is an act of faith in people just like you and in your own ability to deal effectively with the crisis of cancer.

Cancer support networks exist for you—to be joined, organized, and cultivated. Their members are eager to share their experiences with you and to learn what they can from you. This chapter will help you make the most of this valuable resource.

PEER SUPPORT IN THE CANCER SURVIVORSHIP MOVEMENT: A BRIEF HISTORY

Cancer is only one of many life situations that motivate people to create peer-support networks and mutual-aid groups. Historically, those who have shared political, social, medical, and other mutual concerns have worked together to create resources to meet their needs. Alcoholics Anonymous is one of the oldest and best known of these peer-support networks.

The United Ostomy Association is another peer-support organization with a long and effective history. In 1949, five people who had ostomies (surgery to construct an artificial opening in response to colon cancer and other illnesses) met in Philadelphia to share their experiences and knowledge. In 1975, the organization joined the International Ostomy Association, which now has chapters in 40 countries. By 1996, the United Ostomy Association had 36,000 members and 539 chapters in the United States alone.

Although many of the United Ostomy Association members have had cancer, the organization's primary focus is on the common experience of having an ostomy. Other peer-support organizations concentrating exclusively on cancer issues began to evolve in the early 1970s. Two of the oldest organizations are Make Today Count and the Candlelighters Childhood Cancer Foundation.

Make Today Count was founded by Orville Kelly in 1974 to address the emotional needs of people with cancer. It eventually expanded to address the needs of those with other life-threatening illnesses. It flourished in the late 1970s and early 1980s with more than 400 local chapters, providing practical information and emotional support to survivors and their families. Although Make Today Count no longer has a national office, over 100 local Make Today Count organizations are still active.

In 1970, parents of children who had cancer founded the Candlelighters Childhood Cancer Foundation to address the needs of their families. By 1996, Candlelighters had become an international organization with over 400 local chapters. On a local level, Candlelighters chapters provide opportunities for sharing experiences and information about the needs of children with cancer and their families. On a national level, the organization serves as a clearinghouse for information on childhood cancer, develops resources to address members' concerns, and advocates for adequate funding for childhood cancer research and treatment and for the legal rights of childhood cancer survivors. Candlelighters also has three newsletters, the *Candlelighters Quarterly* for parents, the *Candlelighters Youth Newsletter* for children who have cancer, and *The Phoenix* for adult survivors of childhood cancers.

Cancer-related peer-support programs provide support by cancer survivors and their families for survivors and their families. However, many organizations that offer education and support programs have both a professional and a peer-support component. The largest of these organizations is the American Cancer Society, founded in 1945.

In addition to its other activities, such as funding cancer research and promoting cancer prevention and early detection, the American Cancer Society distributes information about cancer to the public and to cancer survivors and their families. One of its most popular educational programs is I Can Cope, an eight-session educational program for newly diagnosed survivors and family members. The program was founded in 1977 at North Memorial Hospital in Minneapolis by two oncology nurses, Judi Johnson and Pat Norby.

Over the years the American Cancer Society has developed many peer-support programs, such as Reach to Recovery and CanSurmount. Reach to Recovery was started in 1952 by Terese Lasser, a breast cancer survivor from New York. The program provides a first step to rehabilitation through peer support to women who have had breast cancer surgery and to their families. Through referral,

Reach to Recovery offers hospital or home visits by veteran breast cancer survivors, literature about breast surgery, and a temporary breast form.

CanSurmount was founded in 1974 by a Denver oncologist, Paul K. Hamilton, MD, and one of his patients, Lynn Ringer. CanSurmount helps survivors deal with the emotional impact of cancer through one-on-one, veteran-to-newcomer support. Most often a CanSurmount coordinator within a hospital setting arranges for a trained volunteer to visit someone who has just undergone cancer surgery.

THE EMERGENCE OF THE NATIONAL COALITION FOR CANCER SURVIVORSHIP – Although cancer survivors always have exchanged mutual aid, the peer-support movement began to gather momentum in the early 1980s. In 1986, the National Coalition for Cancer Survivorship (NCCS) was started to coordinate and encourage communication among developing survivor-driven activities, most notably, among the growing number of peer-support programs. When survivors and their groups across the country began to communicate, it became clear that a grass-roots social movement was evolving. NCCS was the first to identify this "survivorship movement" and to develop a national survivorship agenda.

Initially working out of the offices of People Living Through Cancer, an Albuquerque peer-support organization, the NCCS was the first successful attempt at providing a national organization to represent the concerns of all cancer survivors, their loved ones, and their organizations. In 1991, the NCCS moved its office to Washington, DC, where it has become the primary organization advocating on behalf of cancer survivorship.

In the early 1990s, cancer survivors in organizations like the NCCS and the National Breast Cancer Coalition became the cutting edge of a new wave of cancer survivor organizations with a primary mission of advocacy. These organizations are raising the visibility of cancer issues and demanding that more of the nation's resources be dedicated to eradicating the disease.

THE VALUE OF PEER SUPPORT

It may not seem like it now, but there are worse things than having cancer, and facing cancer alone is definitely one of them. That is why one of the most important things you can do for yourself when going through a cancer experience is to find people who will give you adequate emotional support. Support can come from many different places, but perhaps the most abundant and most natural source is the vast population of cancer survivors and their loved ones.

> **SHARING THE JOURNEY**
>
> Interdependence
> not independence
> is the reality of this world.
> I have a shared destiny
> touching the lives of countless others
> as ripples in a pond
> fan out in even widening circles.
> We live in
> one another's company.
> Together we can diffuse the pain
> and multiply the
> joy
> of being.
>
> *Brenda Neal © 1985*
> *People Living Through Cancer Journal*

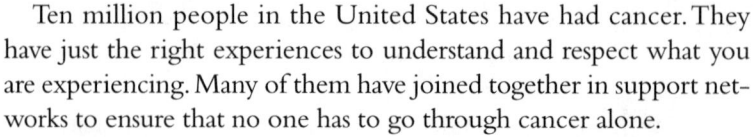

Ten million people in the United States have had cancer. They have just the right experiences to understand and respect what you are experiencing. Many of them have joined together in support networks to ensure that no one has to go through cancer alone.

Even survivors with very supportive friends and families often feel they need more—they want to talk with someone who knows what they are experiencing. For many, relationships with family members and friends become strained and uncomfortable after a cancer diagnosis. At the very time the need for support increases, old support systems often are unable to respond adequately.

People facing cancer seek out peer support for different reasons. Most often, they simply want to feel better—to ease emotional distress caused by the diagnosis. Support networks offer inspiration from the courage of others as well as increased motivation to fight for your life. They offer role models who can help you accept a changed life, a new identity, and an uncertain future. Networks can provide a venue to gain control of some aspects of your life again and a place to vent and validate feelings. They offer hope—sometimes hope for cure or improved health, sometimes hope for a good life, and sometimes hope for a good death.

Usually people know what to expect from peer support, but some people are looking for absolute optimism about regaining health and control over the course of the disease. They are likely to be disappointed because people in support networks not only inspire and motivate each other, but they face difficult issues together and share one another's pain and disappointment.

Survivors and their family members also reach out to peers for information or for help in making difficult decisions. Cancer veterans have a wealth of knowledge that can help others find their own path through the cancer experience.

THE VALUE OF SHARING YOUR STORY – Telling your story and listening to others' stories can be the foundation for both personal healing and building a sense of community. Sharing your story is healing because it breaks through isolation and allows you to express your feelings to others. Hearing others' stories connects your life to theirs and helps you sort out which of your responses are natural reactions to the stresses of dealing with cancer and which might be signs of special problems deserving professional attention.

Sharing stories also builds a foundation for advocacy. It helps survivors understand survivorship in the broader sense—beyond just their own unique experience. It helps identify the kinds of problems that survivors and family members face, and it prepares them to work with others for necessary changes.

PEER SUPPORT ISSUES – Many issues surface after a cancer diagnosis, and peer support groups can help individuals work through those issues. Examples of the topics discussed include the following.

- Emotional, social, spiritual, and financial issues including—
  feelings of fear, depression, and anger;
  isolation;
  reclaiming a sense of control over your life;
  strained relationships with family and friends;
  loss, grief, and facing the possibility of death;
  changing values and beliefs;
  financial, insurance, and employment issues.

- Treatment issues such as—
  side effects: immediate, long-term and delayed;
  effective use of medical resources;
  relationships with health-care providers;
  pain management;
  complementary and alternative therapies.

- Wellness issues including—
  changes in physical appearance and body image;
  sexuality;
  diet and nutrition;
  long-term health maintenance.

HOW PEER SUPPORT DIFFERS FROM PROFESSIONAL COUNSELING

Peer support is a process of sharing feelings and practical information learned through personal experiences—sharing between "peers" who have similar life experiences. Professional counseling promotes personal exploration and change and is guided by a counselor or therapist who has been trained formally to help others. The chart on page 144 summarizes these two approaches in a group setting.

Many cancer survivors and family members benefit from both kinds of help and find that peer support and professional counseling are complementary. Support group members commonly encourage each other to get professional help. Counselors and therapists often recommend peer-support groups.

Sometimes peer support is mistakenly perceived as a stop-gap measure, implemented because professional counseling is not available. But peer support is not a substitute for professional counseling; it has a distinct value of its own. It builds a sense of community and empowers people through creating social structures that provide opportunities to improve their own survivorship and to help others.

How Peer-Support Groups Differ from Professional Counseling and Therapy Groups

This chart describes some of the basic attributes of peer-support and therapy groups. The groups do not always fall precisely under either type.

Peer-Support Groups	Professional Counseling Groups
Leader	
• contributes to the group from personal experience	• has special expertise founded on professional, theoretical schooling
• balances flow and content of exchanges; keeps the group safe	• directs flow and content of exchanges; keeps the group safe
• comes from within the group, on the same path as other members but may be further along	• usually not from group; trained to maintain professional distance
• nonprofit orientation	• usually has a fee-for-services agreement with group
Purpose	
• helps members manage their lives, cope with emotional and other issues, and educate themselves	• helps members with personal exploration and with change of basic perceptions and behaviors
• social support is a means and end; therapeutic results are by-product	• therapy is purpose; social support is by-product
Process	
• self-governed: goals and format established by group	• group goals and format are set by leader before group meets
• members accept responsibility for themselves; no expectation of others	• leader guides and encourages members to set personal goals and to move toward those goals
• usually ongoing, open-ended	• usually time-limited
• new members may be added at each meeting	• restrictions on adding new members after group begins

THE ROLE OF HEALTH CARE PROVIDERS IN PEER-SUPPORT ORGANIZATIONS

Health care providers have always been valuable advocates, contributors, and supporters of peer-support groups. But some peer groups have a philosophy that endorses peer leadership only. Health care providers need to be sensitive to these views; they might ask how a group views the role of professionals when providers offer their assistance, since the group's identity will change if peers lose ownership.

Maintaining the balance between peer ownership and taking advantage of valuable services offered by professionals is difficult. "Professionalization" of peer networks deserves careful thought both by the peer network leaders and by the health care providers since peer-support networks look to professionals for help in a variety of ways, including direct referrals, consultation, technical assistance, and help with educational programs. Professionals can also help peer groups by advocating on their behalf to other health-care providers.

PEER-LED SUPPORT GROUPS VS. PROFESSIONALLY-LED GROUPS

> I want to be my own expert. Having a health-care provider as the group leader implies that they are an expert and, somehow, that reduces my own expertise. For me, it changes the group process into fixing something that is wrong, instead of learning to live through this difficult life experience with others who share the experience.
> Julie Reichert, breast cancer survivor,
> Albuquerque, NM

Peer-support groups have two models: (1) "pure" peer-support groups, where everyone in the group, including the leader, shares the cancer experience, and (2) peer-support groups led by health-care providers—such as social workers, nurses, counselors, psychologists and psychiatrists. Professionally led peer-support groups are not therapy groups and more closely resemble the description of peer groups on the left side of the chart on page 144. In these groups, the leader takes on the role of facilitating the peer-support process between group members.

Some survivors prefer "pure" peer-support groups that are led by others who share the cancer experience. They believe groups that are peer-led function differently from groups that are led by health-care providers who have not had a personal or family cancer experience. One reason may be because the level of intimacy in a group is affected by whether everyone in the group, including the leader, shares personal feelings and experiences.

Although professional therapists and counselors have a helpful theoretical understanding of healing during and after a cancer experience, peer leaders can be living examples—proof that one can heal and feel whole again. Peer leaders are valuable models showing successful resolution to the search for meaning behind the cancer experience.

Sometimes people dealing with cancer prefer to join support groups with peer facilitators as evidence of their confidence that they can handle their own lives. Some feel that it is more comfortable and more empowering to belong to a group without the guidance and oversight of an outside expert. After medical experiences in which they have felt a significant loss of control of their lives—and with little choice but dependence on outside experts—they want to reclaim control and see peer support as a tool for doing just that.

At times, survivors and family members need to express anger and frustration with health-care providers and the health-care system. The expression of these feelings may be inhibited by the presence of a health-care provider, although a skilled and sensitive professional may be fully aware of the deficiencies in the system and may be sympathetic toward this kind of anger and frustration.

On balance, both peer-led and professionally led groups have their merit. One way to benefit from the best of both peer support and professional expertise is to have the group led by a health-care professional who also has a personal cancer history.

Choosing the Right Peer-Support Program

You are the only one who knows what is best for you. Different kinds of peer support are appropriate for different people, or even for one person at different times in his or her survivorship. Do some careful thinking and researching before you decide when and where to go for peer support. Your decisions should be based on your own values and beliefs, as well as on your physical and financial situation. Think about your experience with giving and receiving support in previous difficult situations. Trust what your experience tells you about your own style of seeking help; at the same time, do not be afraid to try something new.

If available, you may want to look for a group that focuses on your particular kind of cancer, especially if you have a more common diagnosis like breast cancer or prostate cancer; or, you might decide to attend a group that includes people with all kinds of cancer, one that includes survivors and family members, or perhaps a specialty group, like one for long-term survivors or young adults.

Consider your own personal needs over everything else. Are you looking for emotional support to relieve feelings of isolation and fear, or are you hoping to find information and strategies for dealing with the medical system and the decision-making process? Are you looking for the inspiration of meeting others in your situation who are coping well? Whatever your reasons for seeking support, remember that your needs may change, and allow yourself to respond to that change.

No single source will have information about all of the peer-support resources available to you. For this reason, it is probably wise to inquire about support resources from more than one of the following places:
- Social service departments or discharge planners at local hospitals or treatment centers;
- National organizations like
  NCCS at (301) 650-8868 (Maryland)
  Cancer Care, Inc. at (800) 813-HOPE
  The National Alliance of Breast Cancer Organizations at (212) 719-015 (New York)
  Us Too International (for prostate cancer groups) at (800) 808-7866 (Illinois)
  Candlelighters Childhood Cancer Foundation at (800) 366-2223 (Washington, DC);
- Cancer Information Service of the National Cancer Institute at (800) 4-CANCER;
- American Cancer Society at (800) 227-2345;
- State self-help clearing houses;
- Yellow pages of the telephone directory under "social service organizations" or "support groups;" or the white pages under "cancer;"
- Psychologists, counselors, social workers, or clergy;
- Newspaper listings of support groups and help-lines;
- Reference libraries;
- Public health offices and mental health associations.

If you decide to try a peer-support group, call ahead, if possible, to talk with the group's contact person. You can also ask to speak with group members and ask for print material with a description or history of the group. Some groups list only a time and location for meetings, in which case you will have to save questions until you meet someone from the group.

You may want to ask the group's contact person the following questions:
- How many people attend the group's meeting and what is the make up of the group (survivors, family members, age range, kind and stage of cancer diagnoses, etc.)?
- How long is each meeting?

- Is the group limited to a certain frequency or number of meetings?
- Does the group have an established core of members who generally attend meetings?
- How long has the group been meeting?
- Who leads the group sessions and what is his or her experience or training?
- Do group leaders have a personal experience with cancer?
- What is the format of the group meetings?
- Is the primary focus sharing feelings and experiences or sharing information?
- Are there any group guidelines or ground rules?
- What kinds of subjects are discussed? Are there any subjects that are off-limits?
- Are group members asked to share a particular philosophy or approach to cancer?

These questions have no right or wrong answers. But the responses should give you a feeling for whether the group is for you and whether its leaders are thoughtful about providing a quality group that is responsive to group members' needs.

Have You Found the Right Group?

When you first try out a cancer support group, look for the following:
- The atmosphere is welcoming to newcomers.
- The group's process encourages constructive solutions and does not dwell only on problems.
- Group members participate actively in supporting each other and do not look to the group leader as the expert.
- The group has a sense of shared ownership; one or two members do not dominate the group process.

Remember, groups have different personalities. Not everyone is a good match for every group, no matter how well a group functions. Does the group feel comfortable to you? Trust you own instincts, but give a new group a second and third try, unless you are absolutely sure it is not for you. One or two meetings may not be enough to get the feel of a group. If you decide the group is not for you, check out another group, if possible. It may be a better fit. When you find the right group, it should feel a little like coming home.

Guiding Principles of Effective Peer-Support Groups

At the present time, no universally accepted standards guide the quality of peer-support or mutual-aid groups, so the quality varies

greatly. Many cancer veterans, however, look for several simple guiding principles in peer-support groups as well as in other peer-support programs:
- *All participants should be asked to give nonjudgmental support* and to respect others' rights to make their own decisions based on their own values and lifestyles. This principle is reflected in acceptance of different approaches to dealing with cancer and an expectation and appreciation of diversity among those in the support group or network.
- *All information shared will be kept confidential.* Confidentiality enhances honesty and openness, the most basic requirements for adequate support.

These two ground rules should be discussed as part of orienting new members to groups, and the rules should be repeated to all group members on a regular basis.

Rewards of Giving Back to Your Support Group

It takes time and energy to sustain a group. When you are ready, consider giving back to the group with your time, energy, and financial contributions. Be willing to help sustain and improve the group as needed so it will be around for others.

Perhaps the most important way to give back is to become part of the core of people who attend regularly. This core is vital to the group's effectiveness, and core members develop deep and powerful friendships with one another. The longer you stay, the greater will be your understanding of the cancer experience.

When a group has developed a mature core of cancer veterans, it is in a unique position to be of enormous help to group members, even those in great distress. Few things in life can equal being part of this kind of human experience.

Creating Your Own Peer-Support Group

In your search for peer support, you may find that none exists in your community, or that existing ones do not meet your needs. As a result, you may consider creating your own.

LOOK BEFORE YOU LEAP – Before creating a new organization, your first task is to look at what already exists. Creating a survivorship program can be both energizing and exhausting. To both begin and sustain an organization demands personal energy as well as financial resources. These are limited commodities in the cancer community, and they need to be conserved. Since a new group may even undermine existing groups by competing for group members and resources, consider working within an existing network rather than creating a new one. Making the decision to start a new group should be done only if you are sure your new program does not duplicate existing services.

In order to determine whether a new resource is truly needed, make a thorough search of the peer-support resources in your community. Then determine what needs, if any, they do not address, and what services, if any, they do not provide. Does your community need a telephone hot line, a support group, a newsletter, a hospital visitation program, or some other service? Are only certain populations within the cancer community served by existing programs? If you are a 65-year old man with prostate cancer, support groups that cater to young adults or women with breast cancer may be of little value to you.

Other organizations can serve as models, but as the creator, you will have to determine what will work for you and your particular community. The requirements for a program in a large city where people live close together, have access to transportation, and may have a defensive mistrust of strangers, will be different from the requirements for a new organization in a rural area, where transportation problems are balanced by a strong sense of community trust.

Before you begin the difficult task of founding a new organization,

---

WEAVING STORIES INTO THE FABRIC OF SURVIVORSHIP

In a support group, one story after another describes the very personal experiences of survivors and family members—the feelings and problems, the hopes and disappointments. Each person's unique cancer story tells of the profound life-changing impact of cancer. At first, group members know cancer only through their own experiences. Although they know it intimately, their understanding is limited. Often these experiences are so all-consuming that they isolate survivors from the people around them.

As the stories are shared, common themes and common bonds evolve and begin to weave the stories together. Like individual threads stretched side by side in a loom, the stories are woven into a strong fabric. The same powerful experiences that once isolated survivors now link them to others, with whom they share their experiences. Their stories become part of the fabric of survivorship, and the survivors gain strength from one another.

The story tellers also have gained a much broader understanding of the cancer experience, an understanding that allows group members to heal and help each other, as well as build a foundation for advocacy.

clearly define the concerns your group will address and be sure that others share those concerns. In addition, your group must be accessible to prospective members. Find the best way to link people to your resource. Many cancer survivors who want to participate in your group may be too busy or too ill to do so. Traditional programs like group meetings can be adapted and expanded to accommodate survivors who are homebound, have mental or physical disabilities, are isolated in rural communities, or have limited financial means.

If you do not have the resources to start a group on your own, then look to other survivors, supportive professionals, and hospitals or other organizations to work with you as a team.

STEPS IN ORGANIZING A PEER-SUPPORT GROUP — What follows are suggestions that have worked for a variety of peer-support groups and might be used as general guidelines. Adapt them as necessary to fit the circumstances in your community.

Getting started — Before you consider starting a cancer support organization, examine the history of peer-support organizations. Even more important than library research, however, is field research. If possible, visit other programs, especially those that serve cancer survivors and their families. Note what you like and dislike, how the group members interact, and how the structure of the group addresses—or fails to address—its goals.

If you are interested in becoming a chapter or an affiliate of an existing organization, first make sure that a similar group does not already have a chapter serving your community. Contact the organization to learn whether it has specific guidelines you must follow. If you want to form an independent group, you may still wish to model your organization on a successful peer-support organization.

Identify a core working group of people who are interested in working with you — To help ensure the success of your group and prevent burnout, it is crucial to develop a "core working group" that includes a few people with commitment to the program. Working-group members can be survivors, family members, oncology professionals, and experienced community organizers. Look for individuals who have strengths that complement yours and who can assist in everything from designing the organizational structure to addressing envelopes.

The first meeting — The first meeting of your group will set the tone for the future. Before you determine the structure of the first meeting, the core members must decide what services you want your group to provide. A group whose purpose is to offer emotional and social support to a limited group of participants may start with an informal gathering in a member's home. If your goal is to provide education about surviving cancer, you may wish to begin with a meeting to plan a community-wide program, such as a conference on a current survivorship topic.

Tasks in planning the first meeting should be shared by working group members. They may include arranging the meeting space, preparing a presentation, and advertising the meeting to your target audience. You can attract participants by advertising in local newspapers; placing flyers at community, health, and religious institutions; speaking with survivors in other cancer programs; and encouraging local health care providers to tell their patients about your plans.

Planning for the future – At the close of the first meeting, the group should reach a consensus on whether and how to continue. Future meetings must strike a balance between focusing on the purpose of the group (for example, emotional support) and tending to the business of developing the structure of the organization that will sustain the program. Participants should be invited to contribute time or resources to the group.

In planning the future of your group, you should resolve the following questions to ensure that the purpose of the group is defined clearly and that the means exist to work toward that purpose.

- What are the specific goals? Are the goals useful, or should they be changed?
- Who may be a member of your group? Anyone? Only cancer survivors and their families? Only survivors of a specific type of cancer?
- When, where, and how often will you meet?
- How will you publicize the group?
- Will group discussions be facilitated by a cancer survivor, a health-care provider, or both?
- What will be the focus of your first activities? Support group meetings? A newsletter? A public education program? An editorial in the local newspaper?
- How will you handle the business aspects of your group? Will you charge a membership fee? Will you elect officers? Will you adopt bylaws? Will you seek federal tax-exempt status so that donors can deduct their financial contributions from their income taxes and so that group purchases will not be subject to a sales tax? How will you finance the group's activities?

Future troubleshooting – Expect the group to experience a natural flux in attendance and enthusiasm. New problems and issues will arise. What do you do if members of the group disagree about its purpose? How do you handle a member who dominates the discussion? Where do you go if you lose your meeting space? What do you do if a fundraiser is a flop? Be prepared to respond to these and other problems in a way that supports the goals and unity of the group.

On a regular schedule, evaluate the effectiveness of your group. Have you accomplished your initial goals? Have your goals changed? Are your services still needed? Does the group need midcourse redirection? Are the members of the core group working together, or is all the work falling on the shoulders of one or two people? It may take longer than you plan for the program to attract members on a consistent basis. Give your new group sufficient time to develop, grow, and become known in your community. Three things will help you maintain enough members for your group:
- Consistent, long-term, and wide-spread promotions of the group to sustain a large pool of new members;
- Careful cultivation and support of group members to encourage attendance; and
- Skillfully led group meetings.

For open-ended, long-term groups, two kinds of members need to be developed:
- A core of members (including the group leader) who attend regularly and who have been in the group long enough to form close and caring relationships; and
- New group members who are in more immediate need of the support that the group is formed to provide.

Groups with these two kinds of members can create a dynamic group process that keeps participants interested and feeling fulfilled with a potential to make a very real difference in group members' lives.

Peer-support programs are rather complex creatures and take skill, experience, and savvy to sustain and to develop consistent quality. But they are worth everything it takes, and they can make a tremendous difference in the lives of those who lead and those who participate.

Resources to Help You Build and Sustain Your Group

You are not alone in your effort to create a survivorship organization. The first place to turn for help is in your own backyard. Medical centers, churches, synagogues, community centers, and private businesses may provide space and advisers. Ask your oncologist, social worker, or nurse to help. In addition to providing meeting space, your community may be a source of enough donated materials and personal assistance to get you started. An instant-print company may donate flyers that advertise your meetings or a business supply company may give you office equipment. A social worker or an accountant may offer advice for free or at a discount.

NCCS CAN HELP – The National Coalition for Cancer Survivorship offers technical assistance to individuals who want to start a local cancer support organization. The NCCS draws from its experience as a bridge between peer leaders and health care providers to provide a balanced list of suggestions to new organizations.

The NCCS helps new groups in four ways. First, it helps leaders of new groups explore successful models represented by other cancer organizations. Second, it links new and established groups with other local, regional, or national groups that have similar survivorship programs. Third, it sponsors conferences at which leaders of community groups can discuss their programs and learn from people with years of experience. And, fourth, the NCCS collects and disseminates information on organizing survivor networks at the community level.

Other important resources include self-help clearinghouses—nonprofit organizations that help callers locate mutual-aid organizations and provide assistance to peer-support networks. They sponsor training, conferences, newsletters, speakers, and consultation on developing and maintaining groups, development of resource materials, assistance with coalition building, and outreach efforts with professionals and the media. Make sure your group is listed with your regional self-help clearinghouse so they can refer survivors to your programs.

The American Self-help Clearinghouse has some of the best available material on managing support groups, including—

- Guidelines for starting groups and a list of self-help clearinghouses nation-wide (free if you send a self-addressed stamped envelope), and
- *The Self-Help Source Book,* which has lists of all kinds of national peer-support groups and detailed "how-to" materials with lots of practical help for the development and management of support groups. The book is available for $9.00, postage paid from
    American Self-Help Clearinghouse
    Northwest Covenant Medical Center
    Denville, NJ 07834-2995
    (201) 625-7107

GETTING DOWN TO BUSINESS – One of the most difficult tasks in creating a new organization is managing the business aspects. Should you obtain tax-exempt status? How should you raise funds? Should

---

for more information
contact

AMERICAN SELF-HELP CLEARINGHOUSE

Northwest Covenant Medical Center
Denville, NJ
07834-2995

201/625-7107

Self-Help Source Book

you rent an office or work out of your home? When should you risk replacing that old typewriter with a computer? Should you have an all-volunteer or a paid staff? The Support Centers of America can help you answer these questions.

Founded in 1971, the sole mission of the Support Centers of America (SCA) is to increase the effectiveness of nonprofit organizations. The SCA provides management information, training, and consulting services. The SCA has thirteen regional offices and an international office. For a catalogue of services in your area, call (415) 974-5100, send a request by e-mail to sca@supportcenter.org, or visit the SCA web site at http://www.supportcenter.org/sca/. For information about the Support Center of America closest to your community, contact

The Support Centers of America
706 Mission Street, 5th Floor
San Francisco, CA 94104
(415) 974-5100

for more information
contact

THE SUPPORT
CENTERS OF
AMERICA

706 Mission St
5th Floor
San Francisco, CA
94104

415/974-5100

sca@Supportcenter.org
www.supportcenter.org/sca/

catalog of services in your area

PEER SUPPORT WITH A MULTI-CULTURAL FOCUS

Cancer peer-support programs are adapted easily to different cultural groups. In the early 1990s, peer support networks began to emerge in minority communities as a result of the limited success that predominantly white groups had in reaching the minority or economically disadvantaged populations. A growing number of minority survivors have established networks, including the African-American Breast Cancer Alliance of Minnesota in Minneapolis, Nueva Vida in Washington, DC, and A Gathering of Cancer Support, a program of People Living Through Cancer, serving Pueblo Indians in New Mexico.

ESTABLISHED PEER-SUPPORT ORGANIZATIONS

The cancer survivorship movement represents the diverse experiences of hundreds of peer-support organizations. Older, more established groups serve as models for newer ones. Anyone considering starting a peer-support organization can benefit from the successes and failures of these pioneers.

Some national peer-support organizations encourage the development of local chapters. Two of the most established of these organizations are Y-ME and US TOO. Both are based in the Chicago area where Y-ME's successful peer-support programs influenced both the US TOO name and the peer-support model they developed.

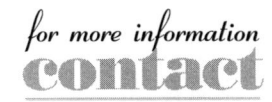

Y-ME – This organization has chapters in seventeen states, although it is probably best known for its national peer-support hot line. In 1978, Y-ME was founded by Mimi Kaplan and Ann Marcou in order to meet with other women who had been through treatment for breast cancer. Twelve women met at the YWCA in Park Forest, Illinois for Y-ME's first support group meeting. The following year, the organization established a 24-hour hot line, at first offering local help, and then expanding to a national service in 1987. The national hot line now has a Spanish-English bilingual line and a men's line for partners of women diagnosed with breast cancer. All of the more than 100 trained volunteer telephone counselors are breast cancer survivors or, in the case of the men's line, partners of breast cancer survivors. Y-ME also has educational brochures and in some states sponsors "open-door groups" that have an educational component often followed by a "rap session."

US TOO – In 1990, responding to patients' requests, a Chicago urologist, Gerald Chodak, MD, brought together a group of his prostate cancer survivors. As a result of this meeting and inspired by the Y-ME model, US TOO was founded by five prostate cancer survivors: John De Boer, Ed Kaps, John Moenck, Edward von Hoist, and Vincent Young.

Just six years later, the organization had grown to four hundred local chapters, mostly in the United States, but also in Australia, Turkey, England, Canada, and other countries. Its formal name is now

QT ALUMNI

In 1950, Mount Sinai Hospital in New York had two wards, Q and T, for patients recovering from life-saving ileostomy surgery. Although surgeons had learned how to perform ileostomies successfully, living with them was quite another matter. People living with ileostomies faced a lack of adequate appliances to collect bodily waste and to prevent its corrosive nature from injuring the skin around the ileostomy. Not content to live with appliances that leaked and fell off, patients on both wards began to share ideas about how to improve the quality of the appliances.

Once they returned to their homes, QT alumni and ostomy patients from other cities kept in touch. Driven by a need to create better appliances, some group members made models of improved appliances in their garages. They shared their discoveries with others as their ideas developed from drawing-board sketches to effective appliances.

The QT alumni were pioneer survivors who had in common practical adversity and, sometimes, social isolation. The drive to find practical solutions to mutual problems led to the first peer-support network for people with ostomies, and laid the foundation for the development of other health-related mutual-aid organizations.

US TOO International, Inc.: A Prostate Cancer Support System. Its stated mission is "to help survivors of prostate cancer and their families lead healthy and productive lives—physically, mentally, and spiritually—by offering fellowship, shared counseling, and discussions pertaining to updated medical options and a positive mental outlook." US TOO has a leadership manual, a booklet on how to start an US TOO chapter, and regional coordinators who help establish local chapters.

The following are examples of four other types of cancer support organizations: a Houston, Texas, group offering one-on-one support through cooperative efforts with local religious congregations; a comprehensive peer-support organization offering a variety of services in New Mexico; an all-volunteer support organization in Port Angeles, Washington; and a peer-support program affiliated with a treatment center in Stanford, California.

CAnCare, Houston, Texas: A Volunteer Cancer Service – CAnCare of Houston is an ecumenical volunteer cancer service rooted in the religious community. In partnership with Houston area congregations, CAnCare recruits and trains volunteers who work one-on-one with cancer survivors and their families. All volunteers have had a cancer diagnosis or have coped with cancer in a family member. After extensive training, CAnCare volunteers are matched with referrals according to cancer site, age, gender, and family situation. The service is unique in that volunteers provide one-on-one, face-to-face support and encouragement based on shared experience. The formation of a caring, nonthreatening friendship creates an atmosphere in which the survivor can be comfortable releasing and clarifying feelings, examining relationships, and struggling with faith issues that surround a cancer experience.

CAnCare was founded on the premise that God enters into the suffering of people and that human life is holy and precious and should be measured in richness and impact—not only in length. CAnCare's primary goals are (1) to improve the quality of life for cancer survivors and their families; (2) to form a network of congregations that concentrate their efforts on caring for those with cancer and helping them live as well as possible for as long as possible; and (3) to spend quality time talking with cancer survivors and their families about the cancer experience, understanding that it affects all aspects of people's lives—physical, emotional, and spiritual.

CAnCare's services include—
- one-on-one support by a trained volunteer;
- educational events and information services;

- a "Library of Hope;"
- volunteer training, annual volunteer retreat and continuing education programs;
- a newsletter, *"About Life;"*
- a speaker's bureau;
- interfaith networking of resources;
- an interdisciplinary and interagency networking of services.

CAnCare of Houston was founded in 1990 by Anne Shaw Turnage, a long-term cancer survivor. The organization began with 13 volunteers, one member congregation, and one part-time staff person. By 1996, CAnCare had trained approximately 400 volunteers who represented 102 Houston area congregations. It had four full-time and two part-time staff positions. CAnCare has a working board of directors composed of 38 members who represent the 27 member congregations.

For more information on CAnCare contact
   Anne Shaw Turnage, Director
   CAnCare of Houston
   9575 Katy Freeway, Suite 428
   Houston, TX 77024
   (713) 461-0028; fax (713) 461-0704

PEOPLE LIVING THROUGH CANCER, ALBUQUERQUE, NEW MEXICO: COMMUNITY-BASED PEER-SUPPORT ORGANIZATION – People Living Through Cancer is a peer-support organization offering comprehensive support and education services to New Mexican families facing cancer. The organization's goals are (1) to foster a community of people who have personal or family cancer histories; (2) to work together within that community to define the problems and potentials of cancer survivorship; and (3) to develop programs to address those problems and to enhance survivorship. People Living Through Cancer does not endorse any one approach to managing life after cancer, but it supports its members in making informed choices based on their own beliefs, values, and experiences.

People Living Through Cancer's peer-led and peer-support programs serve around 1,500 families each year. In 1996 they included—
- fifteen ongoing cancer support groups in Albuquerque and surrounding areas;
- one-on-one support;
- an American-Indian support and education program serving nine pueblos;

- a telephone LifeLine, providing immediate support, information, and referrals;
- the *Living Through Cancer Journal*, a quarterly publication;
- New Mexico's largest library of cancer-related materials for health-care consumers;
- an annual state-wide survivorship conference;
- training sessions on support group facilitation and organizational development, including a national training program for American Indians.

People Living Through Cancer was founded in 1983 by Catherine Logan-Carrillo, a cancer survivor. It began with a founding board of five cancer survivors and no funds, facility, or paid staff. It operated programs in members' homes and in churches. By 1996, it had grown to an organization with five full-time employees working from offices in Albuquerque and Santo Domingo, New Mexico, hundreds of volunteers, a working board of directors, and a sophisticated committee structure.

People Living Through Cancer has a strong commitment to reach underserved populations, and its leadership is culturally diverse. The organization sponsors Hispanic and African-American support networks and has programs that reach New Mexico's Pueblo Indian populations. The Pueblo Programs developed as an independent program in rural New Mexico. In 1992 its founder, Mary P. Lovato, requested that People Living Through Cancer adopt her program.

People Living Through Cancer played key roles in establishing a number of other cancer survivor organizations, including the National Coalition for Cancer Survivorship, the New Mexico Breast Cancer Coalition, and the Prostate Cancer Support Association of New Mexico. People Living Through Cancer was the physical agent and it provided a variety of other services for these organizations until they became independent nonprofit organizations on their own.

For more information on People Living Through Cancer contact
    Catherine Logan-Carrillo, Executive Director
    People Living Through Cancer
    323 Eighth Street, SW
    Albuquerque, NM 87102
    (505)242-3263

OPERATION UPLIFT, PORT ANGELES, WASHINGTON: AN ALL-VOLUNTEER PEER-SUPPORT ORGANIZATION – Operation Uplift is a nonprofit, grass-roots, community-based organization that encourages people to make informed decisions and to participate in their own health care. The organization does not promote any particular kind of cancer treatment and supports people in the decisions they make.

The organization encourages a positive approach to cancer that is based on a belief that "there is substantial evidence that attitude directly affects the body's ability to cope with disease." This positive approach includes providing support, education, and information.

Operation Uplift's program is open to those with any type of cancer and to those who care about cancer survivors. The services provided include—
- peer-facilitated support meetings;
- one-on-one support through a 24-hour phone line;
- volunteer training;
- literature, including information on cancer, treatment, coping, and nutrition;
- bimonthly newsletters;
- limited financial assistance;
- community cancer education programs;
- annual free breast health clinics;
- workshops on cancer-related subjects;
- free, temporary breast prostheses and wigs, turbans, and scarves for those in chemotherapy;
- annual celebrations of life.

Operation Uplift has no paid staff. The organization is entirely volunteer-driven under the direction of a twelve-member board of directors. It was founded in 1983 by two breast cancer survivors, Denise Heassler and Donna Willits. It began as a breast cancer support organization and in 1988 expanded to serve survivors of all kinds of cancer.

For more information on Operation Uplift, contact
   Liz Zenonian, Director of Administrative Services or
   Linda Williams, Director of Patient Services
   Operation Uplift
   P.O. Box 547
   Port Angeles, WA 98362
   (360) 457-5141

STANFORD HEALTH SERVICES, STANFORD, CALIFORNIA: PEER-SUPPORT SERVICES ASSOCIATED WITH A TREATMENT CENTER - Stanford Health Services (formerly Stanford University Hospital) sponsors both peer-support and professional psychosocial services. It was one of the first treatment centers to sponsor peer-support programs for its cancer patients.

Stanford's peer-support programs include—
- support groups for those in treatment: young adults, long-term survivors and family members, and breast cancer survivors; and
- *Surviving!*, a newsletter by and for those dealing with cancer.

In addition to these peer-support programs, Stanford also provides professional services including individual social work counseling; coping-skills classes that teach cognitive and behavioral therapy including skills such as relaxation techniques, assertiveness training, and planning positive activities.

In 1980, two peer-support groups were formed, one for younger patients and one for older patients. The groups merged the following year and now meet weekly for 90-minute sessions facilitated by Pat Fobair, a clinical oncology social worker. Discussions focus on treatment issues for Hodgkin's disease (for which a majority of Stanford patients are treated) as well as for other types of cancer.

In 1983, at the request of long-term survivors who sought peer support, Ms. Fobair began a support group for follow-up patients. This group meets for three hours once a month, and its newest focus is recovery issues and "after-care" concerns, encouraging patients to search out and integrate all complementary therapies into their well-being. Both groups serve the San Francisco Bay area, as well as Stanford patients. Three times a year, Stanford also sponsors support groups for primary (early stage) breast cancer survivors.

But perhaps Stanford's best-known program is its newsletter, *Surviving!*, created by cancer survivors for the benefit of survivors and their friends and families. The publication is dedicated to the problems of treatment and long-term survival and helps patients regain a sense of control. First published in 1984, it now is distributed nationally to subscribers four times a year and is now available on the Internet.

> "Even in our first meeting we were like old acquaintances at a reunion, although we had not met before."
> —Founder of a cancer peer-support group in Pennsylvania

> "I needed to find someone immediately who knew my terror; someone I could talk with on a personal—rather than clinical—level; someone who had been there. I needed to find a survivor."
> —Janet Morrison, lymphatic-cancer survivor, *Washington Post*, March 9, 1983

For more information contact
   Pat Fobair, LCS., MPH
   Clinical Social Worker/Director of Rehabilitation Services
   Stanford Health Services
   Patient Resources Center, Room H0103
   Division of Radiation Oncology
   300 Pasteur Drive
   Stanford, CA 94305
   (415) 723-7881

THE ROLE OF PEER-SUPPORT NETWORKS IN THE CULTURE OF SURVIVORSHIP

A Mayan shaman once described culture as a blessing from our grandfathers and grandmothers—the ancient ones. Culture is passed down by tradition and through the teachings of the elders. It combines wisdom and knowledge and the tools developed by many generations. Everything from the value of honesty and compassion to learning to light a fire for warmth and even the convenience of a twist-top cap is passed down so we do not have to discover them all over again. What we must do is cultivate these gifts, add our experiences, and pass along an even richer culture to our children and grandchildren.

Survivor organizations and peer-support networks have flourished only for a few decades, but they already have begun to develop a culture of survivorship in much the same way. Wisdom and knowledge, as well as practical techniques to solve difficult problems, have been gleaned from the shared stories and experiences of thousands who lived well and thousands who have died well after a cancer diagnosis. Everything from the wisdom of living in the moment to learning how to get your medical records is passed along from veteran to rookie.

All of us who participate in peer support benefit from this culture of survivorship. We add our own experiences and pass along even more to those who come after us.

Survivor organizations and peer-support groups are the guardians of this survivorship culture—fostering it, improving it, and passing it along. You can tap into this survivorship culture through these groups, benefit from it, and add your experience to it. It is found wherever survivors and their loved ones spend many long hours together sharing their stories.

RADIATION PILOT

I fly like a figure
Drawn by Chagall –
Past the sun with arm raised
To feel the golden rays of the sun
Enter first one side of my breast
Painted and marked red like an Indian
Or Cleopatra
Then turned to a right angle
Again I cross in front of the sun
With a steady raise of hand
Saluting over my head
Like a fugitive soldier from the star system
Stealing sunrays again
As I pass by
Patching up health
With an unseen magical beam
Repairing my flying machine

– Susan Roberts

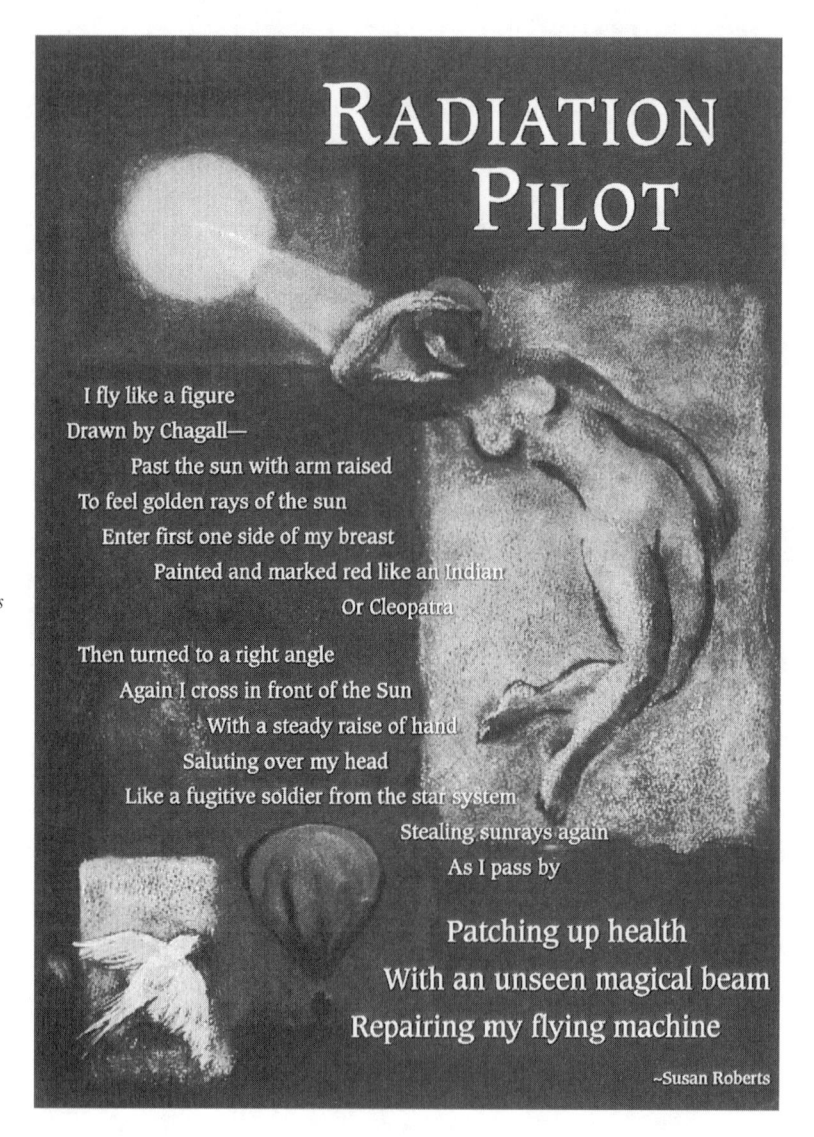

Part Three

Taking Care of Business: Insurance, Employment, Legal, and Financial Matters

Straight Talk about Insurance and Health Plans..................167

Working It Out: Your Employment Rights 205

Legal and Financial Concerns 237

Chapter Eight

Straight Talk about Insurance and Health Plans

by Kimberley Calder, MPS
and Irene C. Card

"Thanks largely to NCCS, lawmakers and other decision-makers are more sensitized to survivors' concerns…."

Kimberley Calder, MPS

"As someone who lost her mother to cancer, and who has managed the business office in an oncology practice, I understood the problems people had with insurance and knew they needed help. I am pleased to be able to work with NCCS in providing information and guidance to cancer survivors."

Irene C. Card

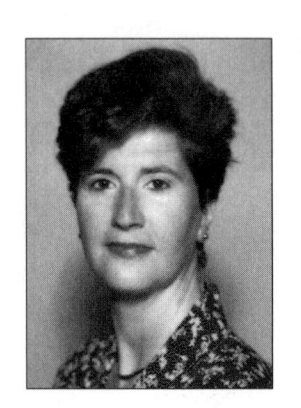

KIMBERLEY CALDER, MPS, is the director of public policy for Cancer Care, Inc., serves on the staff of Cancer Care's Public Policy Committee and as their representative and spokeswoman in all governmental and patient advocacy activities. She chairs the Steering Committee of New Yorkers for Accessible Health Coverage (NYFAHC) and is a founder of the National Breast Cancer Coalition. Ms. Calder serves on the governing boards of Empire Blue Cross Blue Shield, the NYS Cancer and AIDS Pain Initiative, and Affording Care. She is also active on the Public Affairs Committee of the American Pain Society. Ms. Calder has published and made presentations on pain management, access to investigational therapy, managed care, patient advocacy, and other topics.

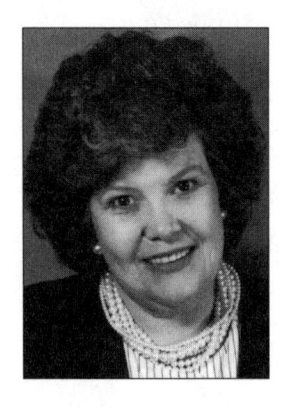

IRENE CARD is the president and founder of Medical Insurance Claims, Inc., a health claims processing company that serves individuals and physicians, and she serves as the insurance adviser to the National Coalition for Cancer Survivorship and to the Post-Treatment Resource Program of Memorial Sloan-Kettering Cancer Center. She is the author of a weekly newspaper column, "Understanding Your Health Insurance." Ms. Card is the consumer representative serving on the Board of Directors for the Oncology Nursing Certification Corporation. She is in frequent demand as a speaker on all aspects of health insurance and is recognized as an advocate for cancer survivors.

No law guarantees that all cancer survivors can buy adequate, affordable health and life insurance. A number of laws, resources, and helpful suggestions, however, can make your search for insurance more productive. This chapter is intended to guide you through your right to health, disability, and life insurance. It is organized in sections to give you descriptive information and to provide easy access to topics of special interest. Terminology you may not be familiar with is defined in the glossary at the end of the chapter. In addition to the glossary, "Resources," beginning on page 283 includes additional organizations and information, and a list of state insurance departments.

INTRODUCTION—HEALTH INSURANCE IN TRANSFORMATION

The health insurance market is in a state of flux. Some of the information presented here may become outdated quickly by new state and federal laws and trends within the commercial insurance and managed care industries.

In general, insurance is a commodity for sale to groups or individuals whom private companies determine to be a sufficient economic risk. Most companies consider cancer survivors to be a high risk. Cancer survivors often feel trapped and confused by the insurance system and can feel resentful toward a system which seems to prioritize cost controls. Obstacles to obtaining, collecting on, and keeping insurance can hinder cancer survivors' efforts to receive needed medical care. Cancer survivors have to be very savvy consumers to make the system work for them. You must arm yourself with information about your rights and options for you and your dependents.

The good news is that state and federal officials are increasingly aware of the need to reform the health insurance system so that cancer survivors and others can be assured it will include them and their health-care needs. That is why you need to investigate thoroughly the implications of any decision to purchase insurance or to change your coverage in any way. You may find it useful to consult with an advocacy or patient service organization, an attorney or financial planner, your state insurance department, or other governmental agencies.

Types of Health Insurance

The market offers many different types of health insurance: fee-for-service or indemnity policies (what most people think of as traditional, private insurance); health maintenance organizations and their variations, known collectively as managed care plans, and public health insurance programs (Medicaid and Medicare).

Fee-for-Service (or Indemnity) Policies

Fee-for-service is traditional insurance which pays providers on a fee-for-service basis. Individuals under age 65 should have a basic and a major medical insurance policy. In lieu of basic and major medical policies, you may have a comprehensive policy, which includes the benefits of basic and major medical in the same policy. Basic insurance covers your very minimum expenses, usually only the hospital bill and a very small portion of the doctor's bill when he or she sees you in the hospital. For that reason, you must have major medical to pick up where basic leaves off.

All major medical policies have a policy deductible and a lifetime benefit maximum (or cap). Generally, the higher your deductible, the lower your premiums. Once you meet your policy deductible, the major medical policy will cover bona fide (medically necessary) medical expenses according to the terms of the policy. Usually these policies pay 75 percent or 80 percent of reasonable and customary (R&C) charges (rather than a stipulated amount), and you pay the remainder. However, most major medical policies have a stop loss feature; this is the point at which out-of-pocket expenses cease and the major medical policy pays 100 percent of your claims for the remainder of the calendar year. Most major medical policies cover prescription drugs, durable medical equipment, limited mental health coverage, private duty nursing when medically necessary, and other medical expenses.

Catastrophic Insurance and Medical Savings Accounts

Catastrophic policies are like major medical policies in that they cover the costs of serious (expensive) illnesses. These policies tend to be attractive to people with no chronic health problems, but can be helpful to people with cancer in certain circumstances. For example, if you have a major medical plan with low lifetime maximum benefits, or a cap on a certain illness, such as cancer, a catastrophic policy can be helpful as a supplement to your major medical policy. Catastrophic coverage by itself, however, is inadequate coverage if you have cancer or another condition likely to result in ongoing medical expenses. Catastrophic policies are relatively inexpensive and usually have a very high deductible (usually $10,000 or more). Once you reach the deductible, even if those expenses are paid by your major medical policy, the catastrophic policy will pay 100 percent of your expenses. However, few insurance companies currently offer catastrophic policies.

The promotion of medical savings accounts (MSAs) could make catastrophic policies more common in the future. MSAs are similar to flexible spending accounts. Instead of buying a traditional insurance policy, you purchase a catastrophic policy to cover very high medical expenses, and you may be able to finance lower cost medical expenses and deductibles through a tax-free savings account dedicated to that purpose. If an MSA becomes an option for you, be sure you understand completely what will happen to the money you do not spend from your account. This concept can sound attractive (to healthy people especially), but is frowned upon by health-care economists and others. If federal legislation makes MSAs more accessible, some fear that healthier people will gravitate toward catastrophic policies combined with MSAs, leaving less healthy people in traditional health insurance. Clearly, the drain on the traditional insurance funds would result in higher premiums for those people who need insurance the most.

If you are considering buying a catastrophic policy, make sure it will apply to its deductible any expenses paid by your other health

CANCER INSURANCE

Some insurance companies market "cancer policies," policies that pay benefits only for cancer treatment. Such policies generally are sold only to people who have no previous history of cancer. Because of the many disadvantages of cancer policies, many states have banned or restricted their sale. Most insurance experts recommend buying good basic and major medical plans instead of disease-specific policies for five reasons:

1. Major medical plans usually cover the costs of cancer treatment; additional cancer policies usually duplicate other policies and are an unnecessary expense.
2. Premiums are very high for limited benefits.
3. Cancer policies often exclude coverage of complications from cancer treatment.
4. Some policy salespersons try to mislead consumers and prey on their fears about cancer.
5. Sales and administrative expenses for cancer policies tend to be much higher than other policies.

insurance plans. You want as many of your medical bills applied to the deductible as possible because the sooner your expenses reach the deductible, the sooner the catastrophic policy will pay some of your expenses. Avoid a catastrophic policy that applies only your out-of-pocket expenses to the deductible.

DISABILITY INSURANCE

Disability insurance is a type of indemnity health insurance. Disability insurance provided as an employee benefit, or as a policy you purchase yourself, will pay you a cash amount representing a percentage of your regular income should you become unable to work due to illness. However, many provisions of these policies can differ quite dramati-

ANALYZING AND EVALUATING DISABILITY INSURANCE

FEATURE	VERY GOOD	FAIR	POOR
Elimination period	1–3 mos.	6 mos.	12 mos.
Benefit period	lifetime, or to age 65	5–10 yrs.	1–2 yrs.
Noncancellable?	Yes		No
Guaranteed renewable?	Yes		No
Benefits for partial disability?	Yes	Yes, following total disability	No
Contract definition of disability	Inability to perform the major tasks of your occupation	Inability to engage in any occupation for which one is reasonably suited by education, training, and experience	Unable to engage in any occupation
Taxable income?	No	Partially	Yes
Pre-existing condition exclusion?	None	All preex. conditions excluded 6–12 months	Requires 12 months treatment-free period
A.M. Best Rating	A+, A	B+, B	C or lower

Excerpted and copied with permission of Affording Care.

cally; you will want to comparison shop. The chart on page 170 can help you compare different plans.

Managed Care Plans

Although the term "health maintenance organization" (HMO) was not coined until the 1970s, HMOs were first established in the United States before World War II to serve as both an insurer and a provider of medical care for their members. Today, many variations of the classic HMO model exist and new forms are emerging continually, although all HMOs can be characterized as various types of managed care.

In very traditional, highly structured managed care plans, members may receive health services only from the health professionals and hospitals under contract with the managed care plan. Health professionals may be employees of the plan or under contract with the plan as a member of the plan's "network." Enrollees have all of their care coordinated through their primary care provider, or "gatekeeper." The newer types of managed care arrangements (such as preferred provider organizations or independent practice associations) are typically less rigid. For example, they may not require enrollees to obtain preapproval from their primary care provider in order to see a specialist in the network.

Managed care plans can be sponsored by the government, medical schools, hospitals, employers, labor unions, consumer groups, insurance companies, or hospital medical plans. In comparison to indemnity insurance, the advantages of membership in a managed care plan include lower premiums, no claim forms for enrollees to file, coverage of "preventive" care services (such as cancer screenings), and very low copayments for visits to plan-affiliated providers. Another variation of managed care, point-of-service (POS, also called hybrid) plans allow enrollees to use all health providers or institutions in the network, but also allow you to go outside the network for services for an additional fee. In these plans, when you choose to go a provider outside the network, you first must file claim forms, wait to be reimbursed, and pay any portion of the bill not covered by the insurer. Because these plans let you choose your own provider, they are becoming increasingly popular. The premiums for these plans are higher than for traditional HMOs, however. Out-of-pocket expenses are considerably higher— higher deductibles and coinsurance.

FINDING THE RIGHT MANAGED CARE PLAN - Shopping for the best managed care plan to care for you and your family can be difficult under the best of circumstances. Managed care plans may restrict your access to the best oncology care tailored for your needs. These organizations also are notorious for their unwillingness to disclose information about their plans before a contract has been signed. Information about which health care providers and hospitals are in their networks, however, can be critically important to cancer survivors. Some states have passed laws imposing requirements on managed care organizations to make information available to the public to help prospective customers choose a plan. Before choosing a managed care plan, review the pros and cons of Medicare HMOs on page 180, and consider the following suggestions:

Look for a network where your physicians practice – If you have a choice between managed care plans, ask your doctor which managed care plans he or she has joined. Ideally, your entire health-care team has joined a managed care plan at the same time. Thus, that plan may guarantee you coverage of services provided by any member of the team at less cost than you were paying under traditional fee-for-service insurance. Ask your doctor and his or her office staff, who often have had more experience with the plan's administrators than the doctor, about their opinion of the plans.

Try to find out if the services and specialists you may need at some point during your treatment are included in the plan – These could include a comprehensive cancer center; a selection of board-certified oncologists, including at least one who is particularly experienced in treating your type of cancer; conveniently located radiation therapy services; pain specialists; and home care, mental health, and prescription drug coverage. If any of these features are not guaranteed by the plan, you may want to choose a point-of-service (POS) plan that provides coverage for services outside the network of approved providers.

Determine what requirements the plan will impose on you – Will you have to select a primary care provider who must preapprove all of your care, even during chemotherapy or radiation therapy, or will the plan allow your oncologist to act as your care coordinator during a course of treatment? Who will monitor you after your treatment?

Determine if the plan guarantees coverage of a specialist or service outside of the network if no provider in the plan can provide that service.

What percentage of your premiums actually goes toward medical care versus administrative fees? – The term for this in the insurance industry is medical loss ratio. For example, if the loss ratio is 80 percent, 20 percent of the premiums are being used to conduct the business of administering the plan, and 80 percent goes toward medical care.

Typical loss ratios in traditional insurance are in the 70 to 80 percent range, although some nonprofit insurers maintain ratios closer to 90 percent.

What specifically is excluded from the plan? – What are your rights and responsibilities if you wanted to appeal a decision by the plan that denied coverage of something your doctor recommended?

Is the plan accredited by the National Committee for Quality Assurance (NCQA)? – Arguably, NCQA accreditation does not guarantee that it is the best plan for you and your family, but it may indicate a better plan than a competing plan that does not have NCQA accreditation. The most telling piece of information about NCQA accreditation may be if the plan has been turned down for it. See page 199 for information about NCQA.

What provisions or limitations would the plan impose if you needed medical care when traveling?

HOSPITAL INDEMNITY POLICIES

A hospital indemnity policy pays a daily benefit for each 24-hour period that you are in a hospital. These policies are a source of extra cash during an illness because benefits are paid directly to you in cash for you to use as you see fit. Hospital indemnity policies are relatively inexpensive and simple; you only need to submit proof of how many days you were hospitalized to collect. A fixed amount is paid for each day you were in the hospital, regardless of the actual charges, although some policies may not pay for the first few days. Try to find a policy that pays benefits starting the first day of your hospitalization. An inpatient hospital policy is a "nice little extra" for high-risk individuals who are very likely to be hospitalized numerous times. Many of these policies have a two-year waiting period for persons with preexisting conditions. The American Association of Retired Persons (AARP) will sell hospital indemnity policies to anyone 50 years of age or older. Their policies have only a three-month waiting period for preexisting conditions.

LONG-TERM CARE INSURANCE

Limited health insurance offering coverage of home care and nursing home care is known as long-term care coverage. Long-term care insurance, however, is medically underwritten, so as a cancer survivor, you may not find an insurer that will issue you a policy. Even if you obtain a policy, the premiums will be determined by both your health risk and your age. Your state insurance department will have information about insurers that offer long-term care insurance.

MEDICARE

Medicare and Medicaid are sometimes referred to as "public health insurance." Medicare is health insurance provided by the federal government and funded through the Social Security program. Any person who meets any of the following criteria qualifies for Medicare:
- Sixty-five years or older and entitled to either Social Security, Widow's, or Railroad Retirement benefits;
- Totally disabled and, regardless of age, collecting Social Security benefits for at least 24 months;
- Legally blind; or,
- On renal dialysis regardless of age.

Medicare Part A covers the hospital bill and charges from other health-care facilities if eligibility requirements are met. Part A, which has no premium, is provided free and paid through the Social Security program (as long as you are 65 or older and have at least 40 Social Security quarters.) If you are 65 or older but have made fewer than 40 quarters' worth of contributions to Social Security, you are eligible for Medicare Part A, but you will have to pay a premium.

For example, in 1996, the inpatient deductible was $736 per benefit period. A benefit period consists of 60 days. If you are out of the hospital for more than 60 days, a new period begins and you must meet the deductible all over again. If you reenter the hospital within 60 days of your last discharge date, you do not have to meet the deductible again. After the deductible-per-benefit period, Part A will pay the hospital bill in full for the first 60 days. From the 61st to the 90th day in 1996, you paid $184 per day for inpatient days. Also in 1996, use of any of your 60 lifetime reserve days would have cost you $368 per day.

Medicare Part B covers your medical expenses, durable medical equipment, and certain other supplies. In 1996, the Part B deductible was $100 per calendar year. The premium ($42.50 per month in 1996) is deducted directly from your Social Security check.

Part B Medicare will pay for most medically necessary services rendered, but will not pay for—
- Routine annual physicals unless you have a diagnosis.
- Experimental treatment.
- Any services rendered outside of the United States, unless the individual is close to a border (Canada or Mexico) and the nearest hospital is outside of the United States.

- Prescription drugs, with one exception: chemotherapy drugs that are injected intravenously or by intravenous pump are covered by Medicare. If the doctor provides the drug, Part B will cover it. If the doctor gives the patient a prescription to get filled and the patient takes the drug to the office for injection, a copy of the actual prescription must be sent to Medicare with the pharmacy receipt.
- Syringes or insulin for diabetic patients.

Areas of coverage of special interest to those with cancer include—
- Mammography—routine mammogram screening is covered every two years. If the individual is in a high-risk group, mammography will be covered more frequently.
- Physical and occupational therapy—a fixed amount is covered per year ($900 in 1996).
- Ostomy patients—incontinence products for ostomy patients are covered if you specify on the documentation that they are for an ostomy patient. In some states, Medicare pays 100 percent of the approved amount.

Clinical laboratory procedures—such as blood tests, urinalyses, and cultures are covered. If the doctor processes the blood and receives the results, he or she must accept assignment, and Medicare will pay the doctor 100 percent of whatever it approves. Doctors who draw blood at their offices can charge $3.00 for collection and interpretation. In most cases, the doctor draws the blood and sends it to an outside laboratory. The laboratory must then bill Medicare, and Medicare pays the laboratory 100 percent of the approved amount. Many times laboratories are not notified that the patient is on Medicare. If you receive a bill from a laboratory, you should simply write your Medicare number on the bill and send it back to the laboratory.

A participating physician accepts assignment on all Medicare patients. The physician can charge only what Medicare approves. Medicare pays 80 percent of the approved amount and you are responsible for 20 percent of the approved amount. When the doctor accepts assignment, Medicare mails the check to the doctor.

A nonparticipating physician does not accept assignment. You are responsible for the entire charge. However, the doctor is not allowed to charge you more than 15 percent above that which Medicare approves for the service, although some states require you to pay a smaller percentage. Nonparticipating doctors can still choose to accept assignment on a case-by-case basis. On no-assignment claims, the Medicare payments are mailed directly to the patient and the patient is responsible for paying the doctor.

Straight Talk about Insurance and Health Plans – **CHAPTER EIGHT**

for more information
contact

DEPARTMENT OF HEALTH AND HUMAN SERVICES

Health Care Financing Administration

6325 Security Blvd.
Baltimore, MD 21207

Guide to Health Insurance for People with Medicare

TEFRA/DEFRA – TEFRA is the Tax Equity Fiscal Responsibility Act. DEFRA is the Dependent Equity Fiscal Responsibility Act.

If you continue to be employed actively 30 hours per week or more for a company with 20 or more employees, your group insurance is primary and Medicare is secondary. If you are retired and your spouse is employed 30 hours or more per week by a company with 20 or more employees, and you are covered under your spouse's health insurance policy; the group insurance plan is primary and Medicare is secondary.

If you are TEFRA/DEFRA eligible, you probably do not require Part B Medicare. Once you or your spouse decides to retire, however, the employer must write a letter to the Social Security Administration giving your Social Security number and the effective date of your retirement, stating you will no longer be covered under the group insurance plan as primary insurer. Take this letter to your Social Security office. This is very important so that you may obtain Part B (medical) benefits effective the date of your retirement. If you neglect to do this, you can purchase Part B Medicare only during the open enrollment period in January, February, or March of each calendar year, and the benefits become effective July 1 of that year. In addition, you will have to pay a 10 percent increase in premium for each year you did not have Medicare. You can save this added expense and waiting period by having your employer notify the Social Security Administration in writing of your retirement or your spouse's retirement. If this is done, your Medicare benefits are effective immediately and you are not penalized by having to pay additional premiums.

MEDICARE SUPPLEMENTAL OR "MEDIGAP" PLANS – Medigap policies are intended to supplement your Medicare coverage since even Medicare Parts A and B combined may not cover everything you need. Prescription drug coverage is particularly important to cancer survivors and is not covered by either Medicare Part A or B. When a person retires from employment, the employer's group coverage may end. Medicare supplements are needed by those who can no longer continue their major medical benefits.

Congress has standardized the Medigap market. Since 1992, insurance companies that sell Medigap policies can sell only standard Medigap plans identified as Plans A through J. Each state insurance commissioner determines which of the ten plans will be available for sale in their state. Plan A consists of the very basic benefits and Plan J the most deluxe, including up to $3,000 in prescription benefits. For complete details on the ten standard plans and the benefits provided by each, you should request a copy of the *Guide to Health Insurance for People with Medicare* from the U.S. Department of Health and Human Services, Health Care Financing Administration, 6325 Security

MEDIGAP PLAN BENEFITS

CORE BENEFITS	A	B	C	D	E	F	G	H	I	J
Part A hospital (days 61–90)	X	X	X	X	X	X	X	X	X	X
Lifetime reserve (days 91–150)	X	X	X	X	X	X	X	X	X	X
365 Life hosp. days - 100%	X	X	X	X	X	X	X	X	X	X
Part B coinsurance	X	X	X	X	X	X	X	X	X	X
ADDITIONAL BENEFITS										
Skilled nursing facility coinsurance			X	X	X	X	X	X	X	X
Part A deductible		X	X	X	X	X	X	X	X	X
Part B deductible			X			X				X
Part B excess charges						100%	80%		100%	100%
Foreign travel emergency			X	X	X	X	X	X	X	X
Recovery at home				X			X		X	X
Prescription Drugs★								1	1	2
Preventive medical care					X					X

★*Two plans provide some prescription drug benefits: Plans H and I offer a basic benefit with $250 deductible, 50 percent coinsurance, and a $1,250 maximum annual benefit. Plan J has a $250 annual deductible, 50 percent coinsurance, and a $3,000 maximum annual benefit.*

Core benefits pay the patient's share of Medicare's approved amount for physician services (20 percent) after 100 percent annual deductible, the patient's cost of a long hospital stay, and charges for the first three pints of blood not covered by Medicare.

Boulevard, Baltimore, MD 21207.

Congress has mandated that the benefits be identical on all of these plans regardless of where you purchase the policy. The only variables will be the premium and the service you receive from the companies. Some companies waive any waiting period for preexisting conditions if you buy the supplement the month you turn 65, and some waive the waiting period for preexisting conditions if the policy is replacing another Medicare supplement or other medical coverage. Congress has further mandated a six-month open-enrollment period for buying Medicare supplemental health insurance. This law guarantees that for the six months immediately following enrollment in Part B, persons age 65 or older cannot be denied Medigap insurance due to their health status or history. This means you must be issued a Medigap policy regardless of your health, and the waiting period for preexisting conditions cannot be longer than six months.

Each of the ten plans has a letter designation ranging from "A" through "J." Insurance companies are not permitted to change these designations or to substitute other names or titles. They may, however, add names or titles to these letter designations. While companies are not required to offer all of the plans approved for sale by the individual states, they all must make Plan A available if they sell any of the other nine plans in a state.

Medigap policies can be problematic for people who are on Medicare because of a disability and are under age 65. If you are under age 65, you may have a hard time finding a company to sell you a policy. If your prescription drug needs are very extensive, Medigap plans will not provide you enough coverage. This is an increasing problem for people with chronic and expensive illnesses who are disabled, and health policymakers are slowly beginning to address it by mandating that insurers sell individual comprehensive policies to people in these situations. Contact your state insurance department or Medicare Beneficiaries Defense Fund at (212) 869-3850 for the current status of your state law.

MEDICARE HMOs – Due to the rising cost of Medicare Part B and Medigap policies, many Medicare recipients will find enrolling in Medicare HMOs increasingly attractive. Medicare HMOs contract with Medicare to provide the full range of Medicare-covered services to Medicare beneficiaries. To be a member, you must continue to pay your Part B monthly premium to Medicare, and Medicare, in turn, pays the HMO for providing you with health care. Certain HMOs also require you to pay some additional fees. Most Medicare HMOs are risk-based HMOs, meaning the HMO will receive a set fee from Medicare for each enrollee, regardless of the number of services received or the cost of delivering those services. The HMOs assume the "risk" that caring for you will not cost more than they receive from Medicare to do so.

As a Medicare risk member, you will pick a primary care physician who will coordinate your care, and in conjunction with plan administrators, decide when it is appropriate for you to see a specialist or go to the hospital. Like traditional HMOs, in Medicare HMOs, you will be able to use only the health professionals in the HMO network. HMO's offer some clear advantages and disadvantages to cancer survivors.

POSSIBLE DISADVANTAGES OF MEDICARE HMOS:
- You will lose some control over your health decision-making.
- You will be covered only for health-care services received through the HMO, except in emergency and urgent care situations. Generally, if you take long trips or spend part of the year outside the HMO plan area, or expect to be away for more than 90 days, joining an HMO is not in your best interest.
- You will not be able to see a specialist or be admitted to the hospital (except in emergencies) without authorization from your HMO primary care physician.
- No system exists to measure the quality of treatment options paid for by HMOs. An HMO will limit your freedom of choice and may present a compromise in the level of care you receive.

ADVANTAGES OF MEDICARE HMOS:
- You may receive coverage for services that Medicare does not cover. HMOs generally offer free checkups and other preventive care services; they may also offer limited routine eye care, limited hearing care, free transportation to and from the HMO and limited prescription drug coverage.
- You will not need Medigap insurance.
- You will not have to pay the Medicare deductibles or coinsurance.
- You will not have to deal with Medicare paperwork.

MEDICAID

Medicaid is a jointly financed federal-state insurance program for low-income families. The federal government administers Medicaid through the Health Care Financing Administration (HCFA) of the Department of Health and Human Services. Each state has a single agency (usually the Department of Social Services or the Department of Public Welfare) that administers Medicaid in that state.

Although Congress is considering changes, the federal government requires certain basic benefits; each state then determines what additional benefits it will provide and who is eligible. Because states have some role in determining who is eligible for Medicaid and what benefits are paid, Medicaid coverage varies widely from state to state. All states, however, must give you a fair hearing before its state agency if your Medicaid claim is denied. The types of expenses covered by Medicaid may include hospitals, physicians, prescription drugs, and home aids. For more information about Medicaid, contact your state public welfare department.

MEDICARE/MEDICAID DUAL ELIGIBILITY – Through the Qualified Medicare Beneficiary (QMB) or "Medicare Buy-in" Program, Medicare beneficiaries can get Medicaid to pay their Medicare premiums, deductibles and coinsurance. However, not all physicians will agree to accept the Medicaid reimbursement rates. If a doctor does not accept Medicaid, Medicare will pay 80 percent and you will be responsible for any unmet deductible and the 20 percent coinsurance. Under the Specified Low-Income Medicare Beneficiary (SLMB) program, Medicare Part B premiums for those living between 100 and 120 percent of the federal poverty level will be covered by the program. For more information about both programs call the national Medicare hot line at (800) 638-6833.

for more information
contact
MEDICARE HOT LINE
800/638-6833
information about programs

OBTAINING AND MAINTAINING HEALTH COVERAGE

Nearly 40 million Americans have no health insurance, and an additional 50 million have insurance that is insufficient to meet medical expenses for a serious illness. Although recent efforts to provide all Americans with a legal right to health insurance have been unsuccessful, many lawmakers in Congress and state legislatures are seeking ways to reform the laws governing the health insurance market to make it more accessible and affordable. Although most Americans obtain health insurance through their jobs, more than two-thirds of the uninsured are employed or the dependents of employed individuals. Cancer survivors represent a disproportionate number of these uninsured and under-insured Americans.

Because most adults in the United States obtain health insurance through their employment, the loss of employment often results in lost or decreased health insurance. Survivors who are not covered by group policies, which spread the risk among a large applicant pool, are the most vulnerable to insurance problems.

Roughly one in four cancer survivors is unable to obtain adequate health insurance. For example, it is not uncommon for an insurance company to double premiums once it learns that a subscriber has a cancer history. Insurance companies construct barriers to health insurance by rejecting new applications, canceling policies, reducing benefits, increasing premiums, requiring long waiting periods before preexisting conditions are covered by the insurance, and excluding coverage for certain preexisting conditions.

Health insurance reform is popular in many states. Some states have passed legislation making it easier for individuals with preexisting conditions to obtain health insurance. Before you move to a another state, contact the insurance department of the state to which you plan to relocate to ensure that you will be able to obtain health insurance with little or no waiting period for preexisting conditions.

Your Legal Right to Health Insurance

As long as it otherwise complies with state and federal law, (and some states now have very progressive insurance laws) an insurance company can decide what type of insurance it will sell and to whom it will sell a plan. The insurance company can decide what type of risk it will insure as long as it applies the same standards to all similar risks. Except in some states that have outlawed the practice, when you apply for an individual or small group policy, the company will probably "medically underwrite" you. This means that the company considers your medical history in deciding whether, and at what cost, to insure you.

Health insurance premiums that are determined through underwriting are called experience rated because they are based on the history of claims submitted or on the "experience" of the individual or group seeking coverage. Premiums based on the collective experience of all the individuals or groups purchasing comparable policies from the same company are known as community rated. Community rating, which removes the discriminating effect of charging "high risk" individuals or groups more due to their history of illness, is a goal of many insurance reforms because it is considered fairer than experience rating.

In general, you do not have a legal right to adequate health insurance. Whether termination from a plan, denial of benefits under a plan, or refusal to issue insurance violates a law is determined by two factors: the terms of the policy and the applicable law (federal law and state law).

Contractual Rights – An insurance policy is a contract between you (the insured) and your insurance company (the insurer). Your obligations under the contract are to pay your premiums on time and to provide your insurance company with the information it requests to process your claim. Your insurance company's obligations are to pay you benefits and provide other services as spelled out in the policy. If you meet your obligations, but your insurance company refuses to pay benefits (or perform another duty, such as renew your policy) in accordance with the terms of the policy, you may be able to sue your company for breach of contract. In addition to your contractual rights conferred by your insurance policy, you have other rights to health insurance under federal and state laws.

FEDERAL LAWS – No federal law guarantees a right to adequate health insurance. Four laws—the Health Insurance Portability and Accountability Act of 1996, COBRA, ERISA, and the Americans with Disabilities Act (ADA)—however, provide cancer survivors opportunities to keep health insurance they obtain at work, even after they are no longer employed. (See page 212 for an explanation of how the ADA applies to health insurance.)

THE HEALTH INSURANCE PORTABILITY AND ACCOUNTABILITY ACT OF 1996 - In August, 1996, President Clinton signed a modest health insurance reform law that should help cancer survivors retain their health insurance in the following ways:
- Alleviates "job-lock" by allowing individuals who have been insured for at least 12 months to change to a new job without losing coverage, even if they previously have been diagnosed with cancer. In addition, for previously uninsured individuals, group plans cannot impose preexisting condition exclusions of more that 12 months for conditions for which medical advice, diagnosis, or treatment was received or recommended within the previous six months.
- Prevents group health plans from denying coverage based on health status factors such as current and past health, claims experience, medical history, and genetic information. Insurers may, however, uniformly exclude coverage for specific conditions and place lifetime caps on benefits.
- Increases insurance portability for people changing from a group policy to an individual one.
- Requires insurers of small groups to cover all interested small employers and to accept every eligible individual under the employer's plan who applies for coverage when first eligible.
- Requires health plans to renew coverage for groups and individuals in most cases.
- Establishes a demonstration project for medical savings accounts for small employers and self-employed individuals (see page 171) for a description of medical savings accounts).
- Increases the tax deduction for health insurance expenses available to self-employed individuals.

The Act, however, does nothing to ensure the affordability of health insurance or to provide coverage to the millions of Americans who do not have health insurance. Most provisions of the Act take effect July 1, 1997.

COBRA – The Comprehensive Omnibus Budget Reconciliation Act (COBRA) requires employers to offer group medical coverage to employees and their dependents who otherwise would have lost their group coverage due to individual circumstances. Public and private employers with more than twenty employees are required to make continued insurance coverage available to employees who quit, are terminated, or work reduced hours. (Some states require employers of fewer than twenty employees to provide the same benefits as COBRA. Check with your state insurance department to see if your state has a so-called mini-COBRA.) Coverage must extend to surviving, divorced, or separated spouses, and to dependent children.

By allowing you to keep your group insurance coverage for a limited time, COBRA provides valuable time to shop for long-term coverage. Although you, and not your former employer, must pay for the continued coverage, the rate you pay may not exceed by more than two percent the rate set for your former coworkers. Continuation of coverage must be offered regardless of any health conditions, such as cancer.

Eligibility for the employee, spouse, and dependent child varies under COBRA. The employee becomes eligible if he or she loses group health coverage because of a reduction in hours or because of termination due to reasons other than gross employee misconduct. The spouse of an employee becomes eligible for any of four reasons:

1. the death of spouse;
2. termination of a spouse's employment (for reasons other than gross misconduct) or reduction in a spouse's hours of employment;
3. divorce or legal separation from a spouse; or
4. a spouse becomes eligible for Medicare.

The dependent child of an employee becomes eligible for any of five reasons:

1. the death of a parent;
2. the termination of a parent's employment or reduction in a parent's hours;
3. a parent's divorce or legal separation;
4. a parent becomes eligible for Medicare; or
5. a dependent ceases to be a "dependent child" under a specific group plan.

The continued coverage under COBRA must be identical to that offered to the families of your former coworkers. If your employment is terminated for any reason other than gross misconduct or if your hours are reduced, you and your dependents can continue coverage for up to 18 months. A qualified beneficiary who is determined to be disabled for Social Security purposes at the time of the termination of employment or reduction in employment hours can continue COBRA coverage for a total of 29 months. Your dependents can continue coverage for up to 36 months if their previous coverage will end because of any of the above reasons.

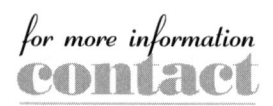

Continued coverage may be cut short if—
- your employer no longer provides group health insurance to any of its employees;
- your continuation coverage premium is not paid;
- you become covered under another group health plan; or
- you become eligible for Medicare.

for more information
contact

DEPARTMENT OF LABOR

PENSION AND WELFARE BENEFITS ADMINISTRATION

Room N-5658
200 Constitution Ave. NW
Washington, DC 20210

202/523-8521

COBRA complaints

The employee or family member has the duty to inform the group health plan administrator of a change in family status. The employer is responsible for notifying the group health plan of an employee's death, termination of employment, or reduction in hours. Employees and beneficiaries are given sixty days from the date they would lose coverage to make a decision about continued coverage.

COBRA is enforced by the Pension and Welfare Benefits Administration of the United States Department of Labor. The first step to resolving a COBRA complaint is to try to work out a settlement with your employer. If no adequate solution can be reached, you should write the Department of Labor at Pension and Welfare Benefits Administration, U.S. Dept. of Labor, Room N-5658, 200 Constitution Ave. NW, Washington, DC 20210; (202) 523-8521.

In certain cases, the Department of Labor may try to negotiate a solution before your case is filed in federal court.

ERISA – Another major federal law that may affect your coverage is the Employee Retirement and Income Security Act (ERISA). This is the federal law that regulates employee-benefit or self-insured plans. Employee benefit plans are defined broadly, and include any plan with the purpose of providing "medical, surgical, or hospital care benefits, or benefits in the event of sickness, accident, disability, death, or unemployment."

Unlike commercial insurance plans that employers purchase to provide health insurance as a benefit for their employees, self-insured plans are funds set aside by employers to reimburse employees for their (allowable) medical expenses. The claims employees file to obtain their reimbursement through these plans are likely to be administered by commercial insurance companies, so most people covered through self-insured plans do not even realize their health insurance is somewhat different from insurance purchased by an insurance company. Generally, large employer groups or unions find it to their benefit to self-insure, while smaller employer groups choose to finance employee health benefits through commercial insurers. Employee-benefit plans are regulated by federal law (ERISA) only, and are not subject to state insurance laws and regulations.

ERISA may provide a remedy to an employee who has been denied full participation in an employee benefit plan because of a cancer history. ERISA prohibits an employer from discriminating against an employee for the purpose of preventing him or her from collecting benefits under an employee benefit plan.

Some employers fear that the participation of a cancer survivor in a group medical plan will drain benefit funds or increase the employer's insurance premiums. A violation of ERISA may occur when an employer, upon learning of a worker's cancer history, dismisses that worker for the purpose of excluding him or her from a group health plan.

If an employer fires an employee for the purpose of cutting off the employee's benefits, regardless of whether the employee is considered disabled under the statute, the employer may be liable for a violation of ERISA. An employer also may violate ERISA by encouraging a person with a cancer history to retire as a "disabled" employee. Most benefit plans define disability narrowly to include only the most debilitating conditions. Individuals with a cancer history often do not fit under such a definition and should not be compelled to so label themselves.

Under certain circumstances, ERISA may provide grounds for a lawsuit to workers with a cancer history. ERISA covers both participants (employees) and beneficiaries (spouses and children). Thus, if the employee is fired because his or her child has cancer, the employee may be entitled to file a claim. ERISA, however, is inapplicable to many victims of employment discrimination, including individuals who are denied a new job because of their medical status, employees who are subjected to differential treatment that does not affect their benefits, and employees whose compensation does not include benefits.

ERISA is enforced by the Pension and Welfare Benefits Administration of the United States Department of Labor. The first step to secure your benefits is to file for all the benefits to which you are entitled under the plan. Your plan administrator must provide you a summary of the plan that tells you how the plan works, what benefits it provides, how they may be obtained or lost, and how you can enforce your rights under ERISA.

You must be notified within 90 days whether your claim for benefits is accepted or rejected. If you are not paid benefits to which you

WHO REGULATES YOUR INSURANCE POLICY

IF YOUR INSURER IS...	IT IS REGULATED BY...
Private company (nonprofit like Blue Cross and Blue Shield; for-profit company like Prudential)	State Department of Insurance
HMO	Several state and federal agencies. Start with your State Department of Insurance or State Department of Health
Private employer or union self-insurance or self-financed plan	U.S. Department of Labor (Office of Pension & Welfare Benefits)
Medicaid (sometimes called other names, for example "MediCal" in California)	State Department of Social Services
Medicare Supplemental Security Income Social Security Benefits	U.S. Social Security Administration
Veterans Benefits CHAMPUS	Department of Veterans Affairs

are entitled within 90 days, you may request a review of the denial, unless the plan administrator requests additional time to respond to your claim. You have at least 60 days from the date of denial to decide whether you will appeal the decision. If you do appeal and your claim is denied upon review, you must be told the reason for the denial and the plan rules upon which the decision was based.

If you are still dissatisfied with the decision, you may file a complaint in federal court. You do not have to have an attorney to file a complaint in federal court, but the assistance of an attorney at this stage usually is beneficial. The federal government does not have an informal administrative procedure to handle appeals from denial of benefits. Information about how to enforce your rights under ERISA may be obtained by writing the Department of Labor at Pension and Welfare Benefits Administration U.S. Dept. of Labor, Room N-5658, 200 Constitution Ave. NW, Washington, DC 20210.

STATE LAWS – Every state has an insurance commission or department that enforces state regulation of insurance companies. The commission determines what types of policies must be offered and when rates may be raised. States regulate insurance sold by insurance companies; they do not regulate self-insured employee benefit plans. State regulations cover all aspects of health insurance, including rates, policy conditions, termination or reinstatement of coverage, and the scope of coverage and benefits.

HEALTH INSURANCE FOR INDIVIDUALS AND DEPENDENTS

Insurance companies traditionally have avoided selling insurance to individuals for two reasons: they know individuals in need of their own insurance are more likely to be high risks (poor business), and administering many individual contracts requires a lot of time and labor on the part of the insurer. As a result, finding insurance to purchase if you are looking to cover only yourself and your dependents can be difficult. Many states have passed laws to assure that individuals can purchase health insurance when they are barred from the marketplace due to their medical history or other circumstances, or to ease the burden for people with preexisting conditions. The status of state laws and programs are changing rapidly. Check with your state insurance department to determine all of your options and to obtain written information on how the laws and programs work in your state.

Your group plan may give you the right to convert to an individual plan. If you do convert from a group to an individual policy, expect an increase in your premiums, and probably, a reduction in your benefits.

High-risk pools require major insurers to participate in the plan and share the "risks" or costs of coverage for individuals in the pool. Risk pools usually provide a package of benefits with a choice of deductibles. Although the premiums are higher than those for individual insurance, most states impose a cap on the amount that can be charged. Most states also have a waiting period for individuals with a preexisting condition, during which you must wait for a period after the policy is issued until the policy will pay benefits. A waiting period of six months for preexisting conditions, such as cancer, is common. For example, if you are receiving cancer treatments in January and you join a high-risk pool with a six-month waiting period, some or all of your medical bills will not be covered by the plan until the following July. Some states, however, will waive the waiting period if you pay a specified premium surcharge. All aspects of these pools vary from state to state.

As of March 1996, most states, but not all, have laws assuring the right of individuals leaving group coverage to convert their policy to an individual plan. The provisions of these laws differ, so be sure you find out your rights and responsibilities before you convert your policy. Most importantly, conversion may not be your only, or best, option. A converted policy rarely resembles the group policy.

Open enrollment or guaranteed issue programs assure that individuals can purchase health policies despite their medical histories or claims experience. The specific rules for these programs, such as exclusions for preexisting conditions, differ from state to state.

Some states have laws requiring carriers to limit preexisting wait-

STATES WITH GROUP CONVERSION RIGHTS

Arizona
Arkansas
California
Colorado
Florida
Georgia
Illinois
Indiana
Iowa
Kansas
Kentucky
Louisiana
Maine
Maryland
Minnesota
Missouri
Montana
Nevada
New Hampshire
New Mexico
New York
North Carolina
Ohio
Oklahoma
Oregon
Pennsylvania
Rhode Island
South Carolina
South Dakota
Tennessee
Texas
Utah
Vermont
Virginia
Washington
West Virginia
Wisconsin
Wyoming

Straight Talk about Insurance and Health Plans – **CHAPTER EIGHT**

STATES WITH OPEN ENROLLMENT

Idaho
Iowa
Kentucky
Louisiana
New Hampshire
New Jersey
New York
Ohio
Utah
Vermont
Washington

(source: Blue Cross Blue Shield Association)

STATES WITH PORTABILITY PROVISIONS

California
Connecticut
Idaho
Indiana
Iowa
Kentucky
Louisiana
Maine
Minnesota
New Hampshire
New Jersey
New York
North Dakota
Ohio
Oregon
Rhode Island
South Carolina
Utah
Vermont
Virginia
Washington
Wyoming

(source: Blue Cross Blue Shield Association)

ing periods to a specified number of months following the effective date of coverage. These so-called portability laws require carriers to credit the time a person was covered by previous coverage in determining whether a preexisting condition waiting period has been satisfied. Again, the provisions of these laws will vary from state to state.

ADDITIONAL TIPS FOR PURCHASING HEALTH INSURANCE — Make sure any policy you purchase is guaranteed renewable. Be sure to read and understand the exclusions (some policies will refer to the exclusions as omissions).

Study the definitions listed in the insurance plan pamphlet and make sure that you understand them — The company from whom you purchase a policy should be rated A or A+ by A.M. Best and Co., which rates all insurance companies. Best's annual directory is in the reference section of most public libraries.

Be certain your agent and the agency with which you are dealing are both licensed by your state insurance department to sell health insurance — See the Resources section for state insurance departments.

Never make a check payable to an individual agent — Checks should be made payable either to the agency or the insurance company.

Before signing the insurance application, make sure any preexisting conditions are listed on your application and that all information is correct — False information or misrepresentation of health conditions on your application may result in the denial of benefits or cancellation of your policy. If you find a mistake, ask the agent to complete a new application. If you find a mistake after the application has been forwarded to the insurance company, notify the insurance company in writing, with a copy of your letter to your insurance agent.

If you are replacing an existing policy with a new one, do not cancel your current policy until you are sure that you have been approved by the new company and your coverage is in effect — In nearly all cases, your new policy will have a waiting period for preexisting conditions. You should understand completely the definition of a preexisting condition as stated by the company from which you are considering making a purchase. Do not drop your current policy until the waiting period for preexisting conditions under the new policy has expired.

Study your new policy carefully when it arrives — Many states have a law that allows you 10 to 30 days to examine a policy once it has been issued. If you return the policy during that period of time, you will get a full refund of any premiums you have paid. Take advantage of this time period to study the new policy. A copy of your application will be included in the new policy and you should check it again for errors. Your state insurance department can tell you how many days you have to review an individual policy in your state.

Check with the Medical Information Bureau (MIB) prior to applying for insurance to make sure the information they may have on file for you is accurate — The MIB is a Boston-based data bank that has medical and nonmedical information on nearly 15 million Americans to protect the insurance industry from fraud. It is comparable to a credit report. It is a nonprofit association with 800 North American insurance industry members who share information through the data bank. They legally enter encoded information from insurance applications into the data bank and consult it when applications are pending before them.

You have the right to verify the information in your MIB file to ensure its accuracy. You can do so by contacting the Medical Information Bureau, Inc., P.O. Box 105 — Essex Station, Boston, MA 02112; (617) 426-3660.

Ask for a form to request disclosure of any information in your file. It also will tell you how you may correct any inaccurate information. MIB charges a small fee for this service.

Pay premiums quarterly rather than monthly, if you are paying your own. This will save you a little in processing.

for more information
contact

MEDICAL INFORMATION BUREAU

P.O. Box 105
Essex Station
Boston, MA 02112

617/426-3660

verify the accuracy of information in your MIB file

GETTING THE MOST OUT OF YOUR HEALTH INSURANCE

Cancer treatment often involves numerous bills from a variety of parties: the hospital, physicians (such as surgeons, anesthesiologists, oncologists and radiologists), support services (such as nurses, social workers, nutritionists and therapists), a radiology group, a pharmacy (drugs and medical supplies), and consumer businesses (for items such as wigs, breast inserts, and special clothing). Your insurance company will pay some of these parties directly, in part or in whole. You must pay other bills and submit copies to your company for reimbursement. If you have more than one policy, you must submit the right bill to the right company in the right order.

Keeping track of dozens of expenses, which can amount to tens or hundreds of thousands of dollars, can be confusing and exhausting.

The key to collecting the maximum benefits to which you are entitled under your insurance policy is to keep accurate records of your medical expenses.

Collecting Health Insurance Benefits

SUBMITTING CLAIMS - *Submit your claims in a timely fashion* – Most insurance companies have a time limit for submitting claims. It could be one year from the date of service or it could be all of the preceding calendar year plus the current year. Make sure you know what your policy defines as the time limit.

Keep accurate records – This is essential to collecting maximum benefits. If you have a large number of bills, work on this chore frequently. Do not let the bills pile up for so many months that it becomes an unmanageable task. If you find this chore overwhelming and simply cannot figure out where to begin, you may be better off financially in the long run to hire a health claims processing service to do this for you.

Use an accountant's worksheet pad (available in your local stationery store) – Assign a number to each bill and apply that same number to each insurance explanation of benefits that you receive relative to that particular claim.

Make copies of all of your bills – Keep originals for follow-up unless your carrier is one of the few that insists on having the originals; in that case, keep very good copies for your records.

Submit in the proper order – The patient's insurance is always primary, the spouse's is secondary.

WHY CLAIMS ARE REJECTED:
- Insurance identification number is incorrect on the claim.
- Information is incomplete on claim forms.
- Diagnosis is missing or incomplete; the diagnosis must always be consistent with the services offered. For example, if your doctor does a glucose tolerance test and the only diagnosis is cancer of the breast, insurance will not pay for the glucose tolerance test because it is not required for diagnosis of cancer of the breast. If the diagnoses are diabetes and cancer of the breast, insurance will pay for the glucose tolerance test.
- Date the services were provided is missing.
- First name of the patient is missing.

- Superbill is not legible.
- Reasons for multiple visits made in one day are not stated.
- Date is incorrect or the year is missing.
- Charges are not itemized.
- The insurance carrier wants additional information—be sure to study the explanation of benefits and send them what they want.

WHEN THE INSURER DOES NOT PAY ENOUGH OR DENIES YOUR CLAIM – *Send the claim back again* – When you send a claim back for review, it is not necessary to complete another claim form. Always send the explanation of benefits (EOB) with your notation written on it and a copy of the bill or whatever documentation is required.

Do not take "no" for an answer – Study the EOB form that comes with or without a check. Do not be satisfied with a greatly reduced amount of money for the claim.

Make sure that you are right – If your policy requires precertification, it means that if an 800 number is not called before you are admitted to a hospital, the policy will pay at a greatly reduced rate. It is your responsibility to tell your doctor to call the 800 number. Make sure you know whether your policy requires precertification. If yours is an emergency admission, you will have approximately 48 to 72 hours to report the admission. In extenuating circumstances, you may be able to get the insurer to pay at the normal rate, even though the precertification number was not called.

Make sure the total charges agree with the total amount of your bill – Do this by studying the EOB. Often, the insurer may forget to include one of the services rendered. When this happens, make a copy of the EOB and write on it exactly what happened. Then send the EOB and a copy of the actual bill back to the insurer.

Justify your doctor's charges – If the insurance greatly reduces the "reasonable and customary (R&C)" charge, it may be up to you to prove to the insurance company that your doctor's charge was reasonable, or that he or she was justified in charging that particular fee. First, ask your doctor to write a letter to the insurance company documenting and justifying the charge. Be sure the doctor sends the letter to you so that you can keep a copy for your records. If the insurer still fails to reduce its R&C fee, you may have to do your own research. The easiest way to do this is to verify the R&C for the particular service rendered by checking the *Physicians' Fee Reference*. This compendium of

R&C rates, adjusted for different parts of the country, is not easy to find, however. At $129 per annual issue, you may only find it through an advocacy organization or medical library. Otherwise, call at least ten of the same specialists in the same geographic area (county) and ask what they charge for the same procedure. Make sure you identify the procedure with the insurance company along with the results of your research in a letter. Note on the EOB that you are attaching a letter. In your letter, make reference to the EOB, the claim number, and your policy number.

Resubmit the claim and hope that a different claims examiner will process and pay it without question – Keep in mind that claims for durable medical equipment, prosthetic bras and implants, and chemotherapy wigs always require a copy of the prescription in addition to the bill.

Ask for a review of the denied claim – Simply write the following sentence on your EOB. "Please review—I think you should have paid more." If they still reject the claim, write on the EOB, "I would like to request a review of this denial of coverage by the peer review physicians." Do not take no for an answer. Fifty percent of the time, claims that are rejected the first time are paid the second time around. You may have to send a rejected claim back for review five times before you finally get the answer you want.

Always get the name of the customer service representative or claims examiner with whom you speak in a phone conversation – Keep a file on this particular claim, along with the date and the subject that was discussed. If you receive no response, as a final effort, you may have to write a letter to the general counsel of the insurance carrier explaining everything that has happened to date.

Be persistent! – If you are unable to resolve your claim with your insurance company, consider contacting
- the state or federal agency that regulates your insurance provider. (See page 188 for a chart that describes which agency regulates your insurance. See page 308 for a list of state insurance departments.)
- a cancer advocacy or peer-support organization. Some organizations, such as the Candlelighters Childhood Cancer Foundation, offer ombudsman programs to help survivors and their families maximize insurance reimbursement.
- an attorney. If your claim is not settled informally, consider filing a complaint in small-claims court or hiring an attorney to sue your insurance company.

COVERAGE OF INVESTIGATIONAL OR EXPERIMENTAL THERAPIES

Cancer survivors who have health insurance may find some of their claims rejected because the insurance policy does not cover "experimental treatment." Unfortunately, what your doctor considers the best treatment for you may be considered "experimental" by your insurance company. For example, oncologists often use chemotherapy drugs to treat their patients for cancers other than the specific type of cancer indicated on the package insert. Although the Food and Drug Administration permits doctors to prescribe approved drugs for any use, some insurance companies and self-insured plans refuse to pay for chemotherapy that is used in a way not listed on the "package insert." As of March 1996, twenty states have laws requiring insurers to cover these so-called "off-label uses" of anticancer drugs provided sufficient evidence of their usefulness against that type of cancer can be found in standard lists of drugs. Unfortunately, because these are state laws, self-insured plans need not comply.

The other major forms of cancer treatment that insurers may consider experimental are drugs and devices or procedures still under study and therefore not "standard" therapy. For example, bone marrow and peripheral stem cell transplants are procedures considered experimental as treatment for certain types of cancer and therefore often are not covered.

If you participate in a clinical trial to test a new treatment, your insurer may refuse to cover the patient care costs involving that trial. These costs, which will include the hospital and physicians' bills, can be so expensive that patients are prevented from receiving the anticancer treatment their oncologist recommended for them.

If you are in this situation, appeal your insurer's decision, and with the help of your physician, exhaust every remedy, including possible legal action against your insurer. Many survivors have found that appeals reviewed by the medical department of the insurance company are overturned in their favor.

Others have found that they needed to involve an attorney before the insurer agreed to provide the coverage. Do not delay in seeking the help of an attorney. If you need a bone marrow transplant, insurance company delay tactics can waste critical time. Sometimes it takes little more than a letter from an attorney to persuade the insurance company to "rethink" its position. Before you spend any money to retain an attorney, make sure he or she is experienced in handling these kinds of cases. Contact the *Bone Marrow Transplant Newsletter* at (708) 831-1913 for the name of an experienced attorney in your area. Although every appeal is not successful, each appeal further encourages your insurance company to pay for the most current and promising treatment as determined by your physician.

STATES WITH LAWS MANDATING COVERAGE OF OFF-LABEL ANTICANCER DRUGS (MARCH 1996)

Alabama
Arkansas
California
Connecticut
Florida
Georgia
Hawaii
Illinois
Indiana
Maryland
Massachusetts
Michigan
New Jersey
New York
North Carolina
Ohio
Oklahoma
Rhode Island
Virginia
Washington

Note that the provisions of these laws differ among the states.

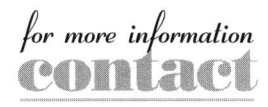

for more information
contact
BONE MARROW TRANSPLANT NEWSLETTER
(708) 831-1913
attorney referrals

LIFE INSURANCE AND "LIVING BENEFITS"

> There have certainly been times when I have felt greater uncertainty about my long-term survival than I have at other times. In each of the last three autumns, I have wondered whether to plant the tulip and daffodil bulbs for the spring bloom or not to bother. Now again this past spring, a glory of living color rewarded me, and once again I have planted for next spring's blooming.
> —Robert M. Mack, M.D., lung cancer survivor, "Lessons from Living with Cancer," *New England Journal of Medicine,* Vol. 311, No. 25, p. 1640, December 20, 1984.

for more information
contact

AFFORDING CARE
212/371-4714

referral to a guaranteed-issue life insurance plan

Life insurance provides two types of benefits: replacement of wages if a wage-earner dies and replacement of retirement income if a retired family member dies. Although most people agree that life insurance is practical protection in the event of unforeseen tragedy, many are confused about who needs life insurance and why. Insurance experts recommend buying life insurance when—

- you have young children (all adult wage earners in the family should be covered);
- you have a family without young children, and one spouse would suffer financial hardship if the other spouse died suddenly; and
- you are supporting an aged parent who depends on you for income.

When you apply for life insurance, your medical history becomes of vital interest to the insurance company. Very few insurers sell life insurance policies to "high risk" individuals. Contact Affording Care at (212) 371-4741 for referral to a guaranteed-issue life insurance plan.

Some companies market policies for people with serious health problems. Before buying such a policy, read it carefully. The benefits often are limited (you might have no coverage for the first two policy years) and these policies can be relatively expensive.

Although the questions asked on applications vary, common questions which affect the chance of cancer survivors securing life insurance include—

Have you been treated for cancer in the past twelve months?

Has any other insurance company ever rejected you, and if so, why?

You must answer these questions honestly. If you do not, and the company discovers the truth, it may cancel your policy or deny some or all of the benefits. If the company is suspicious about your medical history, it may check your file at the Medical Information Bureau.

The company may ask you to submit to a medical exam, paid for by the company, so it can further evaluate your health. It may also conduct an investigation of your daily habits and medical history.

Once the company has collected the information it requires, it determines whether it will issue you life insurance, and if so, what rate it will charge you. Different companies have different systems for determining what your rate will be.

The following suggestions may increase the cancer survivor's ability to obtain adequate life insurance.

Try large companies that carefully grade the type and stage of cancer.

Obtain estimates from several companies – An efficient way to do this is to have an independent agent (one who does not work for a particular company) shop among the companies in your area to obtain the best possible plan for your needs. You may get a list of all licensed insurance brokers in your area from the state insurance department.

Consider a graded policy if you are unable to obtain a life insurance policy with full death benefits – If you die from cancer within the first few years of the policy (usually three years), a graded policy returns only your premium plus part of the face value of the policy to your beneficiaries. If you die after the waiting period has passed, the company will pay the full face value of the policy.

Try to obtain life insurance through a group plan – Many employers and organizations that offer group health insurance also offer group life insurance. The insurance company does not make an individual evaluation of the health of each plan member of a large group; however, your health may be considered if you participate in a plan with a small number of members (for example, if you are one of 30 workers). If your health is considered, you may be excluded from the plan, denied full benefits, or required to pay an extra premium.

Whether you will be able to buy life insurance and what rate you will pay will depend upon the type of cancer you have, when you were diagnosed, and your prognosis. When you apply for life insurance, you are rated and assigned a risk factor. If you are rated within a short time of being diagnosed with a malignancy, the company may decline to issue you a policy at all. If your prognosis improves, you may be issued a policy, but you may be charged an extra premium. The amount of this premium varies depending upon your individual medical history.

How do companies determine these figures? Large companies and reinsurers publish risk selection guides based on reports by their medical staffs. Underwriters then use these guides to evaluate your medical files and determine what policy, if any, it will issue you. Some companies, however, do not differentiate substantially between different types and stages of cancer.

LIVING BENEFITS – Life insurance can provide a needed source of cash to the terminally ill. The term living benefits is used to describe two separate methods for accessing most the of the face value of your life insurance policy if you are terminally ill. While these benefits are beneficial to some, selling your life insurance is a decision to be made cautiously and with full knowledge of its advantages and disadvantages. You may wish to consult a personal financial planner, accountant, or lawyer to help you and your family determine if this is the best use of your life insurance funds.

The following are two basic methods for accessing living benefits.
1. "Accelerate" the death benefit of your policy through your insurer directly by purchasing a rider to your policy. Typically, you must have a life expectancy of six months or less, or be permanently confined to a nursing home. You can expect to receive approximately 80 percent of the face value of the policy through acceleration of your death benefit.
2. "Viaticating" your policy, or literally selling it to a third-party viatical settlement company. These companies typically pay 50 to 75 percent of the face value of your policy in exchange for designation of the company as beneficiary upon your death. The advantage of viaticating is that the companies' terms are more generous than riders on life insurance policies. You will be eligible to viaticate if your life expectancy is 24 months or less, thus providing a potential source of cash while you are still ambulatory and enjoying a good quality of life. Anticipate that the longer your life expectancy at the time you apply for viatication, the lower the cash award you will receive. Generally, you must keep paying premiums on the policy until your death even after you have viaticated.

Some important considerations before obtaining living benefits include the following.

Both accelerated benefits and viatical settlements currently qualify as income for tax purposes and for determination of eligibility for SSI and Medicaid – If you did not viaticate or accelerate, benefits paid to your beneficiary(ies) after your death would not subject them to income tax liability.

EVALUATING YOUR INSURANCE OPTIONS
NATALIE DAVIS SPINGARN AND NANCY CHASEN, JD

In evaluating insurance plans, you may want to check the *Consumers' Guide to Health Plans*, published in 1995 by the non-profit consumer organization, Center for the Study of Services. This book rates 250 health care plans nationwide based on survey responses of 90,000 consumers. It is available for $12 (including postage and handling) from the center at 733 Fifteenth St., NW, Suite 820, Washington, D.C. 20005.

A number of managed care plans have funded a private organization, the National Committee for Quality Assurance (NCQA), to evaluate managed care plans for accreditation. Measuring each against certain standards, the NCQA prepares a scorecard of plans it reviews, granting full or partial accreditation or denying the NCQA accreditation altogether.

Because it is not a regulatory agency, the NCQA cannot take any action against plans that do not meet its standards, but many employers and organizations do refer to the scorecard in deciding which plans to offer. To date, only 35 percent of the 208 HMOs reviewed have been fully accredited, with 14 percent receiving outright denial. The NCQA scorecard is available by writing to 2000 L St. NW, Suite 500, Washington, D.C. 20036, or it may be accessed on the Internet at http://www.ncqa.org.

Present day accreditation is a useful indicator in choosing among managed care plans, but it should not necessarily be the deciding factor. Not every accredited plan will be right for you. Indeed, some still unaccredited plans reportedly have earned high marks from consumers.

Until rating systems are fine tuned to include the patient's point of view, you may also want to check with, the Foundation for Accountability (FACCT). FACCT is a consumer-friendly organization that develops yardsticks to help you evaluate plans from the patient's point of view. For example, it reports how competing plans have helped patients limit disease progression, and how satisfied patients feel about various services received. You can reach FACCT at (503) 22-FACCT, or by writing to FACCT at 220 NW Second Avenue, Suite 725, Portland, OR, 97209.

Any funds you receive while living means less money for your beneficiaries after you die – For this reason, you should carefully weigh the benefit of accessing living benefits

Comparison shop – A wise consumer will do a lot of comparison shopping. Companies will vary in their terms. Affording Care recommends obtaining bids from at least six companies when considering viaticating. Know that past abuses of vulnerable consumers have occurred, leading to calls for state regulation of the viatical settlement industry.

Your life expectancy and other detailed medical information must be verifiable with your physician(s) – If you ask several firms to bid on your policy, they will all contact your doctor for verification. Inform your doctor's office that they may receive several requests so they are prepared.

Obtain professional advice if you encounter obstacles – Obtaining living benefits from a group life insurance policy can be more complex because more parties are involved, (such as employers and plan administrators) but not impossible.

When you viaticate, expect four to six weeks from the time you start the process until you have your cash.

Demand up front that the viatical settlement company whose bid you have accepted put the funds in a third party escrow account.

Conclusion—When All Else Fails

Survivors often must overcome considerable obstacles to obtain and keep health, disability, and life insurance. If all of your attempts to secure insurance fail, talk with your doctor. Most doctors want to help you. Explain your financial status to your doctor and anyone else who will listen, such as the office manager or billing secretary. When the doctor knows your financial situation, he or she will be more apt to work with you.

Glossary Of Insurance Terms

In order to maximize your benefits, you should have a clear understanding of the following health insurance and managed care jargon.

AGENT: An insurance company representative licensed by a state to sell insurance.

ASSIGNMENT: The transfer of one's rights to collect an amount payable under an insurance contract—assignment of benefits.

BASIC INSURANCE: Coverage of hospitalization costs only.

BENEFIT: An amount payable by the insurance carrier.

BENEFIT PERIOD—MEDICARE: The period of time that begins the first day a person enters a hospital or skilled nursing facility and ends 60 days after discharge without being readmitted to either type of facility.

BROKER: An insurance solicitor, licensed by the state, who places business with a variety of insurance companies and who represents the buyer, not the company.

CARRIER: An insurance company that "writes" the insurance.

CATASTROPHIC INSURANCE: A type of limited health insurance that serves the purpose of covering very high medical expenses. The deductibles are very high ($10,000 or above) and the premiums are low.

CARRY OVER: A provision in many major medical policies to avoid two deductibles if expenses are incurred toward the end of one calendar year, and illness continues into the new year. Usually October through December charges toward the deductible will count in the new year.

CERTIFICATE OF INSURANCE: Document given to employees to explain their group insurance benefits. In some cases it may be a benefits booklet.

COINSURANCE: The portion of the bill for which the insured is responsible.

COMPREHENSIVE COVERAGE: Insurance is either comprehensive or limited. Comprehensive means broader coverage and/or higher indemnity payments than limited coverage.

COMMUNITY RATED: A method for determining premium amounts based on the claims experience of all covered individuals with the same coverage and the same insurer. It is the opposite of experience rated.

CONVERSION: The exchange of one insurance policy providing temporary or group coverage for another individual policy—for example, when a person ceases working and an individual policy is issued to replace employer group coverage. No evidence of medical insurability is required.

COORDINATION OF BENEFITS: A group health policy provision designed to eliminate duplicate payments and provide the sequence in which coverage will apply when a person is insured under two contracts.

COPAYMENT: In managed care plans, the insured must pay directly to the provider of the service. It is typically five to fifteen dollars.

CPT-4-CURRENT PROCEDURE: Codes describing every procedure a provider can give a patient. Codes are used for billing purposes.

DEDUCTIBLE: The amount of money the insured must pay out of pocket before benefits begin. Deductibles are usually on a calendar year or policy year basis. Some policies have deductibles per diagnosis—the least desirable—or family deductibles. A policy may have a $250 deductible per individual with a $500 deductible per family. This means that when two individuals have each satisfied a $250 deductible, the remaining family members will not have to meet any deductible.

DIAGNOSIS RELATED GROUP (DRG): A system of paying hospitals based on the patient's diagnosis rather than on the total amount of service provided during their hospitalization.

ELIMINATION PERIOD: The first days of an illness that are not covered by insurance.

EXPLANATION OF BENEFITS (EOB): One of these forms comes with or without an insurance check to explain what portion of the submitted bill was covered and why. If you have more than one policy covering you, this is your proof of what your primary coverage paid.

EVIDENCE OF INSURABILITY: Under medically underwritten insurance, this is proof of a person's physical condition or occupation determining his or her acceptance for insurance.

EXCLUSIONS: Specified illnesses, injuries, or conditions listed in the policy that are not covered. Experimental therapies, cosmetic surgery, and eyeglasses are common exclusions.

EXPERIENCE RATED: A method for determining premium amounts based on the claims experience of the contract holder (which is most often the employer group). It is the opposite of community rated.

FEE-FOR-SERVICE: See indemnity insurance.

GUARANTEED ISSUE: Insurance carrier will issue the policy regardless of the health risk of the individual. In other words, no evidence of insurability is required.

HEALTH MAINTENANCE ORGANIZATION (HMO): The first and most traditional type of managed care plan. Like other types of managed care, HMOs are organizations that both finance health care (provide insurance) and provide the care by collecting fees in advance.

HMOs employ or contract with many physicians and other providers from whom the enrollee may seek care.

HYBRID INSURANCE: See point-of-service plans.

ICD-9: Codes used in describing diagnoses referring to the International Classification of Diseases.

INDEMNITY INSURANCE: Traditional insurance which pays providers on a fee-for-service basis.

LIFETIME MAXIMUM: Total benefits that the insurance company will pay per individual over a lifetime.

MAJOR MEDICAL INSURANCE: Coverage of expenses excluding the hospital fee.

MANAGED CARE: Organizations that function as both insurer and provider of health care simultaneously. HMOs were the first type, but variations include preferred provider organizations and independent practice associations. HMOs tend to operate with stricter rules than their variations.

MEDICALLY NECESSARY: What the insurer (managed care or indemnity) determines was truly necessary care and will therefore cover.

OPEN ENROLLMENT: Insurance that is issued regardless of one's health status or risk, but may be limited to a certain period of the year.

PARTICIPATING PROVIDER: A health care provider who has joined a managed care plan and is willing to accept its contracts.

PORTABILITY: Insurance that can be retained even if one leaves employment or the group plan.

PREEXISTING CONDITION: A health condition that existed before a policy was purchased. Companies' definitions of preexisting condition vary, but usually anything for which you have seen a doctor during the previous 12 months is a preexisting condition and will not be covered during the waiting period, which is typically six to twelve months after the effectiveness date of coverage.

POINT-OF-SERVICE PLANS: Managed care plans that give the insured the option of seeing providers within the network and paying the copayment amount only, or seeing providers out of the network and getting reimbursed as you would under an indemnity policy. Although these plans are increasingly popular because they allow for choice of providers, the premiums are higher than plans that give you no coverage for providers outside the network.

PRIMARY CARE PROVIDER (PCP): Sometimes referred to as the gatekeeper, PCPs are nonspecialist physicians in many managed care plans that enrollees choose to serve as their coordinator for all the services they may need. PCPs must preapprove all referrals to specialists and use of services, including emergency room care.

PROVIDER: The supplier, physician, psychologist, pharmacist, or other health care professional providing a service to the insured.

PUBLIC HEALTH INSURANCE: Medicare or Medicaid.

REASONABLE AND CUSTOMARY (R&C): In medical insurance, an approach to benefits under which the policy agrees to pay the "reasonable and customary" charges for a service or procedure, rather than a stipulated amount. Customary means the amount charged by a significant number of providers for a given service in a statistically similar geographical area. Reasonable means the usual or customary charge, whichever is less.

RELEASE OF INFORMATION: A form signed by the patient before information may be given out to an insurance company or third party.

RIDER: A legal document that modifies protection of a policy. It may either increase or decrease the payable benefits, or eliminate the condition entirely.

SCHEDULE OF BENEFITS: The list of benefits to which the insured is entitled.

SERVICE BENEFIT: An insurance benefit that fully pays for specific hospital or medical care services rendered.

STOP LOSS: The point during a calendar year when your insurance policy pays 100 percent of costs for the remainder of the year. Thus, your out-of-pocket expenditures, or losses, stop. Most policies pay 80 percent and the individual pays 20 percent. If the policy has a $5,000 stop-loss point, 20 percent of that equals $1,000. This means that when you have spent $1,000 out of your pocket plus your deductible, the policy will pay 100 percent rather than 80 percent.

SUBSCRIBER: A person who holds an insurance policy. Also known as the enrollee, the insured, the certificate holder, or the policyholder.

SUPERBILL: An itemized billing statement given to the patient so that he or she may submit the claim directly to the insurance carrier.

THIRD PARTY PAYER: An insurance carrier other than the doctor or patient which intervenes to pay hospital or medical bills.

UNDERWRITING: The process by which an insurance company determines whether and on what basis it will accept an application for insurance.

WAITING PERIOD: Time after the beginning of a policy date when benefits are not payable.

WAIVER: An agreement attached to a policy which exempts from coverage certain disabilities or injuries that are normally covered.

WAIVER OF PREMIUM: A provision included in some policies that exempts the insured from paying premiums if he or she is disabled during the life of the policy.

Chapter Nine

Working It Out: Your Employment Rights

by Barbara Hoffman, JD

"As a disability rights advocate and Hodgkin's disease survivor, I had been searching for a means to provide survivors with information about their legal rights. NCCS–and now this book–have empowered survivors with knowledge about their employment and insurance rights so that they can advocate to enforce and expand those rights."

Barbara Hoffman, JD

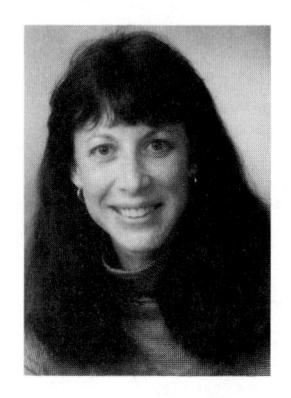

BARBARA HOFFMAN, JD is a cofounder of the National Coalition for Cancer Survivorship, serves as its general counsel, and has testified as an advocate for survivors before federal and state congressional committees. Ms. Hoffman is codirector of the Appellate Advocacy Program at Seton Hall University School of Law, where she teaches disability law and other subjects. She has provided information on the legal rights of cancer survivors at over 70 conferences and workshops, on television and radio, and in many publications. Ms. Hoffman's publications include *Charting the Journey: An Almanac of Practical Resources for Cancer Survivors,* (Mt. Vernon: Consumer Reports Books, 1990) as coeditor and more than a dozen articles in legal, medical, and consumer publications.

> Work on, My Medicine, work!
> — *William Shakespeare* (Othello)

Work fulfills a critical financial and emotional need for most cancer survivors. In addition to providing income and important benefits such as health insurance, employment can also be a source of self-esteem. Cancer, however, may create barriers to finding and keeping a job, wreaking havoc on your ability to pay your bills and insure your family.

Although an individual's risk for cancer increases with age, cancer often strikes working-age adults. Forty percent of all newly diagnosed survivors are between the ages of 20 and 64. The American Cancer Society estimates that approximately 80 percent of survivors who are employed at the time of diagnosis attempt to return to work. Personal factors such as age and type of cancer affect a survivor's ability to return to work. Many survivors are able to continue to perform their jobs, yet are denied the opportunity to work because of their cancer. Others may be unable or unwilling to perform their previous duties because of the severity of their illness. All survivors have the right to be treated as individuals at work and not as a stereotyped "cancer patient." Yet, in addition to waging a medical battle against cancer, some survivors face another struggle—obtaining and retaining employment.

This chapter describes how cancer affects survivors in the workplace; under what circumstances employment discrimination against survivors may be illegal; how you can avoid such discrimination; and what you can do when faced with such discrimination. This chapter also discusses vocational rehabilitation resources available to cancer survivors.

EMPLOYMENT DISCRIMINATION

EMPLOYMENT PROBLEMS FACED BY CANCER SURVIVORS

Until recently, cancer survivors faced many limits to job opportunities. Medical treatment often could not provide a length or quality of life necessary to work. Employers could discriminate against sur-

> About three o'clock or so I woke up in a total fright. I had been dreaming that I was wandering along the Beltway outside Washington trying to find the Raytheon plant that was located somewhere in those rolling hills. I was applying for a job after being turned down everywhere else. I had to find the plant to submit my resume, but I was hopelessly lost. My cancer had rendered me unemployable, and my family was going to be destitute.
>
> *former United States Senator Paul Tsongas (Heading Home, Vintage: 1986)*

vivors without fear of being sued. In the 1990s, however, cancer survivors can expect to live longer and better after diagnosis (see Chapter 1). They can also enjoy the benefits of many new federal and state laws designed to protect their employment rights. Despite these medical and legal advances, many survivors still find that cancer creates barriers to obtaining and keeping employment.

> A 1992 survey of 200 supervisors found that 66 percent were concerned that employees with cancer could no longer perform their jobs adequately. Nearly one-half said that a current cancer diagnosis would affect their decision to hire a qualified applicant. Of 500 employees surveyed, 13 percent believed that coworkers with cancer probably would not be able to do their jobs. One in four coworkers thought they would have to work harder to pick up the slack.
> —Yankelovich, Clancy, Shulman (1992)

Some employers and employees treat cancer survivors differently from other workers. Workplace problems most frequently reported by cancer survivors are dismissal, failure to hire, demotion, denial of promotion, undesirable transfer, denial of benefits, and hostility in the workplace. Although discrimination can be blatant and arbitrary, cancer-based discrimination is usually subtle and directed against an individual.

Job discrimination affects all cancer survivors, young and old, rich and poor. Nevertheless, some groups of survivors experience higher rates of discrimination than others. For example, studies suggest that blue-collar workers tend to encounter more problems obtaining and keeping a job than do white-collar workers. Survivors of childhood cancer confront different hurdles in the workplace from those faced by survivors diagnosed as adults. Although their employment rates differ little from the general population, survivors of childhood cancer report greater problems obtaining health, life, and disability insurance through work, slightly lower incomes, and fewer opportunities in military careers than do other young adults. One study suggests that survivors who were diagnosed as young children faced less discrimination than those diagnosed as teenagers.

Adult cancer survivors who are denied job opportunities commonly experience stress and anxiety over economic insecurity, loss of independence, and reduced self-esteem. Many survivors who are able to keep their jobs find it difficult to change jobs, to advance, or to change their careers. Since cancer is often considered a preexisting condition, a new employer's health insurance policy may not cover cancer-related medical treatment for months or years after employment begins. Many survivors are unable to take the risk of working without health insurance coverage for cancer-related treatment. As a result, they face "job lock;" they remain in an undesirable job mainly to secure health insurance benefits for cancer treatment.

REASONS FOR EMPLOYMENT DISCRIMINATION

Most employers treat cancer survivors fairly and legally. Some employers, however, erect unnecessary and sometimes illegal barriers to job opportunities for survivors. Most personnel decisions are driven by economic factors, not by charitable or personal considerations. Some employers face increased costs due to insurance expenses and lost productivity. Other employers worry about the psychological impact of an applicant's cancer history on other employees. Some employers fail to revise their personnel policies to comply with new laws. Employers who have updated personnel policies may not properly train their personnel managers to comply with these laws.

Although employers should evaluate cancer survivors on their individual qualifications for a job, some employers permit vague stereotypes and myths about cancer to color their decisions. For example, some people erroneously believe that cancer is contagious. The myth that cancer is contagious may result in physical and emotional isolation of survivors in the workplace. In California, one survivor who applied for a job with a medical emergency services company reported that he was asked by his interviewer, "Cancer, how did you catch that?" Another man reported that he "was transferred from his job in a hotel kitchen for fear that he might 'contaminate' the food." Other misconceptions about cancer, such as "cancer is always a death sentence" or "cancer renders workers unproductive," cause employers to treat cancer survivors differently from other workers. In fact, most cancer survivors who are employed at the time of diagnosis are able to return to work, often within a few weeks after starting treatment.

"I lost my breast, not my brain."

Mastectomy survivor in response to being fired from her job as a paralegal

WHEN CANCER-BASED DISCRIMINATION IS ILLEGAL

Under federal law and most state employment discrimination laws, an employer cannot treat a cancer survivor differently from other workers in job-related activities solely because he or she has been treated for cancer. You may be protected by these laws only if—
- you are qualified for the job (you have the necessary skills, experience, and education), and you can do the essential duties of the job in question; and
- your employer treated you differently from other workers in job-related activities because of your cancer treatment.

FEDERAL LAWS

Four federal laws provide some job protection to cancer survivors:

the Americans with Disabilities Act, the Federal Rehabilitation Act, the Family and Medical Leave Act, and the Employee Retirement and Income Security Act.

THE AMERICANS WITH DISABILITIES ACT (ADA) – *What the ADA Requires* – The Americans with Disabilities Act prohibits some types of job discrimination by employers, employment agencies, and labor unions against people who have or have had cancer. The ADA covers private employers with 15 or more employees, state and local governments, the legislative branch of the federal government, employment agencies, and labor unions. All cancer—regardless of whether your cancer is cured, is in remission or is not responding to treatment—is considered a "disability" under the ADA.

The ADA prohibits employment discrimination against individuals with a "disability," a "record of a disability," or those who are "regarded as having a disability." A disability is a major health problem that substantially limits the ability to do everyday activities, such as drive a car or go to work. Because all cancer survivors, even those who do not consider themselves to be limited by their cancer, fit under at least one of these three groups, all cancer survivors are protected by the ADA from the time of diagnosis. You are covered by the ADA for example, in the following instances.

- Your cancer currently substantially limits your ability to do everyday activities such as not being able to walk up stairs. A temporary, nonchronic impairment, such as a broken bone, is usually not considered a disability.
- At one time your cancer substantially limited your ability to do everyday activities, but no longer does. For example, during your treatment, you could not walk up stairs, but now you can. The ADA protects all cancer survivors who have completed treatment from discrimination based on their medical histories.
- Your employer believes that your cancer substantially limits your ability to work, even if you feel it does not.

The ADA prohibits discrimination in almost all job-related activities, including, but not limited to—
- not hiring an applicant for a job or training program;
- firing a worker;
- providing unequal pay, working conditions, or benefits, such as pension, vacation time, and health insurance;
- punishing an employee for filing a discrimination complaint; or
- screening out disabled employees.

In most cases, a prospective employer may not ask you if you have ever had cancer. An employer has the right to know only if you are able to do the job at the time you apply for it. A prospective employer may not ask you about your health history, unless you have a visible disability and the employer could reasonably believe that it might affect your current ability to perform that job. A job offer may be contingent upon passing a relevant medical exam, provided that all prospective employees are subject to the same exam. An employer may ask you detailed questions about your health only after you have been offered a job.

Your employer must keep your medical history in a file separate from your other personnel records. The only people entitled to see your medical file are supervisors who need to know whether you need an accommodation, emergency medical personnel, and government officials who enforce the ADA.

If you need extra time or help to do your job, the ADA requires an employer to provide you a "reasonable accommodation." An "accommodation" is a change, such as in work hours or duties, to help you do your job during or after cancer treatment. For example, if you need to take time off for treatment, your employer may "accommodate" you by letting you work flexible hours until you finish treatment.

An employer does not have to make changes that would be an "undue hardship" on the business or other workers. Undue hardship refers to any accommodation that would be unduly costly, extensive, substantial, or disruptive, or that would fundamentally alter the nature or operation of the business. For example, if you have to miss a substantial amount of work time and your work cannot be performed by a temporary employee, your employer may be able to replace you.

The ADA does not prohibit an employer from firing or refusing to hire a cancer survivor under any circumstance. Because the law requires employers to treat all employees similarly, regardless of disability, an employer may fire a cancer survivor who would have been terminated even if he or she were not a survivor. For example, a Georgia sheriff's department hired Martin Smith in 1984 to work as an undercover investigator. Mr. Smith had a cancerous eye removed in 1993; however, he did not tell his supervisor that he had cancer. The following month, the department fired Mr. Smith because he had forged a magistrate's signature on a search warrant. A federal court ruled that the department did not violate the ADA because it had the right to fire any employee who forged a judge's signature and because it did not know at the time that Mr. Smith had cancer.

The ADA allows employers to establish attendance and leave policies that are uniformly applied to all employees, regardless of disability. Employers must grant leave to cancer survivors if other employees would be granted similar leave. They may be required to change leave policies as a reasonable accommodation. Employers are not obligated to provide additional paid leave, but accommodations may include leave flexibility and unpaid leave. Additionally, survivors have other rights to medical leave under the Family and Medical Leave Act (see page 215).

The ADA does not require employers to provide health insurance, but when they choose to provide health insurance, they must do so fairly. For example, if your employer provides health insurance to all employees with jobs similar to yours, but does not provide you health insurance, the employer may be violating the ADA. The employer must prove that the failure to provide health insurance is based on legitimate actuarial data (statistics), or that the insurance plan would go broke or suffer a drastic increase in premiums, co-payments, or deductibles. If your employer is a small business that can prove it is unable to obtain an insurance policy that will cover you, the employer may not have to provide you the same health benefits provided to your coworkers.

Most employment discrimination laws protect only the employee. The ADA offers protection more responsive to survivors' needs because it prohibits discrimination against family members, too. Employers may not discriminate against workers because of their relationship or association with a "disabled" person. Employers may not assume that your job performance would be affected by your need to care for a family member who has cancer. For example, employers may not treat you differently because they assume that you would use excessive leave to care for your spouse who has cancer. Additionally, employers that provide health insurance benefits to dependents of employees may not decrease benefits to an employee solely because that employee has a dependent who has cancer. State laws, however, do not protect you if an employer treats you differently because a family member has cancer (see pages 217 and 315 for a discussion of state employment discrimination laws).

How the ADA is enforced – If you believe you have been treated differently by an employer covered by the Americans with Disabilities Act because of your cancer history, you must file a complaint with the United States Equal Employment Opportunities Commission (EEOC) to enforce your rights. You must file a complaint within 180 days of when you learned of the discriminatory act. Although you do not have to hire an attorney to file the complaint for you, an experienced attorney can help you evaluate your chances of obtaining the remedy you desire and can draft the complaint in a way to best represent your claim.

The EEOC will appoint an investigator to evaluate your claim. If the EEOC determines that your rights may have been violated, it will attempt to settle the dispute. If no settlement is reached, the EEOC may sue on your behalf or may grant you the right to file your own lawsuit in federal court. Most ADA complaints are resolved at the administrative level and do not proceed to court.

Your complaint should be filed with the closest regional EEOC office. To obtain the location of your regional EEOC office, call the EEOC Public Information System in Washington, DC at (800) 669-4000. You can obtain publications from the EEOC that explain the Americans with Disabilities Act and how to enforce your rights under the law by calling (800) 669-EEOC or (800) 949-4232.

If you can prove you are qualified for a job but have been discriminated against because of your cancer history, you may be entitled to back pay and benefits, injunctive relief such as reinstatement, equitable monetary damages, and attorney's fees. The Americans with Disabilities Act allows an award for compensatory or punitive damages up to $300,000 for intentional discrimination. Intentional discrimination, however, is difficult to prove. These damages are not available against state or local governments or against a private employer who made a "good faith" effort to accommodate you.

Two percent of all complaints filed under the ADA from July 26, 1992, through June 30, 1995, claimed cancer-based discrimination (1,210 of 49,974 complaints received by the EEOC). Indeed, the first employment discrimination case under the ADA to reach a jury was brought by a cancer survivor. Charles Wessel was fired by AIC Security Investigations, an Illinois security company, when the company's owner learned that the cancer in Wessel's lung had spread to his brain. A federal jury found that Wessel's employer violated the ADA because Wessel was able to perform his job as executive director when he was fired. Wessel was ultimately awarded $50,000 in compensatory damages (one year's salary) and $150,000 in punitive damages. The United States District Court for the Northern District of Illinois found that punitive damages were appropriate because Wessel's employer intentionally fired an excellent worker because he was dying.

THE FEDERAL REHABILITATION ACT – *What the Rehabilitation Act requires* – Prior to the passage of the Americans with Disabilities Act in 1990, the Federal Rehabilitation Act was the only federal law that prohibited cancer-based employment discrimination. The Rehabilitation Act bans public employers and private employers that receive public funds from discriminating on the basis of a disability. The following employees continue to be covered by the Rehabilitation Act, but not by the ADA:

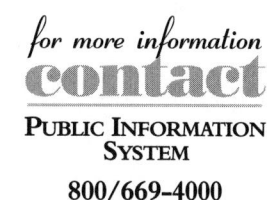

for more information
contact

PUBLIC INFORMATION SYSTEM
800/669-4000

EQUAL OPPORTUNITIES EMPLOYMENT COMMISSION
800/669-EEOC
800/949-4232
regional EEOC office locations

- Employees of the executive branch of the federal government (covered by Section 501 of the Rehabilitation Act).
- Employees of employers that receive federal contracts and have fewer than 15 workers (covered by Section 503 of the Rehabilitation Act).
- Employees of employers that receive federal financial assistance and have fewer than 15 workers (covered by Section 504 of the Rehabilitation Act).

For example, small companies that receive federal grants for research and development, physicians in small groups that receive Medicare Part B funds, and small health agencies that receive Medicaid payments may be subject to the Rehabilitation Act but not to the ADA. The military does not have to obey either the ADA or the Federal Rehabilitation Act, although retired military personnel and civilian employees of the Department of Defense are protected.

Like the ADA, the Rehabilitation Act protects cancer survivors, regardless of extent of disability. The Rehabilitation Act protects only qualified workers and requires employers to provide reasonable accommodations.

The United States Department of Labor regulations that enforce the Rehabilitation Act recognize that people with a cancer history often experience employment discrimination by employers and coworkers based on misconceptions about their illness long after they are fully recovered. The regulations explain that someone who has a history of a medical impairment is covered by the law because, "the attitude of employers, supervisors, and coworkers toward that previous impairment may result in an individual experiencing difficulty in securing, retaining, or advancing in employment. The mentally restored, those who have had heart attacks or cancer often experience such difficulty."

> By amending the definition of "handicapped individual" to include not only those who are actually impaired, but also those who are regarded as impaired and who, as a result, are substantially limited in major life activity, Congress acknowledged that society's accumulated myths and fears about disability and disease are as handicapping as are the physical limitations that flow from actual impairment. Few aspects of a handicap give rise to the same level of public fear and misapprehension as contagiousness. Even those who suffer or have recovered from such noninfectious diseases as epilepsy or cancer have faced discrimination based on the irrational fear that they might be contagious.
> —United States Supreme Court Justice William Brennan
> Arline v. School Board of Nassau County, (1987)

How the Rehabilitation Act is enforced – Cancer survivors have won lawsuits under the Federal Rehabilitation Act. In 1988, a federal court agreed that the Rehabilitation Act protected healthy cancer survivors from employment discrimination. The city of Houston Fire Department had a policy against hiring anyone with a history of lymphoma, regardless of whether the survivor was ill or in complete remission.

Walter Ritchie, who had been successfully treated for lymphoma in 1981, applied in 1985 for a position as a fire cadet. Although Mr. Ritchie passed all of the required tests, the city refused to hire him solely because of his cancer history. A federal court found that the city violated Mr. Ritchie's rights under the Rehabilitation Act by assuming that his cancer history made him unfit for the job. The court required the city to hire Mr. Ritchie and to consider applicants based on their individual abilities, not irrelevant medical history.

To enforce your rights as a federal employee (Section 501), you must file a complaint with the government within 30 days of the job action against you. To enforce your rights against an employer that has a federal contract (Section 503), you must file a complaint within 180 days with your local office of the United States Department of Labor, Office of Federal Contract Compliance Programs. To enforce your rights against an employer that receives federal funds (Section 504), you have up to 180 days to file a lawsuit in federal court or a complaint with the federal agency that provided federal funds to your employer. If you do not know the name of that agency or would like more information, contact the Access Unit, Civil Rights Division, Department of Justice, P.O. Box 66118, Washington, DC 20035-6118. Remedies under Section 504 of the Federal Rehabilitation Act include, but are not limited to, back pay, reinstatement, and attorney's fees, but do not include punitive damages.

for more information
contact
ACCESS UNIT, CIVIL RIGHTS DIVISION, JUSTICE DEPT.
P.O. Box 66118
Washington, DC
20035-6116

THE FAMILY AND MEDICAL LEAVE ACT (FMLA) – In 1993, the Family and Medical Leave Act was enacted to provide job security to workers who must attend to the serious medical needs of themselves or their dependents. The Family and Medical Leave Act requires employers with 50 or more employees to provide up to 12 weeks of unpaid, job-protected leave for family members who need time off to address their own serious illness or in order to care for a seriously ill child, parent, spouse, or a healthy newborn or newly adopted child. An employee must have worked at least 25 hours per week for one year to be covered. The law allows companies to exempt their highest paid workers. Employees may enforce their rights by filing a lawsuit within two years of any alleged discrimination.

The Family and Medical Leave Act affects cancer survivors in the

following ways. It—
- provides 12 weeks of unpaid leave during any 12-month period;
- requires employers to continue to provide benefits—including health insurance—during the leave period;
- requires employers to restore employees to the same or equivalent position at the end of the leave period;
- allows leave to care for a spouse, child, or parent who has a "serious health condition;"
- allows leave because a serious health condition renders the employee "unable to perform the functions of the position;"
- allows an intermittent or reduced work schedule when "medically necessary" (under some circumstances, an employer may transfer the employee to a position with equivalent pay and benefits to accommodate the new work schedule);
- requires employees to make reasonable efforts to schedule foreseeable medical care so as to not to disrupt unduly the workplace;
- requires employees to give employers 30 days notice of foreseeable medical leave or as much notice as is practicable;
- allows employers to require employees to provide certification of medical needs and allows employers to seek a second opinion (at employer's expense) to corroborate medical need;
- permits employers to provide more generous leave provisions than those required by the Family and Medical Leave Act; and
- allows employees to "stack" leave under the Family and Medical Leave Act with leave allowable under state medical leave law.

You have up to two years (three for "willful violations") to file a lawsuit in federal court or to file a complaint with the Employment Standards Administration, Wage and Hour Division of the United States Department of Labor. Check your local telephone book under "United States Government" for your regional office of the Wage and Hour Division.

THE EMPLOYEE RETIREMENT AND INCOME SECURITY ACT (ERISA) – *What ERISA requires* – The Employee Retirement and Income Security Act may provide a remedy to an employee who has been denied full participation in an employee benefit plan because of a cancer history. ERISA prohibits an employer from discriminating against an employee for the purpose of preventing him or her from collecting benefits under an employee benefit plan. All employers who offer benefit packages to their employees are subject to ERISA. (For a more complete description of ERISA, see Chapter 8).

STATE LAWS

STATE EMPLOYMENT DISCRIMINATION LAWS – Most employers have to comply with federal and state employment discrimination laws. Cancer survivors who face discrimination by employers not covered by federal law must turn to state laws for relief. Every state has a law that regulates, to some extent, employment discrimination against people with disabilities. The application of these laws to cancer based discrimination varies widely.

Many state laws have been amended recently to parallel the requirements of the ADA. Most state laws cover cancer survivors because they prohibit job discrimination against persons who—
- have a disability;
- have a record of a disability; or
- are regarded by others as having a disability.

State and federal laws define "disability" in a variety of ways. For example, you may have a "disability" under the ADA, yet not have a "disability" as defined by your state law or the by Social Security Act.

All states except Alabama and Mississippi have laws that prohibit discrimination against people with disabilities in public and private employment. Alabama and Mississippi laws, which have not been amended since the 1970s, cover only state employees. Several states, such as New Jersey, cover all employers regardless of the number of employees. The laws in most states, however, cover only employers with a minimum number of employees. The range is from three (Connecticut) to twenty employees (Delaware).

In states that do not protect individuals with a record of a disability or those who are regarded by others as having a disability, you actually must be disabled by your cancer to be protected by the law. A few states, such as California, the District of Columbia, Florida, Vermont, and West Virginia, expressly prohibit discrimination against cancer survivors.

Cancer survivors have brought successful employment discrimination cases to state courts. For example, Renee Engel was fired from her job as a financial analyst with the Seattle Fire Department after she was diagnosed with ovarian cancer in 1990. She filed a lawsuit in state court in 1992 to reclaim lost wages, five years of lost seniority, health care benefits, vacation, sick leave, and retirement. A jury unanimously ruled in her favor and ordered the city of Seattle to pay her $264,000 for economic damage, back pay, lost benefits, and pain and suffering. The judge also ordered the city of Seattle to pay her attorneys' fees ($58,000).

Any type of employer, including a law firm, may violate state laws regarding cancer survivors' rights. For four years, Jane Karuschkat worked as a capable and loyal legal secretary for a small New York law firm. Then in 1992, she was diagnosed with stage III invasive breast cancer. In an effort to minimize the impact of her illness on her coworkers, Ms. Karuschkat scheduled medical appointments during lunch hours, after work, or on weekends. She even returned to work full-time only ten days after having a mastectomy. Less than two months after her diagnosis, Jessel Rothman, the attorney who owned the law firm, told her that she was fired because he could not "afford" to keep her. At that time, she still had not used all of her vacation and sick days.

Ms. Karuschkat sued her employer in state court for violating the New York Human Rights Act. After a lengthy trial, the State Division of Human Rights ruled in 1996 that Mr. Rothman illegally fired Ms. Karuschkat solely because she had breast cancer, and that he failed to provide her reasonable accommodation (flextime for chemotherapy treatments—one Monday a month for six months). The court ordered Mr. Rothman to pay her $34,679.50 in back pay, $50,000 for emotional distress, pain, suffering and humiliation, and to stop discriminating against his employees based on their disabilities.

Although state discrimination laws vary substantially, they all share one thing in common with the federal law: only "qualified" workers are entitled to relief. For example, a federal court ruled that a nursing home could force Carol Klein, a licensed physical therapist, to retire in 1990 while she was being treated for colon cancer that had metastasized to her brain and lung. The United States Court of Appeals for the Sixth Circuit found that Ms. Klein was not "qualified" to perform her job at the time she resigned because she was unable to perform the "essential functions" of the job, even with reasonable accommodations. The court held that the nursing home did not violate Ms. Klein's rights under either Ohio law or the Federal Rehabilitation Act.

Most state laws prohibit discrimination in "terms and conditions of employment," such as salary, benefits, duties, and promotional opportunities. Some state laws, like the federal ADA, require employers to provide reasonable accommodations for an employee's disability. The most protective laws prohibit employers from asking about your medical history until after they offer you a job.

The type of remedy to which you may be entitled depends not only on the state where you work, but on where your complaint is resolved (state agency or state court). Most states offer some or all of the following remedies:
- An order requiring the employer to "cease and desist" discriminatory activity.
- An offer for a position which you were denied.
- Reinstatement if you were fired or demoted.

- Back pay.
- Lost benefits (such as insurance and seniority).
- Money to compensate you for your injury.
- The costs of filing the complaint (court and attorney's fees).

Most states have a state agency that enforces the state's fair employment practices law. Some states permit you to file a lawsuit in state court to enforce your rights. Others require you to file a complaint with the state agency before or instead of going to court. Under most state laws, you have up to 180 days from the time you learn of the action against you to file a complaint with your state enforcement agency.

More information about the laws in your state is available from—
- your state division on civil rights or human rights commission;
- an attorney who is experienced in job discrimination cases;
- the EEOC Public Information System at (800) 669-4000 for help locating the appropriate state enforcement agency;

Although each state has different procedures, most state agencies will handle a complaint using the following four steps:
1. An investigator will accept a complaint signed by you if you believe an employer has violated your rights under the state antidiscrimination law.
2. The investigator will ask the employer to present his or her side of the story.
3. If the investigator decides that you did not state a claim under the law, he or she will dismiss your case. If the investigator decides that you may have a legitimate claim against the employer, he or she will try to get you and the employer to reach a fair settlement. Most complaints are resolved at this stage.
4. If you and the employer cannot come to an agreement, the investigator may recommend that your case be heard by a judge. Most states allow you or your employer to appeal an unfavorable decision to a court or to a higher level in the state agency.

For example, the New York State Division of Human Rights ruled that a medical institute violated a cancer survivor's rights under the New York Human Rights Law, which prohibits discrimination based on disability. Lisa Goldsmith, MD, applied for admission in 1976 to the New York Psychoanalytic Institute. Three committees had to approve her admission. Two of the committees found that Dr. Goldsmith was highly qualified and gave her excellent evaluations. The third committee rejected her application because of her cancer history. Dr. Goldsmith had been treated for Hodgkin's disease, but had been in remission since April 1974. The Institute allowed reapplications, but turned Dr. Goldsmith down again in 1978.

Dr. Goldsmith filed a complaint with the New York Human Rights Division. The Division found that the Institute's actions were unlawful because they were based solely on Dr. Goldsmith's cancer history.

The Institute appealed the decision to state court. The Appellate Division of the New York Supreme Court affirmed the Division's decision. The court reasoned that the Institute denied a qualified applicant like Dr. Goldsmith the opportunity to enjoy a full and productive life after her cancer experience.

Idaho, Louisiana, and a number of states that have an enforcement agency allow you to enforce the law yourself by filing a lawsuit in state court. You should consult with a private attorney and a state agency before making a choice. Each state has different rules regarding when you may file a lawsuit in state court. Choosing where to file a complaint (state agency or court) involves a number of factors (such as which forum is likely to provide the swiftest solution, what remedies are available, and whether you can maintain an agency complaint and a lawsuit simultaneously). As under federal law, you do not have to hire an attorney to file a state law employment discrimination complaint for you. An experienced attorney, however, can help you evaluate your chances of obtaining the remedy you desire and can draft the complaint in a way to best represent your claim.

STATE MEDICAL LEAVE LAWS – Approximately half of the states have leave laws similar to the Federal Family and Medical Leave Act in that they guarantee employees in the private sector unpaid leave for pregnancy, childbirth, and the adoption of a child. As of 1996, however, only 12 states also provide employees with medical leave to address a serious illness, such as cancer. Of those, only six states (Alaska, California, Connecticut, Maine, Rhode Island and Vermont) and the District of Columbia provide coverage more extensive than the Family and Medical Leave Act:

> Alaska employers with 21 or more employees must grant unpaid leave of up to 18 weeks to care for a seriously ill family member.
> California employers with 50 or more employees must grant unpaid leave of up to four months to care for a seriously ill child, spouse, or parent.
> Connecticut employers with 75 or more employees must grant unpaid leave of up to 16 weeks to care for a seriously ill child, spouse, or parent.

- District of Columbia employers with 20 or more employees must grant unpaid leave of up to 16 weeks to care for a seriously ill child, spouse, or parent.
- Hawaii employers with 100 or more employees must grant unpaid leave of up to four weeks to care for a seriously ill child, spouse, or parent.
- Maine employers with 25 or more employees must grant unpaid leave of up to ten weeks to care for a seriously ill family member.
- New Jersey employers with 50 or more employees must grant unpaid leave of up to 12 weeks to care for a seriously ill child, spouse, or parent.
- Oregon employers with 50 or more employees must grant unpaid leave of up to 12 weeks to care for a seriously ill family member.
- Rhode Island employers with 50 or more employees must grant unpaid leave of up to 13 weeks to care for a seriously ill family member.
- Vermont employers with 15 or more employees must grant unpaid leave of up to 12 weeks to care for a seriously ill family member.
- Washington employers with 100 or more employees must grant unpaid leave of up to 12 weeks to care for a child under 18 years old who is terminally ill.
- Wisconsin employers with 50 or more employees must grant unpaid leave of up to two weeks to care for a parent, child, or spouse with a serious health condition.

These state leave laws vary widely as to when leave can be taken, which employees are covered (most states require an employee to have worked for a minimum period of time), how much notice an employee must give prior to taking leave, whether benefits are continued and who pays for them, and how the law is enforced (state agency or private lawsuit). Contact your state employment antidiscrimination enforcement agency (see page 315 for a list of state agencies) for more information on how to enforce your rights under your state medical leave law.

STATE LAWS GOVERNING ACCESS TO YOUR EMPLOYMENT RECORDS – Employers are entitled to collect all medical information about you necessary to ensure that you are qualified for your job and for health insurance purposes. This may include information about your cancer history. A few states have laws that specify what information an employer may keep in your personnel file. In general, employers may disclose information about your medical history only to persons with a legitimate need to know for a legitimate business reason. Many cancer survivors, however, find that their medical history was revealed improperly by their employer or coworkers to other employees, prospective employers, insurance agents, and creditors.

You can take several steps to decrease the chance your cancer history will be revealed. If you tell your employer or coworkers about your medical history, be specific about whether you want the information to remain private. Ask your doctors, nurses, and social workers not to disclose your medical history to anyone without your written permission. If your employer reveals your cancer history without your permission, you may have a claim for invasion of privacy. (See pages 53 for more information about your medical records and privacy rights.)

How to Avoid Employment Discrimination

Lawsuits are neither the only nor usually the best way to fight employment discrimination. State and federal anti-discrimination laws help cancer survivors in two ways. First, they discourage discrimination. Second, they offer remedies when discrimination does occur. These laws, however, should be used as a last resort because they can be costly, time consuming, and may not result in a fair solution.

The first step is to try to avoid discrimination. If that fails, the next step is to attempt a reasonable settlement with the employer. If informal efforts fail, however, a lawsuit may be the most effective next step. The most constructive efforts against cancer-based discrimination are those that eliminate opportunities for discrimination in the first place. The following are some steps that cancer survivors can take to lessen the chance of encountering employment discrimination.

Do Not Volunteer the Information That You Have or Have Had Cancer Unless It Directly Affects Your Qualifications for a Job – An employer has the right—under accepted business practices and most state and federal laws—to know only if you can perform the essential duties of the job. Unless it directly affects your ability to do that job, you have no obligation to disclose your medical history any more than any other personal or confidential information. Few jobs, for example, require a woman to have two breasts or a man to have a prostate gland.

Do Not Lie On a Job or Insurance Application – If you are hired and your employer later learns that you lied, you may legally be fired for your dishonesty. Insurance companies may refuse to pay benefits or they may cancel your coverage. Federal and state laws that prohibit employment discrimination do not guarantee that all employers will refrain from illegally asking survivors about their cancer histories or about gaps in their education or employment. If you are asked a question that you think is illegal, give an honest (and perhaps indirect) answer that emphasizes your current abilities to do the job.

KEEP IN MIND YOUR LEGAL RIGHTS. – For example, under the Americans with Disabilities Act, an employer may not ask about your medical history, require you to take a medical examination, or request medical records from your doctor before making a conditional job offer. Once an employer has made a conditional job offer, the employer can require you to submit to a medical examination only if it is required of all other applicants for the job. The medical examination may consider only your ability to perform safely the essential duties of that job.

KEEP THE FOCUS ON YOUR CURRENT ABILITY TO DO THE JOB IN QUESTION – Employers may not ask how often you were absent from past jobs, but they can ask if you can meet the employer's current attendance requirements.

If a job interviewer asks you an illegal question, such as "have you ever had cancer?" one way to respond is "That's a very interesting question. I'm a little curious. How does that question relate to the job for which I'm interviewing?" This puts the burden back on the interviewer to ask you only about your current qualifications.

If a written questionnaire asks an illegal question about your medical history, you could respond "I am presently fit to perform the duties of the job for which I am applying," or "I currently have no medical condition that would interfere with my ability to perform the duties of the job for which I am applying."

If you believe it is necessary or desirable to discuss your cancer history, do so in a way that keeps the focus on your current abilities. You should tell an interviewer what you can do (skills, experience), will do (why you want to work there), and how you will fit in with that workplace.

APPLY ONLY FOR JOBS THAT YOU ARE ABLE TO DO – An employer may reject you for a job if you are not qualified for it, regardless of your medical history.

IF YOU HAVE TO EXPLAIN A LONG PERIOD OF UNEMPLOYMENT DURING CANCER TREATMENT, IF POSSIBLE, EXPLAIN IT IN A WAY THAT SHOWS YOUR ILLNESS IS PAST, AND THAT YOU ARE IN GOOD HEALTH AND ARE EXPECTED TO REMAIN HEALTHY – One way to de-emphasize a gap in your school or work history because of cancer treatment is to organize your resume by experience and skills, instead of by date. The American economy in the 1990s resulted in so much upheaval in employment that lengthy gaps became commonplace; periods of unemployment are more commonly attributed to downsizing or technology changes than to serious illness.

OFFER YOUR EMPLOYER A LETTER FROM YOUR DOCTOR THAT EXPLAINS YOUR CURRENT HEALTH STATUS, PROGNOSIS, AND ABILITY TO PERFORM THE ESSENTIAL DUTIES OF THE JOB FOR WHICH YOU ARE APPLYING — Be prepared to educate the interviewer about your cancer and why cancer often does not result in death or disability.

ASK A JOB COUNSELOR FOR HELP WITH RESUME PREPARATION AND JOB INTERVIEWING SKILLS — Practice answers to expected questions such as "Why did you miss a year of work?" or "Why did you leave your last job?" Answers to these questions must be honest, but should stress your current qualifications for the job and not past problems, if any, resulting from your cancer experience.

IF YOU ARE INTERVIEWING FOR A JOB, DO NOT ASK ABOUT HEALTH INSURANCE UNTIL AFTER YOU HAVE BEEN GIVEN A JOB OFFER — Then ask to see the "benefits package." Once you have been offered a job, but prior to accepting it, review it to make sure it meets your needs.

IF POSSIBLE, LOOK FOR JOBS WITH STATE OR LOCAL GOVERNMENTS OR LARGE EMPLOYERS (50+ EMPLOYEES) — They are less likely than small employers to discriminate. Large employers are subject to more federal and state laws than are small employers. Because large employers have a large pool of employees participating in group health insurance, their insurance costs are less likely to be affected by the medical expenses of one employee. Do not rule out small employers, however. One study found that smaller employers tended to provide a family-type atmosphere and were more likely to offer flexible work schedules (1995 study of 422 cancer patients at the M.D. Anderson Cancer Center in Houston, Texas).

DO NOT DISCRIMINATE AGAINST YOURSELF BY ASSUMING THAT YOU HAVE A DISABILITY — Although cancer treatment leaves some survivors with serious physical or mental disabilities, many survivors are capable of performing the same duties and activities that they did prior to diagnosis. With the help of your medical team, make an honest assessment of your abilities compared with the mental and physical demands of the job.

How to Enforce Your Legal Rights

Cancer survivors have numerous options to enforce their legal rights. If you suspect that you are being treated differently at work because of your cancer history, consider an informal solution before leaping into a lawsuit. You want to stand up for your legal rights without casting yourself as a troublemaker.

If you face discrimination, consider the following suggestions.

CONSIDER USING YOUR EMPLOYER'S POLICIES AND PROCEDURES FOR RESOLVING EMPLOYMENT ISSUES INFORMALLY – All state and local government employers are required to have a grievance procedure and a designated compliance officer for civil rights violations of persons with disabilities. Many private employers have formal grievance procedures.

TELL YOUR EMPLOYER THAT YOU ARE AWARE OF YOUR LEGAL RIGHTS AND WOULD RATHER RESOLVE THE ISSUES OPENLY AND HONESTLY THAN FILE A LAWSUIT – Be careful of what you say during discussions so that your employer will not use something you say to hurt your claim should your discussions fail to resolve the problem.

Timothy Calonita, a Long Island attorney and Hodgkin's disease survivor, counseled one survivor through a potential job problem without having to resort to a lawsuit. Another Hodgkin's disease survivor who was eight-months pregnant, took time off from her job at a bank for cancer treatment. After having a healthy baby, she returned to her workplace seeking reinstatement. The bank manager told her that he had no openings, but that another branch several hours away in a less desirable neighborhood could hire her. Instead of taking the less desirable position or immediately filing a legal complaint, the survivor made an appointment with the regional manager of the bank. She brought with her newspaper articles about employment discrimination against cancer survivors. She then praised the regional manager, thanking him for continuing her employment at the bank and for not responding to her cancer like those employers vilified in the newspaper articles. The end result: the regional manager promoted her to a position in her old branch.

IF YOU NEED TO BE ACCOMMODATED IN SOME WAY TO HELP YOU WORK, SUCH AS FLEXIBLE WORKING HOURS IN ORDER TO KEEP DOCTOR'S APPOINTMENTS, SUGGEST SEVERAL ALTERNATIVES TO YOUR EMPLOYER– The following situation suggests one possible reaction to employment discrimination.

> I tried to return to work, but my employer said my old job wasn't there. (It's being filled by two part-time people). I knew things like this happened, but I didn't think it could happen in a small town. Of course you probably know the rest of the story—no job, no health insurance. We shouldn't sit back and let things like this happen, we have to keep fighting.
>
> *James D. Moll*
> *Hodgkin's disease survivor*

You must receive chemotherapy one day a week. Your doctor will give you Friday afternoon appointments. You inform your boss who says, "I'm sorry, but I'll have to let you go because your job demands that you work at least forty hours per week."

One way to respond is, "My doctor and I believe I am able to continue working. Because I can stay at work until 1:00 P.M. on Fridays, I would be pleased to work an extra hour or two Monday through Thursdays to make up the missed time. My doctor anticipates that I will need chemotherapy only for _____ weeks, so I should be back to my regular schedule by _____. I understand that the state human rights law protects my right to work if I am able to continue to perform my job despite my illness."

If your employer offers to accommodate you, do not turn down the offer lightly. Such an offer may be in the employer's favor if the case ends up before a judge. The Job Accommodation Network, a free service of the President's Committee on Employment of People with Disabilities, helps employers fashion accommodations for employees with disabilities. Call (800) ADA-WORK for more information.

EDUCATE EMPLOYERS AND COWORKERS WHO MIGHT BELIEVE THAT PEOPLE CANNOT SURVIVE CANCER OR REMAIN PRODUCTIVE WORKERS – You might, for example, give your employer a letter from your doctor explaining the type of cancer you have or have had, and why you are able to work. More than ten million Americans are cancer survivors, so there is a good chance that some of your coworkers may have had cancer and are now valued employees.

ASK A MEMBER OF YOUR HEALTH-CARE TEAM TO WRITE OR CALL YOUR EMPLOYER TO OFFER TO MEDIATE THE CONFLICT, AND SUGGEST WAYS FOR YOUR EMPLOYER TO ACCOMMODATE YOU.

SEEK SUPPORT FROM YOUR COWORKERS – They have an interest in protecting themselves from future discrimination.

Despite good personal advocacy, sometimes informal solutions fail. Cancer survivors should then take the following steps to preserve their rights to seek a legal remedy:

KEEP CAREFULLY WRITTEN RECORDS OF ALL RELEVANT EVENTS AT WORK – In a lawsuit, positive performance evaluations or good attendance records show that you were qualified for the job. Other events, however, may be evidence that your employer violated your rights, such as, for example, if your employer moves you from a job that has much public interaction to a job that has little interaction with the public after you experience hair loss from chemotherapy. Keep complete notes of telephone calls and meetings (including dates, times, and attendees), letters, and the names and addresses of witnesses. Make written notes as events occur instead of trying to recall the events weeks or months later.

PAUSE BEFORE YOU SUE – Carefully evaluate your goals. For example, do you want your job back, a change in working conditions, certain benefits, a written apology, or something else? Consider the positive and negative aspects of a lawsuit. Potential positive aspects include getting a job and monetary damages, protecting your rights, and tearing down barriers for other survivors. Potential negative aspects include long court battles with no guarantee of victory (some cases drag on for five years or more), legal fees and expenses, stress, a hostile relationship between you and the people you sue (including your employer and former coworkers), and a reputation in your field as a troublemaker.

CONSIDER AN INFORMAL SETTLEMENT OF YOUR COMPLAINT – Someone, such as a union representative, a human resources or personnel officer of your company, or a social worker may be able to assist as a mediator. Your state or federal representative or local media may help persuade your employer to treat you fairly. Keep in mind that the first step most government agencies and companies take when they receive a complaint is to try to resolve the dispute without a costly trial.

OBSERVE FILING DEADLINES SO THAT YOU DO NOT LOSE YOUR OPTION TO FILE A COMPLAINT UNDER STATE OR FEDERAL LAW – You have 180 days from the date of an action against you to file a complaint under federal law with the United States Equal Employment Opportunity Commission. If you work for the federal government, you have only 45 days to begin counseling with an agency equal employment opportunity counselor. Under most state laws, you have 180 days to file a complaint with the state agency. If you file a complaint and later change your mind, you can drop the lawsuit at any time.

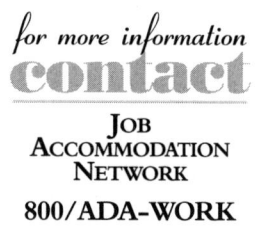

for more information
contact

JOB ACCOMMODATION NETWORK
800/ADA-WORK

If you decide to file a complaint with an agency or in state court, the following suggestions may ease your legal journey:

YOU ARE YOUR BEST ADVOCATE – Federal and state agencies, as well as federal and state courts, handle thousands of cases annually. Litigation can drag on for years. If you have a case in the system, periodically followup on the status of your case with a letter or telephone call, either personally or through your lawyer. Educate your lawyer and the agency or court about your type of cancer and your specific abilities. The more your attorney knows about you, the better he or she can help you.

CHOOSE THE AGENCY MOST RESPONSIVE TO YOU – In some situations, a single act may support a claim of discrimination under more than one law. For example, a cancer survivor who is denied a job by an employer in New York City may have a claim under the New York Human Rights Law (state), the New York City Law on Human Rights (city), and the Americans with Disabilities Act (federal).

If you have a choice of remedies, you may file a complaint with each relevant enforcement agency. One agency may "stay" (not act on) your claim until another agency issues a decision. You may always drop a complaint at any time once you determine which agency is most responsive to your claim. Factors to consider when choosing a resource include the types of remedies available, how quickly the agency responds to complaints (ask them how long the process usually takes), and which office is most convenient to you.

BE PREPARED TO ENDURE THE NUMEROUS STAGES OF LITIGATION – If you file a lawsuit, you have the initial burden of "stating a claim under the law." This means that you must allege facts that, if true, would entitle you to win your lawsuit unless your employer had a legitimate defense. "Stating a claim under the law" does not mean you automatically win. It does mean, however, that you have alleged sufficient facts to have your day in court. To state a claim that your employer violated the law, you must produce facts that show each of the following:
- You have a cancer history (or your employer mistakenly thought you had cancer).
- You were qualified for the job.
- You were denied the position, fired, or treated unfairly despite your qualifications.
- The employer sought to fill or filled the position with someone who did not have a disability or was not regarded as being disabled.

As an example, the following facts would state a claim under the Americans with Disabilities Act:
- You have breast cancer (you have a physical impairment that substantially limits a major life activity).
- You have twenty years experience as an office manager of a company with twenty employees and you always received good performance evaluations (you are qualified for your job).
- You took three weeks off for breast cancer surgery and can receive follow-up treatments without affecting your work schedule (you are able to perform the duties of your job).
- Your company fired you the day you returned to work because it did not want the risk of having to hire a temporary worker should you become unable to work in the future (discrimination because of speculative fear of future disability).

The following scenario would not state a claim under the ADA:
- You work as a receptionist for a company with 13 employees (employer too small to be subject to the ADA).
- You have a laryngectomy and learn esophageal speech, and your employer transfers you to a lower paying job after receiving customer complaints that they can not understand you (you are unable to perform reasonably the essential duties of a receptionist).

Once you have stated a claim, the burden then shifts to the employer to raise a legitimate defense. The most common defenses are—
- you were not qualified for the job;
- we looked at your qualifications, not your cancer history;
- we are reorganizing and dismissed everyone in your department.

If the employer raises a defense, the burden shifts back to you to show that its defense is a pretext to hide the truth.

Most lawsuits, like agency investigations, are either settled or dismissed. If you do go to trial and win your lawsuit, a federal or state judge may order your employer to reinstate you and to compensate you for your harm, including back pay, and your attorney's fees.

BE PREPARED FOR ANY RESULT – Even if your legal rights were violated, there is no guarantee that a public agency or court will provide you a fair remedy. Sometimes a well-financed employer can wear down the plaintiff with seemingly endless motions and appeals. A trained job counselor, social worker, nurse, or clergy may help you deal with the personal issues that result from employment discrimination due to your cancer history.

CHOOSE A LAWYER WHO HAS EXPERIENCE IN EMPLOYMENT DISCRIMINATION – You do not have to have a lawyer to represent you before an enforcement agency or court. However, someone who is represented by a lawyer experienced in job discrimination, especially the legal rights of people with disabilities, is more likely to meet with success.

FINDING A LAWYER

You can receive help in finding a lawyer experienced in employment discrimination by contacting:

YOUR LOCAL BAR ASSOCIATION – Most county and state bar associations have a lawyer referral service that provides the names of lawyers in your area who have experience in job discrimination. Many can also refer you to a local public interest law center. Look in the telephone book under "State" and "County" listings, as well as under "Lawyer Referral Services," "Legal Services," and "Attorneys" and "Lawyers."

YOUR REGIONAL EEOC OFFICE – Some EEOC offices provide attorney referrals.

LOCAL ORGANIZATIONS THAT PROVIDE CANCER SURVIVORS' SUPPORT AND SERVICES – Some local cancer organizations and hospitals keep a list of lawyers who represent cancer survivors in job discrimination cases.

NATIONAL CANCER ORGANIZATIONS
  The National Coalition for Cancer Survivorship
  1010 Wayne Avenue, Fifth Floor
  Silver Spring, MD 20910
  (301) 650-8868
  NCCS provides publications, answers to questions about employment rights, and assistance in locating legal resources.

  Cancer Care, Inc.
  1180 Avenue of the Americas
  New York, NY 10036
  (212) 302-2400 or (800) 813-HOPE
  Cancer Care provides assistance by oncology social workers, including answers to questions about employment rights and assistance locating legal resources.

Candlelighters Childhood Cancer Foundation's Ombudsman Program
7910 Woodmont Avenue, Suite 460
Bethesda, MD 20814
(800) 366-2223
Services to young cancer patients, survivors, and their families include insurance reimbursement strategies, employment discrimination assistance in the context of the Americans with Disabilities Act, enforcement of special education rights under federal and state law, securing and maintaining government benefits including Medicaid and SSI, and a second opinion referral program.

American Cancer Society (ACS)
(800) ACS-2345
Services vary widely from county to county. Some ACS units may be able to help you find a lawyer.

NATIONAL ATTORNEY REFERRAL ORGANIZATIONS.
National Employment Lawyers Association
600 Harrison Street, Suite 535
San Francisco, CA 94107
The NELA is a nonprofit, professional membership organization of more than 2,600 lawyers from around the country who represent employees in employment matters. To request a state listing of employment lawyers, please send a written request and a self-addressed, stamped, letter-sized envelope to the NELA at the above address. Please allow four to six weeks for delivery.

LOCAL PUBLIC INTEREST LAW CENTERS AND DISABILITY RIGHTS ORGANIZATIONS – Many large cities have public interest law centers that can recommend attorneys with experience in civil rights litigation. Some organizations that advocate on behalf of individuals with disabilities, such as the United Cerebral Palsy Association, may offer legal referrals in your community.

WORKER'S COMPENSATION LAWS

Worker's compensation laws provide fixed income and medical expenses to employees or their dependents in case of employment related accidents and illness. The purpose of worker's compensation laws is to compensate workers who are injured on the job without the complexities of litigation. In short, worker's compensation are no-fault health benefits.

Worker's compensation laws are commonly applied to cases where an employee is hurt in an accident at work. Workers who contract occupational cancers (for example, miners, shipyard workers, and nuclear power plant employees) may be entitled to worker's compensation. In some cases, workers have recovered benefits where an injury at work aggravated a preexisting cancerous condition. However, because the cause of cancer often is unknown, cancer is not generally considered an injury caused by work. In most cases, you must obtain expert medical testimony to show that your work caused or aggravated your cancer.

Workers benefit from these laws because, in order to collect compensation, they do not have to prove that their employer negligently harmed them. Employers are strictly liable to their workers who are hurt on the job. Employers benefit because they agree to pay a fixed benefit to an injured employee in return for protection from being sued. Worker's compensation is the only remedy the worker is entitled to receive. A worker who accepts worker's compensation benefits for one injury may not then sue his employer for causing that injury.

Worker's compensation laws are state laws. State laws vary as to the amount of compensation, the types of employment covered, and the duration of benefits. Federal employees are covered by a separate law, the Federal Employees Compensation Act. For information about the law in your state, contact your state Department of Labor or Worker's Compensation Division (look under "State Government" in your telephone book).

Unemployment Disability Laws

Some states provide for unemployment disability benefits for people who are unable to work because of illness or injury unrelated to their jobs. The worker and his or her physician must usually fill out a form provided by the employer in order to receive disability benefits. Benefits (some percentage of the weekly wage) are paid until the disability ends or a fixed period of time has passed. State laws do not guarantee that a worker may return to his or her job. An employer may replace the worker for any legitimate business reason. For information about the law in your state, contact the state Department of Labor or Unemployment Division.

Vocational Rehabilitation

Some cancer survivors, especially those who were physically disabled by their treatment, may benefit from vocational rehabilitation services offered by public and private agencies. Vocational rehabilitation services help people whose disabilities make it hard to find or keep a job. Depending on the agency, services may include financial assistance, job training and counseling, and the provision of special equipment.

One important way in which rehabilitation services help cancer survivors is to suggest job accommodations. A job accommodation is a change in the job or workplace that fairly balances the worker's abilities with the employer's needs.

Cancer survivors can benefit from many types of job accommodations, including flexible work hours to accommodate medical treatments; "borrowing" sick days from future years; changing job duties (such as reducing lifting); redesigning the equipment used to perform a job and retraining a worker for a new skill.

For example, an accommodation for a survivor whose larynx has been removed may include speech therapy and electronic speech aids. Vocational rehabilitation may be appropriate for survivors at different stages of work, including those who are entering the job market for the first time, entering the job market after retraining, or those unable to perform the duties of the previous job.

Resources are available to help your employer create an appropriate accommodation. The Job Accommodation Network, a free service of the President's Committee on Employment of the Handicapped, was established in 1984 to provide information on practical job accommodations (see page 234 for the address and telephone number). The Network has a toll-free number to reach a consultant who can suggest appropriate accommodations for a particular situation. Any company, regardless of size, may call the Network whenever it has a disabled employee whom it wants to promote, help return to work from injury or illness, help perform a present job more easily, or hire for a vacant job.

STATE VOCATIONAL REHABILITATION RESOURCES – Every state has a vocational rehabilitation agency that provides direct services to individuals. You are covered by the agency in the state where you live, not where you work.

The Federal Rehabilitation Act requires state rehabilitation agencies to provide the following minimum services:
- Evaluation of your rehabilitation potential;
- Counseling and guidance;
- Placement services;
- Rehabilitation engineering services if you need physical accommodations, such as a special piece of equipment (the agency is not required to provide you the equipment, but it must help determine what type of equipment would assist you).

In addition to these minimum services, many states offer additional services, such as transportation and special equipment.

You can find your state rehabilitation agency in the telephone directory under one of the following state departments: Labor, Human Resources, Public Welfare, Human Services, or Education. In addition, some states have independent rehabilitation commissions, listed under "Vocational Rehabilitation Services" or "Rehabilitation Services."

FEDERAL VOCATIONAL REHABILITATION RESOURCES – Although the federal Rehabilitation Services Administration does not provide direct services, it is responsible for ensuring that each state agency complies with federal law. If you believe your state agency is unreasonably denying you rehabilitation services, you may file a complaint with

> United States Department of Education
> Rehabilitation Services Administration
> Office of the Commissioner
> Office of Special Education and Rehabilitation Services
> 330 C Street, S.W.
> Washington, DC 20202
> (202) 732-1282

For help in creating an accommodation, your employer may contact

> Job Accommodation Network
> President's Committee on Employment of People with Disabilities
> P.O. Box 468
> Morgantown, WV 26505
> (800) JAN-PCEH (526-7234)

You may choose between filing a lawsuit in court or filing a complaint with the Employment Standards Administration, Wage and Hour Division of the United States Department of Labor. Check your local telephone book under "United States Government" for your regional office of the Wage and Hour Division. Most complaints filed with the Wage and Hour Division are resolved informally.

CONCLUSION

Unlike the cancer survivors of thirty years ago, survivors today have expanding job opportunities. Not only has the quality of life after cancer treatment improved, but new state and federal laws require employers to treat survivors based on their individual abilities and not their cancer history. No longer can employers assume that cancer survivors are unproductive liabilities to be avoided or dismissed. Survivors should be aware of their legal rights—and be willing to advocate for themselves and others—so they can protect their right to be treated with fairness and dignity at work.

Chapter Ten

Legal and Financial Concerns

by Barbara Hoffman, JD

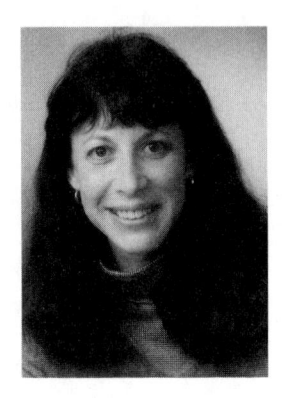

BARBARA HOFFMAN, JD is a cofounder of the National Coalition for Cancer Survivorship, serves as its general counsel, and has testified as an advocate for survivors before federal and state congressional committees. Ms. Hoffman is codirector of the Appellate Advocacy Program at Seton Hall University School of Law, where she teaches disability law and other subjects. She has provided information on the legal rights of cancer survivors at over 70 conferences and workshops, on television and radio, and in many publications. Ms. Hoffman's publications include *Charting the Journey: An Almanac of Practical Resources for Cancer Survivors,* (Mt. Vernon: Consumer Reports Books, 1990) as coeditor and more than a dozen articles in legal, medical, and consumer publications.

Cancer is not only physically and emotionally draining, it can be financially draining as well, and it could affect your legal rights. This chapter takes a look at some financial and legal questions faced by many cancer survivors and provides guidance on resolving some of these unsettling issues.

Financial Costs and Resources

The Expenses of Cancer Treatment

> When I had to give up my Empress Club card with Canada Airlines International, I felt like a spectator watching life from the outside. The loss of the club card, a symbol of my success as a salesman, symbolized my loss of full participation in life.
>
> —a multiple myeloma survivor

Cancer can have a devastating financial impact on survivors and their families. Two types of expenses are associated with cancer care: (1) direct medical costs and (2) related nonmedical expenses, such as travel to and from treatment, childcare, housekeeping assistance, and home care products.

Direct medical costs are those resulting from cancer treatment, such as physician's fees, hospital expenses, and pharmacy bills. Most of these expenses are covered by basic health insurance plans. The extent of direct medical costs to the survivor depends on the type of cancer, the extent of insurance coverage, and the community in which the survivor is treated.

Everyone recognizes that medical care for a serious illness can be quite expensive. Few people, however, are prepared for the nonmedical costs of illness until they are faced with mounting bills. Most nonmedical costs related to cancer care are not covered by health insurance. Depending on the extent of your insurance policy, you may have to pay for such nonmedical items as transportation to and from treatment, childcare, a nurse's aide, a housekeeper, a counselor, or treatment related consumer products, such as wigs or prostheses. In

Legal and Financial Concerns – **CHAPTER TEN**

addition, many survivors find that their insurance premiums are increased and sometimes insurance is discontinued after diagnoses.

Cancer can have an especially harmful financial impact on those survivors who are not employed, do not have adequate health insurance, or do not have savings or other financial resources. The cost of cancer care is particularly high for those who require expensive long-term care, including long stays in a hospital, rehabilitation, or care in a nursing home.

As survivors' costs are increasing, their income is often decreasing. Survivors who are unable to work or those who face employment discrimination may experience a loss of income and insurance benefits. As a result, many cancer survivors must dip into their savings or borrow money to pay for cancer care.

If the costs of cancer care far exceed your resources, you may want to contact a financial counselor to help you plan a budget. Look in the telephone directory under "consumer credit counseling services" for a nonprofit service that can help you manage your bills. A nonprofit service is likely to provide free or inexpensive assistance; a for-profit company will charge you a fee for its services.

If you can not locate a nonprofit service in your community, contact the National Foundation for Consumer Credit, Inc. (NFCC) for the name of a credit counseling service in your area. You can reach the NFCC at National Foundation for Consumer Credit, Inc., 8701 Georgia Avenue, Silver Spring, MD 20901; (301) 589-5600.

If you write the NFCC, include a stamped, self-addressed envelope. The NFCC is a nonprofit umbrella membership organization of more than four hundred nonprofit consumer credit counseling services. The NFCC provides confidential financial counseling for people having trouble managing their bills. No one is turned away because of inability to pay.

Private Sources of Financial Support

A number of organizations provide financial support for the costs of direct medical care and related expenses. For example, some organizations, such as the American Cancer Society, have programs that provide free transportation to and from treatment when a volunteer is available, and "lending libraries" of wigs, hospital beds, wheelchairs and other products. Other organizations offer stipends to families who cannot pay their bills.

The type and amount of financial assistance available varies from community to community. Many of these services are not advertised, but are available for the asking. Organizations to contact for financial assistance include—

- the social service department of your hospital;

---

for more information
contact

NATIONAL FOUNDATION FOR CONSUMER CREDIT

8701 Georgia Ave.
Silver Spring, MD
20901

301/589-5600

credit counseling referral

- cancer organizations;
- labor unions;
- community service organizations;
- religious organizations;
- social and fraternal organizations;
- pharmaceutical companies that offer free drugs to indigent patients;
- a local congressional representative's office; and
- the local public assistance office.

Public Sources of Financial Support

SOCIAL SECURITY BENEFITS — One source of federal financial assistance is Social Security. The Social Security Act creates several programs for providing financial assistance to qualified individuals. These programs include disability insurance benefits, unemployment compensation, and supplemental security income for the disabled. The following section describes each of the major Social Security Programs. For more information about these programs, contact the Social Security Administration's toll-free hotline at (800) 772-1213.

Retirement Benefits — To be eligible for retirement benefits, you need not be disabled or poor. All that is required is that you be of a certain age and have paid into the Social Security system for a specified number of quarters. Under certain circumstances, children of retirees may receive additional benefits.

Spouses', Survivors', and Dependents' Benefits — A widow, a widower, a surviving divorced spouse, and a child or parent of a person who was entitled to Social Security benefits may directly receive those benefits if certain conditions are met.

Supplemental Security Income (SSI) Benefits — The SSI program is designed to provide income to people with income below the federal minimum level and who are 65 or older or blind or disabled. Eligibility is determined by need, not by whether you paid into Social Security as an employee. Although SSI payments can be quite small, in many states an individual receiving SSI benefits will automatically be eligible for Medicaid and may also receive a state supplemental payment.

Disability Insurance Benefits — Disability benefits are designed to provide income to people who are unable to work because of a disability. You are entitled to receive disability benefits while you are disabled before the age of 65 if—

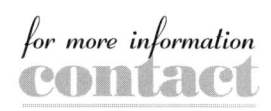

for more information **contact**
SOCIAL SECURITY ADMINISTRATION HOTLINE
800/772-1213
information about Social Security programs

Legal and Financial Concerns – **CHAPTER TEN**

- you have enough Social Security earnings to be insured for disability;
- you apply for benefits;
- you have a physical or mental disability that prevents you from doing any substantial gainful work;
- the disability is expected to last, or has lasted, at least 12 months, or is expected to result in death; and
- you have been disabled for five consecutive months.

In some cases, spouses of disabled claimants are also entitled to benefits.

The amount of disability benefits is based on a sliding scale determined by elaborate and frequently changing formulas based on your age and past earnings. An employed person may not collect benefits. Workers may not receive both workers' compensation and Social Security disability for the same illness. The medical records of individuals who apply for Social Security disability benefits are evaluated according to regulations issued by the Social Security Administration. Individuals who are denied benefits may appeal to an administrative law judge.

To determine whether your cancer is a disability under the law, the Social Security Administration considers the type of cancer you have, the extent of metastasis, and your response to treatment. Small localized tumors that respond to therapy usually do not constitute an impairment. For example, early stage prostate cancer that is successfully treated with surgery is not considered a severe impairment. Cancer that has spread beyond regional lymph nodes, however, usually is considered a severe impairment. Otherwise, your diagnosis is evaluated on a case-by-case basis.

To apply for disability benefits, you must obtain a form from your local Social Security Administration Office (look in the telephone directory under "United States Government, Department of Health and Human Services"). You can apply by mail or telephone if you are physically unable to go to the Social Security office. You should apply as soon as you become disabled because you must wait five months after you file before you begin receiving payments.

After determining that you are eligible financially, the Social Security Administration gives your application to the state disability agency to determine, according to a complex formula, whether you are disabled under the law. If you are denied benefits, you may appeal to a federal administrative law judge. The judge will hold a hearing to consider all of the evidence. If you are found to be disabled (but not permanently disabled), your case will be reviewed at least once every three years. When your condition improves and you are able to return to work, benefits will be discontinued.

VETERAN'S BENEFITS – The Department of Veterans Affairs (VA) offers a variety of benefits to veterans. Although most disability benefits apply to veterans whose disability is service-connected—which cancer seldom is—some benefits are available to cancer survivor veterans.

Depending on when you served, your age, and your income, you may be eligible for a nonservice-connected pension. An additional allowance may be paid if you are in a nursing home, if you need a home aid, or if you are housebound because of your illness.

Hospital care in VA facilities is provided to veterans who meet certain conditions, such as those who are eligible for Medicaid, those who need care related to exposure to cancer-causing substances (including dioxin, Agent Orange, and radiation), have a VA pension, or have a limited income. Outpatient care and medical equipment are also available at VA facilities under certain circumstances.

Additionally, the Department of Veterans Affairs offers a variety of other benefits to qualified veterans, including life insurance, burial benefits, a death pension to dependents if the veteran's death is non-service-connected, and civil service preference certificates for government employment.

For more information, look in the telephone directory under "United States Government, Department of Veterans Affairs," (formerly the Veterans Administration), for the number to reach a VA representative. Toll-free telephone service is available in all 50 states. If you are a beneficiary or policyholder, call the VA Insurance Service, (800) 669-8477, at any time for information about your insurance coverage.

for more information
contact
VA INSURANCE SERVICE
800/669-8477
information about insurance coverage

DEDUCTING MEDICAL EXPENSES FROM YOUR TAXES – Part of the money you spend on medical care for yourself, your spouse, and your dependents may be itemized as deductions for federal income tax purposes. Keep track of physicians' fees, costs of prescription drugs, dental expenses, home nursing fees, hospital bills, medical insurance premiums that you (not your employer) paid, laboratory bills, and transportation and lodging expenses if you sought medical care away from your home.

At the end of the calendar year, add up all of your medical expenses. From this number, you must then subtract a percentage of your gross income (for example, in 1996, you first subtracted 7.5 percent of your gross income). You may deduct the balance from your income subject to federal income tax.

For example, if your gross income was $20,000, and you had $10,000 in medical expenses, you could claim a tax deduction of $8,500 for your medical expenses.

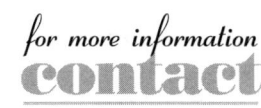

Legal and Financial Concerns – **CHAPTER TEN**

Total medical expenses $10,000
-7.5 percent of gross income   -1,500 (7.5 percent of $20,000)
Medical deduction $8,500

The Internal Revenue Service (IRS) has a number of free publications that describe deductions related to health care. An IRS counselor also will answer your questions about tax regulations over the telephone. You can reach the Internal Revenue Service at (800) 829-1040 (for information) or (800) 829-3676 (for publications).

Of the scores of free publications available from the IRS, the following are of particular relevance to the tax concerns of cancer survivors:

Publication 502 *Medical and Dental Expenses*
Publication 503 *Child and Dependent Care Expenses*
Publication 524 *Credit for the Elderly or the Disabled*
Publication 525 *Taxable and Nontaxable Income*
Publication 529 *Miscellaneous Deductions*
Publication 554 *Tax Information for Older Americans*
Publication 559 *Survivors, Executors, and Administrators*
Publication 721 *Tax Guide to U.S. Civil Service Retirement Benefits*
Publication 907 *Tax Highlights for Persons with Disabilities*

for more information
contact
INTERNAL REVENUE SERVICE

INFORMATION:
800/829-1040

PUBLICATIONS:
800/826-3676

IRS COUNSELOR

PLANNING YOUR PERSONAL AND FINANCIAL FUTURE

The anticipation of death has made it essential for me to give thought to emotional and practical preparations for my children, my mother, my helpmate and partner, and other important people in my life. I have a sense of great satisfaction in having arranged for such practical matters as wills, death benefits, trust funds, and a retirement plan. For the most part, this activity has been associated not with a sense of impending doom or imminent death but with a sense that making these arrangements now frees me from future concern.

—Robert M. Mack, MD, lung cancer survivor,
"Lessons from Living with Cancer," *New England Journal of Medicine* Vol. 311, No. 25, p.1640, December 24, 1984.

Personal and financial planning for the future is important to ensure that your desires for yourself and your property are carried out according to your intentions. Although you may have only limited control over the progress of your disease, with proper planning, you can affect how decisions concerning your medical care and property will be made even after you become incapable of doing so yourself.

PERSONAL PLANNING: ADVANCE HEALTH DIRECTIVES

In the 1990s, a cancer experience often means complicated choices among a variety of complex medical decisions. For one of every two survivors, cancer means facing the reality of death. Because it is your life, you should be the ultimate decision maker about whether to continue medical treatment. Most physicians are trained to provide all reasonable life-sustaining treatment. Because cancer may leave you physically or mentally incapable of expressing your preferences, you should express your desires in advance.

Every state has laws recognizing advance health directives. Advance directives are signed legal documents that inform your family and physicians of your choices for future medical care, including whether you want to stop or not even start life-sustaining treatment. A properly signed and witnessed directive acts as a contract between you and your physician. Your physician must honor your instructions or transfer you to the care of another doctor who will follow your directive. If you have not expressed your desires in advance, your doctors, in consultation with your close relatives, will use their discretion in choosing your medical care. The two most recognized types of advance health directives are a durable power of attorney for health care and a living will.

Durable Power of Attorney for Health Care – A durable power of attorney is a legal document that lets you appoint someone to speak for you. It allows you to transfer your legal right to make health decisions to someone you choose as your "agent" or "proxy." Durable means that your agent can make decisions for you only when you become unable to do so yourself. You can give any adult your power of attorney. Your agent need not be an attorney; most people choose a close family member or friend.

Preparing a durable power of attorney is the best way to ensure that you receive the type of medical care you want. You can specify any type of medical care. Physicians can prolong life with a variety of modern medical techniques, including surgery, drugs, respirators, tube feeding, and kidney dialysis. The more specific you are, the more likely you will receive the care you would have chosen. You should give detailed instructions concerning—

- whether and under what conditions you should receive life-sustaining treatment;
- whether and under what conditions you should have a "do not resuscitate" order (DNR);
- whether and under what conditions you should receive pain medications, artificial nutrition and hydration, or surgery;

- your preference for where you want to receive treatment (hospital, hospice, or home);
- general language that covers unanticipated events in your health, finances, or available medical treatment;
- the names and addresses of the persons you have chosen as your agents.

Avoid vague words such as hopeless, extreme, and heroic. Be specific when using words such as terminal or irreversible. You may consider your cancer terminal if your physician tells you that you are unlikely to live for more than two years; your physician may consider your cancer terminal only when you are within days of death.

Living Will – A living will is a statement that tells your family and your doctor that you do not want your life prolonged by medical procedures if you are near death without any chance for recovery. Similar to your right to refuse medical treatment, you have the right to state in advance of being incapacitated that you do not want to be kept alive by certain procedures.

A living will is not as effective as a durable power of attorney because it simply expresses your preferences to your physicians. Your physician may struggle with medical, legal, ethical, and personal values that conflict with your living will if medical circumstances or pressure from a family member intervene. Your doctor and family may not want to "lose" you, even though you may prefer to die with dignity. A durable power of attorney gives legal authority to a person—not a piece of paper—someone you know and trust to act in your place. Your agent can serve as your advocate to ensure that your wishes are carried out.

How to Make Your Future Health Care Choices - The best way to influence future medical decisions is to complete the types of health care directives recognized by your state and to discuss your decisions with your family and doctors to make sure that they will honor your wishes. Most states recognize both a durable power of attorney and a living will. These laws vary widely as to when and how you may express future medical decisions, how old you must be, and how the law is enforced.

You do not need an attorney to make a durable power of attorney or a living will. Most states provide a form to complete and have signed by witnesses. You may obtain a copy of that language at a law library or from an attorney. In addition, you can obtain state forms and instructions from Choice in Dying. Choice in Dying is a nonprofit organization which serves the needs of dying patients and their families and which is dedicated to protect the rights of the dying. Their address is Choice in Dying, 200 Varick Street, New York, NY 10014-4810; (212) 366-5540 or (800) 989-WILL.

Choose as a proxy someone you are confident will be willing and able to carry out your wishes. You may wish to appoint two proxies, the second to make decisions if the first is unable to do so. Critical medical decisions, such as withdrawing life support equipment, are very difficult. They should be entrusted only to those family members or friends who would make the same decision that you would make about your treatment.

To keep your advance health directive current, you should review it regularly, and write your initials and the date you reviewed it on the document. If you change your mind about an instruction, write in your new instruction, initial and date it. If you decide not to have a directive any more, destroy each copy. Make sure that the people who will be involved in your medical care have a copy of your health care directives. Give a copy to your doctor to keep in his or her files. Discuss your decision with your doctor and ask him or her to continue to be your advocate even if another doctor will be treating you. Keep another copy with your personal papers (not in a bank safety deposit box), so that others can find it if necessary. You may wish to place a card in your wallet that states you have a health care directive and where it can be found.

YOUR RIGHT TO REFUSE MEDICAL TREATMENT - In 1990, the United States Supreme Court ruled that the United States Constitution gives individuals the right to control their own medical care. Nancy Cruzan, 30, was admitted to a Missouri hospital after suffering permanent brain damage resulting from a car accident. Once her physicians concluded that she was in a persistent vegetative state from which she would not recover, her parents asked the hospital to discontinue artificial food and water. The hospital did not want to end treatment and ultimately allow Ms. Cruzan to die because she was incapable of expressing her own wishes.

The Supreme Court ruled that physicians must follow "clear and convincing evidence" of an individual's wishes concerning medical care. Such preferences include the right to die, even if close family members object to withholding life-sustaining treatment. The Supreme Court sent the case back to state court. The state court found clear and convincing evidence that, prior to her death, Ms. Cruzan clearly had expressed her desire not to receive life-sustaining treatment under the circumstances she faced. The court ordered the hospital to withhold treatment. Ms. Cruzan died thirteen days later.

The lesson of Ms. Cruzan is that to protect your rights, you should

for more information
contact

CHOICE IN DYING

200 Varick Street
New York, NY
10014-4810

212/366-5540

800/989-WILL

state forms and instructions for durable power of attorney and living will

Legal and Financial Concerns – **CHAPTER TEN**

provide written "clear and convincing evidence" of your desires in the form of an advance health care directive. The Patient Self-Determination Act, a federal law that took effect in 1991, requires all facilities that receive Medicare or Medicaid, such as hospitals or nursing homes, to discuss health care directives with newly admitted patients. Although it is best to prepare a directive before you go to the hospital, you can obtain your state forms when you are admitted. The law also requires the facility to record your health care directives as part of your medical records.

FINANCIAL PLANNING: PLANNING FOR YOUR PROPERTY

TRADITIONAL WILLS — A traditional will is a written document that states how you would like your property to be distributed when you die. Although contemplating writing a will may cause anxiety (few people are comfortable thinking about their own death), it is essential if you want to control how your property is distributed after your death.

A traditional will is one way for you to ensure that your decisions about your property and family are respected. Even the most simple will should perform three tasks:

1. Explain how your property should be distributed;
2. Appoint someone to take care of your minor and/or disabled children;
3. Appoint an executor (the person you choose to make sure the instructions in your will are followed).

If you die without a valid will, your state will distribute your property according to state probate laws. The result may or may not be the same result you intended. State probate laws are designed to promote fairness and predictability in estate management. They are not designed to protect your family's long term financial needs after your death.

Before you prepare a will, complete the following steps to ensure that your will reflects your carefully considered intentions:

- Discuss long-term financial needs with all family members.
- Make a list of your property (major items such as house, car, insurance policies, heirlooms).
- Decide whom ("beneficiaries") you want to receive what.
- If you have minor and/or disabled children, decide who you want to be responsible for their care and ask that person if he or she is willing to serve as your children's "testamentary guardian."
- Select your will's executor and ask that person if he or she is willing to be responsible for distributing your assets.

You may write your own will; however, your will is more likely to withstand any legal challenge if it is prepared by an attorney. Your state or local bar association can help you locate an attorney with experience in drafting wills. If your will is challenged and declared invalid, the state may disregard your intentions and distribute your property according to its probate laws. The money you save in writing your own will while you are alive may be lost several times over in court battles over your will after your death.

Each state has laws that establish formalities a will must meet to ensure that your wishes are enforced. For example, some states require that two adults witness you sign the will, while other states require three witnesses. Some states recognize a hand-written will, while other states require that it be typed.

Every state requires, at a minimum, the following three elements to recognize a will as valid:

1. If you are preparing a will, you must be capable of making decisions about your property. You must understand what the purpose of the will is, know the nature of your property, know the beneficiaries you name, and be acting on your own free will.
2. Your will must be witnessed by "disinterested witnesses." These are adults who do not stand to gain by your death and who are not named in your will as a beneficiary, executor, or trustee.
3. You must sign and date the will in the presence of the disinterested witnesses. You must also make it known to them that you intend the document to serve as your will and that you are signing it without coercion.

After you prepare a will, you must make certain it remains safe and reflects your current wishes. Give a copy of your will to your attorney and keep a copy for yourself. Because your safety deposit box may be sealed temporarily after your death, an attorney's office is the safest place to keep a will. Also, review your will every few years to determine whether it reflects your current intentions and assets. If you decide to change your will, have an attorney make the changes or write a new will to ensure that your new, and not old instructions, are followed.

TRUSTS AND ESTATES – A trust is a fiduciary relationship in which one party (the trustee) holds title to property for the benefit of another party (the beneficiary). Several different types of trusts accomplish different purposes. Trusts legally may shield your assets to keep you qualified for government benefits such as Social Security and Medicaid. For example, one way to avoid having to "spend down" your money (reduce your assets) to qualify for Medicaid is to give your money to a family member or friend in the form of a trust. Under the terms of such a trust, the family member or friend agrees to spend the money on your care.

By establishing a trust, you may appoint a "trustee" to use his or her discretion in making all decisions about your assets, or you may restrict the types of decisions the trustee may make. Some trusts take effect only once you become disabled, while others transfer decision making powers to a trustee as soon as you sign the documents. You should choose as your trustee someone who is able to make competent financial decisions regarding tasks such as operating your business, borrowing money, managing real estate, and filing your tax returns.

Trusts can be quite complex; they must comply with state laws, and they have a variety of tax consequences. You should contact an attorney to help you draw up such a trust to be certain that it will accomplish the purpose you intend. An attorney or financial adviser could help you determine if you would benefit more from creating a trust or granting a power of attorney. A power of attorney is less complicated and expensive than a trust. A trust, however, it is more flexible than a power of attorney.

POWER OF ATTORNEY – Just as you may authorize an agent to make health-care decisions for you, you may grant another person the right to make financial decisions for you by granting a "power of attorney." This is a simple and inexpensive procedure in which you nominate another person (your "agent") to act in your place and on your behalf.

When you give a power of attorney to your agent, you permit him or her to manage your assets, such as your bank accounts, stocks, and house. Many cancer survivors can relieve themselves of the burden of paying bills and making financial decisions by granting that authority to a responsible person.

Because granting or revoking a power of attorney involves the power to manage your property and must comply with state laws to be valid, you should consult with an attorney for help in preparing the documents that will express your intentions and be accepted by banks and other institutions.

OTHER LEGAL CONCERNS OF CANCER SURVIVORS

MEDICAL MALPRACTICE

Most physicians, hospitals, and other health-care providers give survivors quality cancer treatment that meets professional standards.

Health-care providers have every incentive, from personal to financial, to provide you with quality cancer treatment. In a small number of situations, however, medical care falls below professional standards. In such situations, a cancer survivor may have a claim for medical malpractice.

The 1970s brought a dramatic rise in the number of malpractice cases. Although no evidence suggests that actual malpractice increased during this time, and although the majority of cases are still dismissed without payment to the patient, patients seem to be more willing to sue their doctors for several reasons:

- Patients' expectations have risen as medical care has become more sophisticated;
- Patients no longer view their doctors as infallible;
- Damage awards per case have increased many fold;
- A growing number of attorneys advertise their willingness to handle malpractice cases;
- Courts have recognized greater patient rights.

Cancer survivors are bringing many of these malpractice cases. They sue members of their treatment team for mistakes during surgery, chemotherapy, and radiation treatments. The most common medical malpractice claim is the "failure to diagnose," and the most common of these failures is the failure to diagnose cancer.

For example, Regina Rieger was being treated in Maryland and the District of Columbia for abdominal pain. Although she had a positive hemoccult test and she told her physicians that she had an extensive history of colon cancer in her family, her doctors did not find any cancer. After several months of treatment, Ms. Rieger moved to Mississippi. The same day that she moved, a Mississippi doctor diagnosed her with colon cancer. She had surgery and substantial cancer treatment in Mississippi.

Ms. Rieger sued her previous doctors for failing to diagnose her colon cancer earlier. In 1994, a jury found that her doctors had breached their professional standard of care. A court awarded Ms. Rieger $350,000 for pain and suffering and $18,200 for economic damages.

A patient's claim may be weakened and damages reduced if he or she contributes to the malpractice by failing to follow a doctor's reasonable advice or instructions. For example, Ann Claudet was a patient of Dr. Raymond Weyrich, a Louisiana plastic surgeon. He examined her breasts on a number of occasions. Although he eventually detected a lump in her breast, he did not believe it was cancer. More than once, Ms. Claudet expressed concern to Dr. Weyrich about the lump, but he told her that there was no cause for alarm.

Although Dr. Weyrich advised her to return for a follow-up visit in three months, she waited over one year to return. Subsequently, a biopsy revealed breast cancer.

In 1995, a Louisiana jury found that Dr. Weyrich was liable for malpractice for failing to diagnose Ms. Claudet's breast cancer. The harm resulting from the delay in diagnosis, and resulting delay in treatment, substantially decreased the probability that Ms. Claudet would survive (from 75 percent to 42 percent). The jury also found that Ms. Claudet was at fault for 30 percent of her harm because she failed to follow Dr. Weyrich's advice for follow-up care. The jury determined that Ms. Claudet should be awarded $600,000 for pain and suffering, $180,000 for future lost wages, and $30,000 for future cost of insurance premiums. Because Louisiana law, like many state laws, places a cap on damages, Ms. Claudet would not be allowed to recover all of the damages.

Delay in diagnosis can be reasonable, however, and therefore, not grounds for malpractice. On March 28, 1978, Margherita Henning's doctor examined her for a lump in her breast. He took a mammogram and found no visible difference from the mammogram he took in 1976. He told Ms. Henning to observe the lump and return immediately if she noticed any changes. He told her to return in a month if she noticed no changes. Ms. Henning found no changes and returned to her doctor's office on May 8, 1978. At that time, her doctor suspected a change in the lump and scheduled a biopsy. When the biopsy revealed early breast cancer, her doctor referred her to two oncologists. Ms. Henning's treatment was unsuccessful and she died. A New Mexico court held that her doctor met the duty of skill, knowledge, and care that he owed Ms. Henning under the circumstances, that he diagnosed her breast cancer at the earliest possible stage, and that the one month delay had no effect on her outcome.

RESPONSIBILITY OF CARE – Anyone who provides your medical care has some responsibility for the quality of that care. Hospitals are responsible for their employees, and under some circumstances, for physicians who have admitting privileges. Physicians are responsible for their own work, as well as that of their employees.

All doctors and caregivers have a duty to give their patients reasonable professional medical care. This means that your doctor must act with the minimum level of skill and learning common to other doctors in his or her community and field of expertise. A specialist in one field is measured against other specialists in that same field.

What is "reasonable" depends on professional standards determined by state laws, accrediting agencies, professional societies, hospital rules, expert opinions, and common medical practice. Examples of unrea-

sonable care include the following:
- Your doctor negligently delays diagnosing your cancer, a delay which significantly changes your prognosis and/or treatment.
- Your surgeon fails to remove all malignant tumors that reasonably could be expected to be removed by a surgeon.
- You are harmed by inappropriate radiation therapy or chemotherapy that was given at a frequency, dose, or time considered not medically professional.
- Your doctor prescribed the wrong medication, or you were given the wrong amount of medication.
- Your doctor fails to perform an important test that most other similarly situated doctors would consider essential. For example, your mother and grandmother had breast cancer, and you discover a suspicious lump in your breast, but your doctor decides to wait a few months without performing any diagnostic tests.
- Your doctor was grossly negligent in treating you. For example, he stated that he was an expert in treating your type of cancer, when in fact, you were his first cancer patient.
- Your doctor erroneously and negligently diagnoses a malignancy when in fact none exists, and consequently you are subjected to needless worry or treatment.

Your doctor does not have a duty to guarantee a particular result or to provide you with the most up-to-date form of treatment. Although many patients are unhappy with the outcome of their treatment, very few have a legitimate malpractice claim against their doctor.

BRINGING A MALPRACTICE CASE – Malpractice suits are controlled by state law. Every state sets a statute of limitations, a deadline by which you may file a lawsuit. In most states, you must file a lawsuit within two or three years from either when you were actually injured or when you learned of your injury. A few states provide you only one year to file a lawsuit and a few others provide more than three years.

You can not sue your doctor simply because he or she makes an error in judgment. To bring a malpractice claim against your doctor, you must show three things:
1. Your doctor treated you for a medical condition; and
2. You were harmed by your doctor's treatment; and
3. Your doctor did not exercise reasonable professional care.

> **for more information contact**
>
> **OFFICE OF THE AMERICANS WITH DISABILITIES ACT**
>
> Civil Rights Division
> U.S. Department of Justice
> P.O. Box 66118
> Washington, D.C. 20035-6118
>
> **202/514-0301**
>
> *information on Title III rights*

Your doctor's treatment must actually have caused your injury. It need not have been the only cause of your injury, but it must have been a "substantial factor." In determining the cause of your injury, a court will consider if you contributed to your injury, for example, by smoking or failing to follow your doctor's instructions. Even if you would have died from your cancer regardless of your doctor's mistakes, your family may have a claim for malpractice if your doctor negligently hastened your death.

Like most lawsuits, most malpractice cases are either settled or dismissed. Few result in a trial. If you win a malpractice case, you may be entitled to an award that restores you or your family, at least financially, to the condition you would be in if your doctor had not made a mistake. For example, you may win lost wages, reimbursement for medical expenses, and an award for "pain and suffering." The types and amounts of damages available are determined by state law. If you are considering a lawsuit, you should consult with an attorney who has experience in medical malpractice cases. Your local or state bar association may be able to provide you a referral.

ACCESS TO FINANCIAL CREDIT

Before the 1990s, cancer survivors occasionally faced discrimination in applying for credit, such as educational loans and mortgages. The Americans with Disabilities Act (ADA), passed in 1990, prohibits this type of discrimination.

Title III of the ADA, which took effect on January 26, 1992, provides that "[n]o individual shall be discriminated against on the basis of disability in the full and equal enjoyment of goods, services, facilities, privileges, advantages, or accommodation of any place of public accommodation by any person who owns, leases (or leases to), or operates a place of public accommodation." Banks and other financial institutions are "public accommodations." Cancer survivors are protected as individuals with a disability (see pages 210 to 211 for a discussion of how the ADA covers cancer survivors).

A cancer survivor may not be denied a loan or other financial service solely because of his or her cancer history. A financial institution must consider whether its credit policies screen out individuals with disabilities or unreasonably impede access to credit. A financial institution has the burden of proving that its credit policy is necessary as a sound business practice.

You can file a lawsuit in federal court to enforce Title III of the ADA. The only remedy available through a private lawsuit, however, is an injunction (an order to stop the discriminatory practice). You also may file a complaint with the United States Attorney General, who is authorized to bring lawsuits in cases of general public importance or where a "pattern or practice" of discrimination may exist. In these cases, the attorney general may seek monetary damages and civil penalties. For more information on how to enforce your rights under Title III of the ADA, contact the Office on the Americans with Disabilities Act, Civil Rights Division, U.S. Department of Justice, P.O. Box 66118, Washington, DC 20035-6118; (202) 514-0301.

ADOPTING A CHILD

Some children and young adults who are treated for cancer face fertility problems as a result of their cancer or treatment. Adoption is one alternative for survivors who want children. Survivors should be well prepared before initiating an adoption because some cancer survivors face barriers in adopting a child solely related to their cancer experience.

Domestic and international adoptions can be arranged through private and public licensed adoption agencies or through attorneys. Adoption laws are regulated by state, federal and, when appropriate, international laws.

All prospective adoptive parents must have a preadoptive home study completed by a licensed adoption agency. The home study includes a medical exam by the prospective parents' physician. The physician also must complete a medical report that describes your current health status and history of chronic illness. You should answer all questions in an honest, detailed, and positive manner. An agency is most likely to accept a physician's evaluation if it is sufficiently detailed to present an accurate picture of your current health and prognosis.

Adoption agencies may not discriminate against cancer survivors solely because of their cancer histories. An adoption agency is a "public accommodation" under Title III of the Americans with Disabilities Act. Accordingly, it may not prohibit all cancer survivors from adopting. It must consider survivors on an individual basis and consider their health as they would any other applicant.

An adoption agency must consider whether its criteria to determine who may adopt a child screen out individuals with disabilities or unreasonably burden the adoption process. An adoption agency has the burden of proving that its criteria are necessary to ensure appropriate adoptions. Because the right to equal treatment by an adoption agency is provided by Title III of the ADA, the enforcement procedures are the same as described on pages 212 to 213.

Shop carefully for an adoption agency, physician, and attorney. They must understand the medical and emotional impact of your cancer history and be able to work with you in securing an appropriate adoption. They should work together as your advocates in securing your right to adopt.

Many organizations provide information about coping with infertility and adoption. For information on infertility resources, contact—

>   Resolve
>   1310 Broadway
>   Somerville, MA 02144-1731
>   (617) 623-1156 (business office)
>   (617) 623-0744 (helpline)

Information on adoption, including a list of agencies, resources and local support groups can be obtained from—

>   Adoptive Families of America
>   3333 Highway 100 North
>   Minneapolis, MN 55422
>   (800) 372-3300
>   (612) 535-7808 (fax)

>   International Committee for Concerns of Children
>   911 Cypress Drive
>   Boulder, CO 80303
>   (303) 494-8333

You can obtain a directory of adoption attorneys by state from—

>   American Academy of Adoption Attorneys
>   P.O. Box 33053
>   Washington, DC 20033

LEAF SONG

The leaves ran along
The sidewalk at my feet.
Blown hard and loud
Rushing past like a song.
It was from China
Or Japan or the Far East
A sound like bamboo chimes
A note-filled message of rhymes.
Simply mine and spoken to me
Because I stood and listened
I heard what the wind said
I shall caress and carry thee.
— Susan Roberts

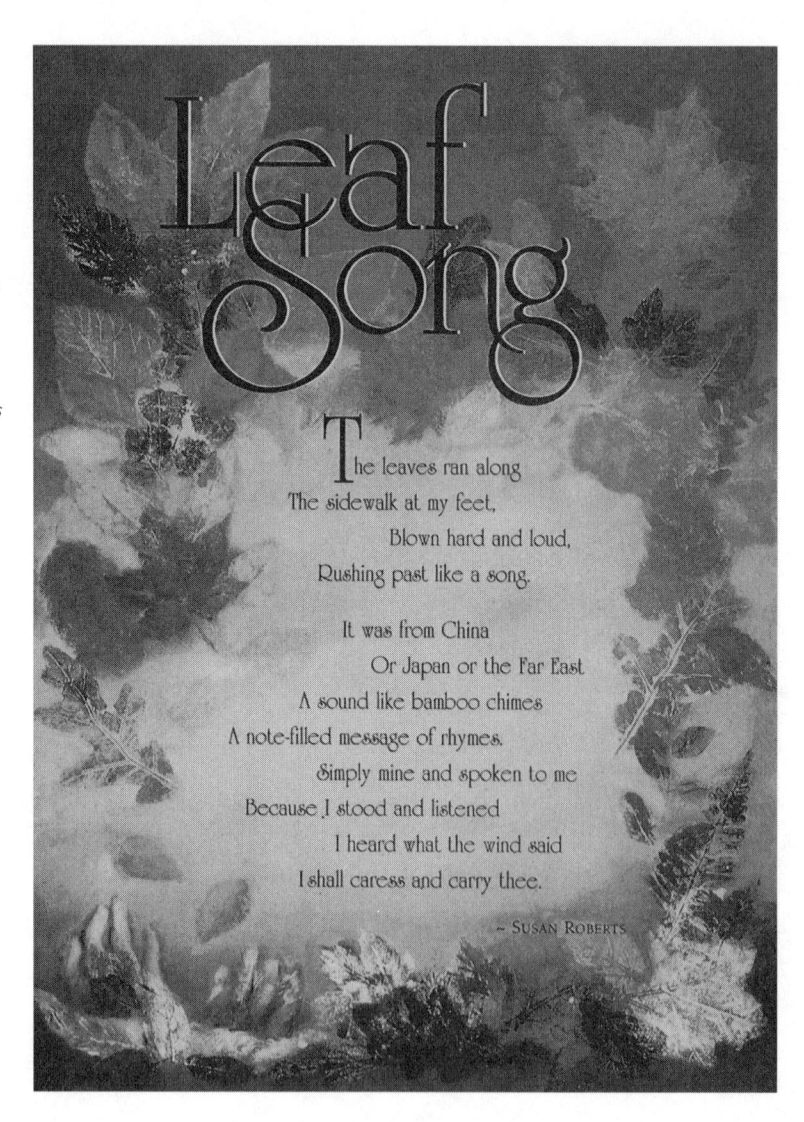

A CANCER *survivor's* ALMANAC

Part Four

Taking Care of Yourself

*Defining Our
    Destiny* 261

*Survivors as
    Advocates* 273

Chapter Eleven

Defining Our Destiny

by Susan Leigh, RN, BSN

"Working with NCCS since its inception has given me a voice for concerns that I had learned to keep to myself; it has provided me strength to handle subsequent cancer experiences and has given me an unsurpassed network of friends who remind me that together we can make a difference."

Susan Leigh, RN, BSN

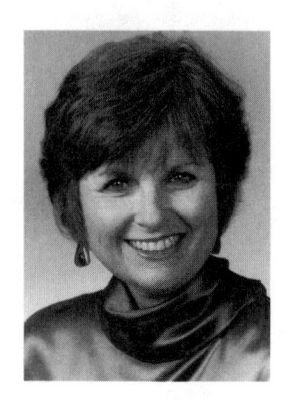

SUSAN LEIGH, RN, BSN is a cofounder of the National Coalition for Cancer Survivorship and served as its president from 1993 to 1995. Drawing on her experience as an oncology nurse and a survivor of Hodgkin's disease, breast cancer, and bladder cancer, she speaks and writes extensively on survivorship issues, with special emphasis on long-term and late effects of disease and therapy.

Ms. Leigh initiated the formation of both the Nurse Survivors Focus Group and the Survivorship Special Interest Group within the Oncology Nursing Society (ONS). She shared the Upjohn Quality of Life Award and the Schering Excellence in Cancer Nursing Research Award at the 1995 ONS Congress. Ms. Leigh served as a lieutenant in the United States Army and completed a tour of duty in Vietnam in 1971. From 1976 to 1989, she worked as an oncology nurse clinician, a pharmacokinetic research nurse, and a study coordinator in Cancer Prevention and Control at the University of Arizona Cancer Center.

"Survival, quite simply, begins when you are told you have cancer… and continues for the rest of your life."
— Fitzhugh Mullan, M.D.

Survivorship in relation to cancer is a relatively new concept. Not long ago these words seemed mutually exclusive because a diagnosis of cancer meant almost certain death. Thankfully, recent advances in technology, science, and the delivery of therapy have changed forever the way we think about cancer.

Cancer survivorship is dynamic as opposed to static; it is not just about long-term survival. It goes beyond the disease and the response—or lack of response—to treatment. Rather, survivorship permeates every aspect of your life after diagnosis.

Approximately ten million people are living today with a history of cancer. About half that number are estimated to have survived five years or more. This growing population is witnessing dramatic changes—both scientific and social—that are helping to dispel myths about cancer and its treatment, redefine the language and stages of survival, and promote the evolution from passive patienthood to proactive survivorship.

CANCER MYTHS

"…if it was not fatal, it was not cancer."
— Susan Sontag, *Illness As Metaphor*

A HISTORICAL PERSPECTIVE — Historically, attitudes about cancer were frequently defined by myths and fears of the unknown, and they paralleled the effectiveness of available treatments. Until we know what causes cancer and how it can be treated effectively, a diagnosis of cancer may continue to be viewed as a death sentence, instilling dread and masquerading as a ruthless, secretive assailant. Even though recent advances in science and medical technology have increased our chances for surviving many types of cancer, the often paralyzing fear of dying from the disease remains a major part of our culture.

When the biology of a disease is not understood, myth and speculation are apt to define the sickness. Cancer continues to be identified as one disease. Rather than understanding that cancer is many diseases with multiple causes and treatments, it frequently is seen as a single entity—the Big C. For example, some people cite stress as a cause of cancer rather than genetic predisposition, dangerous health habits, and environmental carcinogens.

Paired with these myths are other misunderstandings about cancer. In centuries past, cancer was thought to be caused by emotional resignation and hopelessness. Even recently, attempts to identify cancer personalities has become a popular trend. Theories have evolved suggesting that cancer patients must have had too many negative thoughts or repressed feelings. This "pop-psychology" often oversimplifies causation and blames the sick individual for having done something wrong.

Although the blanket paranoia surrounding cancer is gradually diminishing, the disease continues to provoke fear, stigma, shunning, discrimination, and withdrawal of support. Not all myths are rooted in the individual, though. The health-care system, too, is full of myths, misunderstandings, and major changes.

HEALTH-CARE MYTHS – As medical researchers and clinicians focus primarily on curing disease and saving lives, survivors tend to focus on the quality of their lives. Two myths that are rapidly being dispelled because of changes in health care are (1) the all-powerful role of the physician, and (2) the healing environment within our hospitals.

Doctors historically held the power and control in managing patients. That tide is shifting, however, and today the bureaucracy of managed care has created a businesslike atmosphere where decisions are being made by financing and regulatory agencies. Physicians, nurses, and support staff spend increasingly more time on administrative matters, which leaves less time for patient care. People wait longer for appointments and have fewer choices of doctors.

In response to these changes, a new type of health care consumer is emerging. Survivors are encouraged to be more assertive in asking questions and making decisions. They need to become partners with their physicians and other care providers, since long-term survivorship means a long-term relationship with those individuals. In order to effectively use their time together, both patients and physicians need good communication skills (see Chapter 2 for a discussion of doctor/patient communication).

And what has happened to the healing environment? Diagnosis-related groups, cost-containment, utilization reviews, quality assurance, and an overwhelming amount of paperwork have complicated the process and dehumanized the care. While the old system allowed unlimited stays in the hospital and actually encouraged passivity and invalidism, the new system has gone to the other extreme. To reduce expenses, hospitals discharge patients as quickly as possible, and survivors return home sooner and sicker. The home rather than the hospital has become the healing environment. That means greater responsibility for care and recovery is placed on the survivor, family members, or other caregivers. These changing social trends actually are forcing a shift from passive patienthood to a more proactive survivorship, and are thus fueling a consumer-driven survivorship movement.

BIRTH OF A MOVEMENT

The cancer survivorship movement did not happen overnight. It grew out of the collective efforts of individuals and groups who recognized the multiple dimensions of life after cancer, and then identified the unmet needs of survivors within their own communities. The heart and soul of this grassroots movement began with persons who either struggled through their own cancer experience or cared for people with cancer, and who wanted to make the journey a little easier for those who would follow.

As the specialty of oncology emerged, the cancer patient's agenda was often set by health-care providers, especially physicians. Some support programs required physician referrals. Doctors decided what cancer-related information was appropriate for their patients. Support groups were facilitated by nurses and social workers instead of by survivors. Yet as survivors lived longer and the survivor population grew, so did the need for supportive groups and organizations that would deal with issues often overlooked or considered less significant by the medical community.

Eventually, survivors realized that they were more than a disease. Freedom from disease and biomedical longevity were no longer the only standards of success. They were also concerned about psychological and spiritual well-being, social and vocational problems, and economic, legal and end-of-life issues. Concern about the quality of their lives gave rise to a proliferation of support groups, hot lines, educational materials and patient networks that were developed by the people who actually needed these resources. By combining the expertise of allied health professionals with the passion and energies of survivors, the survivorship movement took root.

SURVIVORS UNITE – Some survivors recognized the need to coordinate the independent and diverse nature of this expanding movement. In October, 1986, 22 individuals who shared an interest in cancer survival gathered in Albuquerque, New Mexico, at the invitation of Catherine Logan-Carrillo, Fitzhugh Mullan, MD, and Edith Lenneberg. As founder and executive director of Living Through Cancer (currently People Living Through Cancer or PLTC), Ms. Logan-Carrillo brought a local, grassroots expertise to the meeting. As a physician in the Public Health Service, Dr. Mullan contributed a national and political perspective. As a founding member of the Ostomy Association, Ms. Lenneberg brought the experience of uniting mutual aid groups into a national organization. All shared a vision of unifying the divergent activities around the country, and thus strengthening a fragmented survivorship movement.

Many of the participants in this initial meeting had personal histories of cancer, as well as experience providing a wide variety of services to cancer survivors and their families. At the time, no method or structure existed to link groups, to stimulate the development of new supportive activities, or to share educational materials. While Candlelighters Childhood Cancer Foundation provided an excellent network for children with cancer and their families, no organized group advocated for the overall concerns of adult cancer survivors in the medical, economic, and political arenas.

Discussions during this initial meeting confirmed the need for a national network to coordinate the widespread and diverse activities, to create a comprehensive clearinghouse for survivorship materials, to promote the study of survivorship, and to advocate for cancer survivors on a national level. Thus, the National Coalition for Cancer Survivorship (NCCS) was founded.

THE SEMANTICS OF SURVIVORSHIP

A MEDICAL APPROACH – When cancer was considered incurable, the term "survivor" applied to the family members whose loved one died from the disease. This application of the term was used for years by the medical profession and insurance companies. In the 1960s, our hopes for surviving cancer changed dramatically. The treatment of Hodgkin's disease and childhood leukemias offered the first major glimpse of curing specific cancers. A combination of chemotherapy and radiation therapy, added to the traditional surgery, elevated our expectations about life after cancer. The possibility of cure became a reality.

Once potentially curative therapy became a reality, physicians selected a five-year parameter to define a survivor—either five years from the date of diagnosis or from the end of treatment. If cancer did not recur within this time frame, the patient would graduate to survivor status and, they hoped, regain a normal life expectancy.

Even as the five-year landmark has been modified as a guideline for describing survival, medical professionals seem inclined to categorize anyone receiving therapy or not completely free of disease as a patient, and former patients who are not under treatment or who have no evidence of disease as survivors. This distinction makes sense to many who are oncology professionals, who require parameters for scientific study, or who need to describe recipients of different types of care. Others, however, were uncomfortable with these labels.

A CONSUMER APPROACH – Many people who have histories of cancer feel that survivorship extends far beyond the restrictions of time and treatment. Some people remain alive for over five years but are not cured of their disease. They may require long-term maintenance therapy, or they may periodically change types of treatment. Others experience late recurrences, are diagnosed with second malignancies, develop delayed effects of treatment, or may, in fact, be dying. If survival is considered a process rather than an end point, these people surely are survivors.

Whether on or off treatment, cured or not cured, people with histories of cancer now are describing themselves as victors, graduates, triumphers, veterans, thrivers, activists and, of course, survivors. With the businesslike changes in health care, consumers and customers have joined the list. Meanwhile, all these labels can confuse anyone concerned with cancer care, and have caused many heated discussions among survivors themselves. But as Ross Gray notes in *Persons With Cancer Speak Out,* "The act of defining is an act of power." This is all about the people—the survivors—identifying their own issues and defining themselves rather than relying on the agendas and descriptives of the health-care community.

Any or all of these labels can be considered correct. They simply need to be defined within the context in which they are used. At the NCCS, we maintain the following philosophy:

> From the time of its discovery and for the balance of life, an individual diagnosed with cancer is a survivor.
> —*NCCS Charter*

STAGES OF SURVIVORSHIP

The concept of survivorship helps to bridge gaps of disagreement as to when someone becomes a survivor. While Fitzhugh Mullan was the first to describe survivorship as "the act of living on...a dynamic concept with no artificial boundaries...," Barbara Carter, an oncology nurse and early NCCS board member, further defined this theme as a process of "going through," suggesting movement through phases. With these models, the concept of survivorship can be viewed as a continual, ongoing process rather than a stage or outcome of survival. Survivorship begins at the moment of diagnosis and continues for the remainder of life. It is not just about long-term survival—which is how the medical profession generally defines it—but rather it is the ever-changing process or experience of living with, through, or beyond cancer.

SEASONS OF SURVIVAL

Obviously, cancer survivors have different issues depending upon their individual circumstances and where they are along their cancer journey. In the classic article *Seasons of Survival: Reflections of a Physician with Cancer,* Fitzhugh Mullan was the first to propose a model of survival comprised of different and somewhat distinct stages. These stages, or seasons, are categorized as acute, extended, and permanent.

ACUTE STAGE – The acute (or immediate) stage of survival begins at the time of your diagnostic work-up, and continues through the initial courses of surgery, chemotherapy, and radiation treatments. You commonly are called a patient during this stage, and the primary focus is on physical survival.

Usually, without any prior training, you are required to make sophisticated medical decisions at a time when you feel vulnerable, afraid, and pressured. You often do not understand the scientific basis for selecting one therapy over another and may not feel confident in your ability to make these important decisions. Due to your inexperience, you may rely on your physicians to make treatment-related decisions. You may, however, seek information, explanations, and more effective communication in an attempt to understand your choices.

Supportive services are most available during diagnosis and treatment. Access to the medical team, counselors, patient support networks, resource libraries, hot lines, and family support systems can help you navigate through this stage. The picture changes sometimes dramatically, however, once treatment ends.

EXTENDED STAGE – If your disease responds during the initial course of therapy, you will move into the extended (or intermediate) stage of survival. This stage often is described as watchful waiting, limbo, or remission as you monitor your body for signs that the disease has returned.

Uncertainty about the future prevails as medical-based support systems are no longer readily available. Recovery means dealing with the physical and emotional effects of treatment. Reentry into social roles is often challenged by ignorance and discrimination.

While no longer a patient, you may not feel entirely healthy. You actually may have difficulty feeling like a survivor. Ambiguity defines

---

During treatment, there is an elegant economy to our thoughts. There is no reason to worry about the future. We may not have one.
— Glenna Halvorson-Boyd and Lisa Hunter, *Dancing in Limbo: Making Sense of Life After Cancer*

I was no longer actively engaged in "cancer combat," and a dreadful fear engulfed me: when would the other shoe drop?
—Glenna Halvorson-Boyd and Lisa Hunter, *Dancing in Limbo: Making Sense of Life After Cancer*

this stage as you find yourself afloat in a mixture of joy and fear—happy to be alive and finished with treatments, yet afraid of what the future may hold.

There had been no formal exit from sick to well, no instruction sheet on what to do next with my life. Cancer was my "trial by fire." In surviving it, I had learned many precious lessons.

During this transitional period, many survivors need continued support. Community and peer networks often replace institutional support during this stage. Recovery entails regaining both physical and psychological stamina. A new sense of "normal" gradually replaces what will never be again.

PERMANENT STAGE – A certain level of trust and comfort gradually returns as you enter the permanent (or long-term) stage of survival.

This stage of survival is roughly equivalent to cure or sustained remission. While most survivors experience a gradual evolution from a state of "surviving to thriving," a small number of them must deal with chronic, debilitating, or delayed effects of therapy. As a long-term survivor, you may have no physical evidence of disease and appear to have recovered fully. You never forget, however, the life-threatening experience of having survived cancer. The metaphor of the Damocles syndrome illustrates the apprehension and fear of living under the sword that is dangling by a thread, never knowing if or when it might drop.

Another major problem experienced by many long-term survivors is a lack of guidelines to insure disease-free survival. Pediatric oncology is far beyond adult oncology in the systematic follow-up of long-term survivors that helps to identify potential pitfalls and to institute early interventions. Adults, on the other hand, often feel burdened by what some call the "glorification of recovery"—you are praised for overcoming diversity, yet are made to feel ungrateful if you have continued complaints. The appearance of health can actually hamper the identification of real problems as no one wants to believe that something may be wrong. Medical personnel often think that recovery from a once fatal illness should be reward enough. This feeling that people who survive cancer treatment should simply get on with their lives also frequently is reflected in interactions with family and friends:

> One of the hardest aspects of completing treatment is that the average observer seems to expect you to feel only relief and joy. The average person does not recognize the stress of completing therapy. You may keep your fears and anxieties to yourself to avoid sounding ungrateful or pathologically depressed. Surviving your personal challenge of cancer can be very lonely.
> —Wendy Schlessel Harpham, MD
> *After Cancer: A Guide to Your New Life*

> Staying alive is just the initial challenge; living with the consequences of the disease and therapy become a lifelong responsibility.
> —Carolyn Runowicz and Donna Haupt
> *To Be Alive: A Woman's Guide to a Full Life After Cancer*

> With cancer, people confront death. With survival, they feel an urgency to reexamine how they live the rest of their lives.
> - Glenna Halvorson-Boyd and Lisa Hunter,
> *Dancing in Limbo: Making Sense of Life After Cancer*

Symptoms of distress, both biomedical and psychosocial, must be taken seriously. Despite cost-containment and managed care, survivors need, more than ever, continued access to appropriate specialists.

As the population of cancer survivors increases, attention to long-term survival issues needs to be encouraged. Even if the disease is eradicated, the potential for the development of other cancers, for treatment-related complications, for insurance and employment problems, and for continued psychological trauma from surviving a life-threatening experience must be recognized as barriers to full recovery. (See Chapter 1 for a discussion of the medical problems of long-term survivors.)

Years ago, people with cancer would not question their physicians' orders, request second opinions, seek medical information, talk to others in similar situations, or band together politically. Fortunately, changes in medicine and society have created a new, more savvy health-care consumer. Today, survivors like you and me are more proactive and outspoken. We are developing publications, resource networks, and support programs. We are offering expert advice about quality-of-life issues and are evaluating both local and national cancer programs. In a nutshell, we raising general awareness about cancer survivorship. Partnership is replacing paternalism in the medical arena, and the consumer's voice finally is being heard.

While we all deserve to celebrate our successes, the consequences of surviving cancer must not be ignored. Survivors need—

- cancer therapies that are effective, accessible, and affordable;
- medical insurance that is affordable, obtainable, and portable;
- employment opportunities that are free of discrimination;
- access to continued medical care with doctors who understand our special needs as long-term survivors;
- mental health therapists who understand the psychological trauma of individuals and families who must deal with a life-threatening illness;
- community-based peer support networks that connect newly diagnosed survivors and their family members to the veterans who have "been there;"
- research that is focused on prevention of secondary cancers and the late effects of therapy; and
- education that promotes health, wellness, and advocacy skills.

Survivors and their caregivers, families, and friends have laid the groundwork for survivorship. One of their greatest gifts to today's survivors is knowledge, for knowledge is power. No cancer journey is easy, but with information, understanding, support, and resources, we can work toward dispelling the myths and improving the quality of our lives with, through, and beyond cancer.

Chapter Twelve

Survivors as Advocates

by Ellen Stovall and
Elizabeth Johns Clark, PhD, MSW

"When I learned about NCCS, I found the organization whose ideal–the veteran helping the rookie–validated my own need for peer support. NCCS is *the* organization that gives voice to the issues confronting survivors, and through its programs, publications, and services, makes it possible for countless survivors to live a better quality life."

– *Ellen Stovall*

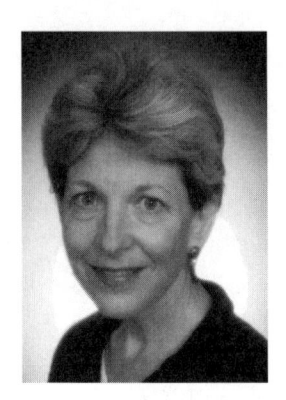

ELLEN STOVALL, a 25-year survivor of two bouts with Hodgkin's disease, has spent 23 years advocating for quality-of-life issues that affect people with cancer and their families. Since 1992, she has served as the executive director of the National Coalition for Cancer Survivorship.

Ms. Stovall has served on advisory panels, working groups, and committees of numerous organizations, including the President's National Cancer Advisory Board, National Cancer Institute, the American Society of Clinical Oncology, the National Cancer Advisory Board, and the Association of Community Cancer Centers. She has given testimony to numerous governmental bodies, including the Senate Appropriations Committee, the House Commerce Committee, the Senate Labor Committee, and the Food and Drug Administration.

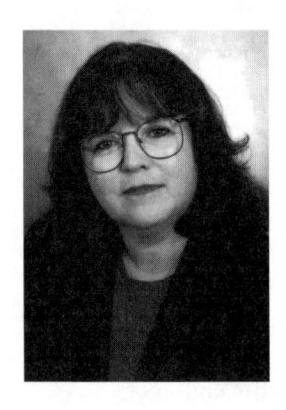

ELIZABETH JOHNS CLARK, PHD is the president of the National Coalition for Cancer Survivorship and was cochair of the First National Congress on Cancer Survivorship, which was held in November, 1995 in Washington, DC. She currently serves as director of Diagnostic and Therapeutic Services at Albany Medical Center Hospital and as an associate professor of medicine in the Division of Medical Oncology at Albany Medical College. She holds a doctorate in medical sociology and master's degrees in both medical social work and public health. Dr. Clark has lectured and published extensively in the areas of social oncology, loss and grief, and hope and burnout.

I have always felt good about my ability to be an advocate for others—for my friends, my family, and for people I don't even know—but when I was diagnosed with cancer, something happened that I would have never expected: I didn't know how to advocate for myself. And even if I had known how, I didn't know what words to use or how to use them. Suddenly, and without any warning, it was as though I were a child but without the blessed innocence that comes with childhood. Like the neophyte child, I had no more than a crude language to use when I spoke. And when I did speak, it was in a primitive way, as if my voice were frozen and stuck—trapped in my throat by a paralyzing fear that I'd never be able to speak up for myself. Would I… could I… ever find my own voice?

—Remarks by a cancer survivor to medical students

As you were growing up, you learned behaviors that gave you a feeling of security when dealing with life's ordinary circumstances. Among these behaviors were communication skills, resourcefulness, problem-solving skills, and negotiation skills. You have used these and other skills in practical ways as you have lived your life. A cancer diagnosis, however, will lessen these skills. For a while, they may disappear altogether.

Experts in psychosocial behavior generally agree that your capacity to be self-reliant, to advocate for yourself, and to move forward, is temporarily diminished by a diagnosis of cancer. They also agree that these skills will reemerge at some point during your cancer experience. When you are in the initial stages of cancer, however, little comfort is derived from hearing that this reduced coping capacity is temporary, predictable, normal, expected, and even natural. Accustomed to being effective, resourceful, and reasonable, nothing about this altered state seems remotely normal or natural. You are in a state of suspended animation. It is as though you are teetering on a highwire—dangling—in a freefall and without a net.

You may be overcome with a fear of having cancer. Fear can paralyze you and keep you from moving forward in a reasonable fashion. Given the magnitude of the consequences—life, quality of life, death—moving forward is essential, but you may not know how to do so. Dr. Martin Luther King, Jr. called this decision-indecision phenomenon a "paralysis of analysis."

While the necessity to take action in the wake of a cancer diagnosis cannot be overstated, it should not be taken as a command to react to each challenge with the same urgency. A fundamental key to achieving effective self-advocacy is to determine a deliberate plan and measurable goals. This plan should begin with information-seeking and developing a clear way to communicate with those who can help you most: your health care team, your family and friends, and other cancer survivors. In summary, you need to become your own best advocate.

Cancer Survivors Can Advocate for Themselves

When diagnosed with cancer, one of the first things that you can do to become an advocate for yourself is to recognize that you are not alone. The National Coalition for Cancer Survivorship's definition of a cancer survivor is "anyone with a diagnosis of cancer, whether newly diagnosed or in remission or with recurrence or terminal cancer." Millions of people have been where you are and are surviving. They have experienced the unwelcome intrusion of cancer into their lives and have had many of the same reactions.

Just like the survivor quoted at the beginning of this chapter, you may feel that you cannot advocate for yourself. Yet, advocacy is "active support on behalf of something." When you begin to act on behalf of yourself, even if not at your peak level, you are involved in self-advocacy.

Other survivors will tell you that through feeling empowered to act on their own behalf, they were able to meet most of their needs on a personal level, and they were able to communicate these needs to their family, friends, and caregivers. An example of an act of self-advocacy is when you seek a second opinion because you have doubts about your diagnosis or treatment plan. Rather than doing nothing about your doubt, or worrying about what your doctor will think about you asking for a second opinion, you actively do something in your own interest. You should be a self-advocate as you deal with your cancer for numerous reasons:
- Advocacy gives you some stability and a feeling of regaining some control of your life.
- Advocacy is confidence building in the way it helps you face challenges that seem insurmountable.
- Advocacy is a way of reaching out to others. It can be as simple as asking your doctor or nurse for the name of someone to talk with who has survived your particular type of cancer.
- Advocacy can improve your quality of life.
- Advocacy for yourself may be the difference that turns feeling hopeless and helpless into feeling hopeful.

Empowered Survivors

Noted author and cancer survivor, Natalie Davis Spingarn, refers to a "new breed of cancer survivors." As Susan Leigh pointed out in the previous chapter, this new breed symbolizes an evolution in medical practice—a moving away from the passive patient model to one that encourages active participation and involvement by patients in making the important decisions that will affect both the length and quality of their lives.

These survivors generally believe in equality in relationships and view their caregivers as partners in their health care. In hospital clinics and physicians' waiting rooms, you can observe survivors who are more outwardly comfortable with self-advocacy. They are equipped with pencil and paper or tape recorders, and are frequently accompanied by a family member or friend. They spend little time in denial or deferred decision making. Rather, they turn their apprehensions and anxieties into energies directed toward obtaining up-to-date information, and becoming more adept at communicating, problem solving, and negotiating.

Empowerment is another important concept for cancer survivors to understand. Individuals who describe themselves as empowered believe that they are capable of understanding their own needs better than others. Yet, it would be misleading to conclude that if you are a competent and capable self-advocate, you are empowered in ways that give you a remarkable advantage over those who are not as adept. Obviously, personality differences, degrees of illness or wellness, and other factors create variables that must be considered. Among these variables are level of education, economic status, social skills, age, and access to care.

No matter what your life circumstances, however, acts of self-advocacy will make it easier for you to make decisions about your care and about healthful living. Self-advocacy will also help you engage in actions to enhance your quality of life.

> A revolution in attitude has finally reached once-passive patients. Civil rights, women's rights, consumers' rights, human rights, growing interest in and candor about medical matters and preventive health—all of these have helped empower survivors, giving them the feeling that they can have at least a hand in their own destiny.
> – Natalie Davis Spingarn

You Can Learn Self-Advocacy

After reading the above, you may not feel that you can identify with the profile of an "active patient." You may think that you are lacking in self-advocacy skills; yet, these skills can be learned. The remainder of this chapter outlines ways that will help you become a more effective advocate—first for yourself, and then for others.

Advocacy skills can be obtained in a variety of ways. One way is through peer support or self-help groups. These groups can provide education about cancer, can help to normalize the cancer experience and can give you a wealth of tips about navigating the health-care system and finding needed information. They also can provide an opportunity for assertiveness training through role playing and other exercises.

The four skills identified in the next few pages have been suggested as essential to cancer advocacy. When used during your diagnosis and treatment, these skills can contribute significantly to your overall well-being and healing.

INFORMATION SEEKING SKILLS – Acting on your own behalf or as an advocate for someone else, you will need basic information about cancer. You will need facts about the diagnosis, all the treatment options available, the expected and possible side effects of treatment, and coping strategies that will be of help to you, all of which have been covered in previous chapters of this book. Informed consumerism is the basic underlying tenet of cancer survivorship, and it provides the best foundation for the other needed self-advocacy skills.

COMMUNICATION SKILLS – Learning communication skills so that you can be a better advocate for yourself with your doctor will be helpful only if both you and your doctor assume equal responsibility for your interactions and for the outcome. Most doctors who treat cancer respect the active patient model and encourage patients to be very involved in planning their care.

A virtual glut of books, magazines, and videotapes about effective communication can be found on the shelves of bookstores and in the self-help section of libraries. A booklet written especially for communication about cancer is available through the NCCS. Entitled *Teamwork: A Cancer Patient's Guide to Talking with Your Doctor*, the booklet includes the following practical suggestions:
- Prepare questions before your doctors appointment and write them down.
- Ask for information in familiar terms (doctors frequently, and unintentionally, lapse into "doctor-speak," using words like "dyspepsia" and "alopecia" to describe loss of appetite and hair loss).
- Make sure you understand what you heard by rephrasing the doctor's responses.
- Take notes or tape record the discussion.
- Ask who in the doctor's office you can call if you have more questions after you leave.

If you feel accomplished in basic communication skills, you may want to explore other areas to enhance your skill level. These include developing better listening techniques, identifying nonverbal cues, getting assertiveness training, and learning new methods of problem-solving and negotiation.

PROBLEM-SOLVING SKILLS – Cancer presents one of life's biggest challenges because it is a predicament that has few clear-cut solutions. As such, it requires a deliberative and strategic decision-making process. If you laid the groundwork during the information-gathering phase of your illness, you probably have lots of information and options to consider. You need to learn how to think through this maze of data, how to sort the information, and how to develop an action plan.

Think about problem-solving techniques that you have used during other crisis periods in your life. Are they applicable when dealing with cancer-related problems? Some people do "pro and con" lists or "if X, then Y" lists for sorting out options. Others talk with people whose opinions they respect and then act on consensus. Still others seek and use expert advice. Do not forget that other cancer survivors are also experts because they may have had similar problems. Their ideas, suggestions, and attitudes may be especially helpful.

NEGOTIATION SKILLS – We use negotiation and bargaining skills in our everyday life. At its simplest, a conversation with a friend about where to have dinner or what movie to see can involve negotiation. More difficult are situations where serious conflicts arise when parties hold different values or opinions about a situation or a problem. Effective negotiation relies on good communication, resourcefulness, keeping an open mind, and knowing your options.

A cancer diagnosis may present situations that require specific and deliberate negotiation and conflict resolution skills. For example, problems related to insurance and employment may be complex and not easily resolved. While these situations may be difficult, practical ways to deal with them often exist. Finding solutions may be as simple as reading about your rights. In cases that are not as easily managed, or where the relationship between the conflicted parties has broken down, a mediator, patient advocate, or legal counsel may be necessary.

Cancer Survivors as Advocates for Others

Whether at age 20 or 80, cancer is a life-transforming—life-awakening—experience. Many survivors want to "give something back" in gratitude for their own recovery or for the help that they have received. The cancer survivorship movement relies on this model of peer support—the veteran helping the rookie concept—to transmit the wisdom of what has been learned from one's own experience to help another.

For example, when people learn you have had cancer, they may call you and ask you to speak to a family member or friend who has

> With communication comes understanding and clarity; with understanding, fear diminishes; in the absence of fear, hope emerges; and in the presence of hope, anything is possible.
> – *Ellen Stovall*

been diagnosed recently. If you are comfortable speaking on a personal level, talking with the newly diagnosed cancer survivor can be an act of advocacy.

Suggestions for other ways in which you may want to use your personal experience to help others include—

- starting a support group in your community;
- volunteering for a local organization's hot line or cancer information line;
- speaking about your cancer experience to community organizations and civic groups;
- making sure your library has a variety of up-to-date resources on cancer, especially those that were helpful to you when you were seeking information;
- speaking to medical students, nurses, social workers, hospital staff, and employers and employees about your cancer experience;
- telling your story publicly to the media or the legislature to help change public opinion and public policy about cancer. In other words, get the message out.

CONCLUSION

While the cancer experience is not unique, each individual's experience with cancer is, and each survivor needs to chart a personal course for survival. The models for self-advocacy exist in the footprints of the millions of survivors who have gone before and are now able to network with their fellow survivors to assist them in resolving the isolating effects of cancer. The wealth of information found in the experiences of veteran survivors can be indispensable to the newly diagnosed. Through effective communication, any cancer experience can become one of hopefulness.

Resources

A CANCER *survivor's* ALMANAC

I. MEDICAL INFORMATION

A. SERVICES OF THE NATIONAL CANCER INSTITUTE (NCI)

CANCER INFORMATION SERVICE (CIS) – Whether looking for information about your particular cancer, treatment options or medical resources, every survivor should know the telephone number of the United States Government's Cancer Information Service (CIS), a network of 19 regional offices supported by the National Cancer Institute: (800) 4-CANCER (for TYY equipment users (800) 332-8615). CIS offices are open Monday through Friday, 9:00 a.m. to 4:30 p.m., local time. The administrative office address is National Cancer Institute, Building 31, Room 10A16, Bethesda, MD 20892. When you reach (800) 4-CANCER, an automated voice will instruct you (in English and Spanish) how to order free NCI publications or how to have your questions answered by a cancer information specialist. Waiting times vary, but it pays to be persistent, as this is an easily accessible and invaluable resource.

CIS information specialists, while not doctors, are trained to answer questions in lay language about cancer and its treatment. They can answer a range of cancer-related questions, from how to quit smoking to how to deal with side effects of treatment. They provide medical information—not medical advice—as well as facts about community resources. Although they cannot make specific referrals, they can provide information about National Cancer Institute-supported programs such as Comprehensive Cancer Centers, Clinical Cancer Centers, Community Clinical Oncology Programs, and the names of hospitals with cancer programs approved by the American College of Surgeons. You can then contact these organizations directly for more specific information about practitioners in your area.

PUBLICATIONS – NCI offers a number of excellent publications on a wide range of cancer topics, such as *Chemotherapy and You, Radiation Therapy and You, Eating Hints, When Cancer Recurs, What Are Clinical Trials All About, Facing Forward: A Guide for Cancer Survivors,* and a series of booklets on specific types of cancer. A free publications list also is readily available.

PDQ – Among the most important tools available to the CIS information specialists is a computerized information service (on line since 1983) called PDQ (Physician Data Query). CIS specialists can access PDQ's up-to-date information about state-of-the-art cancer treatments, methods of dealing with unpleasant side effects of treatment, and summaries of all NCI-funded clinical trials of potentially important new cancer treatments.

You can access the PDQ data base yourself at many public libraries and, if they are open to the public, at medical libraries and other medical institutions. For a $100 membership fee in the NCI's Information Associates Program, you can access the service through your own computer, as many doctors do. The PDQ Member Service Center can be reached at (800) 624-7890 (or (301) 496-7600 outside the United States), Monday through Friday, 9:00 a.m. to 8:00 p.m. EST.

CANCERNET, CANCERFAX – CancerNet, another free NCI service, enables you to get PDQ information summaries and other NCI information on the Internet and other electronic information services. To access CancerNet, send an e-mail message to cancernet@icicc.nci.nih.gov and, in the body of the mail message, enter "HELP" for a response in English or "SPANISH" for a response in Spanish. In just a few minutes, you will receive a listing of publications, updated monthly, covering a wide variety of topics such as prevention and detection, specific types of cancer, and various therapies. You can then order any of these free documents by e-mail.

If you prefer to use a fax machine, you can call CancerFax, a more limited NCI service available 24 hours a day, 7 days a week. Call (301) 402-5874 and an automated voice will tell you how to get CancerFax Contents, a list of information available through this system. This list will include fact sheets on various cancer topics, abstracts from medical literature, information about some investigational drugs, and general information about PDQ and other NCI services and publications.

When you have had a chance to review the list, call again and punch in the necessary information to order the documents you want. The automated system will let you know how long the statement is (from a page or two to over 30 pages). Although the service and the information are free, you may have long distance charges for the calls to Bethesda, Maryland.

B. SERVICES OF THE AMERICAN CANCER SOCIETY

Predominant among the private organizations that provide such consumer information is the American Cancer Society (ACS). The ACS information and referral service number, (800) ACS-2345, offers information about the early signs or symptoms of cancer, appropriate treatments, and ACS publications. This ACS hotline also can refer you to local ACS-sponsored programs, which will help you find transportation, equipment or perhaps others in your area with medical conditions similar to your own.

Following is a list of many of the programs ACS volunteers provide. If you are interested in one of these services, check the telephone directory for your nearest ACS office. If you cannot find one, contact the national office at 1599 Clifton Road NE, Atlanta, GA 30329-4251.

- *Reach to Recovery* – Women just starting down the road to recovery after breast surgery are provided with one-on-one consultation by a volunteer who has been through breast cancer and has made a successful recovery.
- *Ostomy Visitor Program (in collaboration with United Ostomy Association)* – Trained volunteer visitors assist patients who have had bowel or bladder surgery and offer emotional support and practical advice on adjusting to life with an ostomy.
- *CanSurmount* – One-on-one visitation program for cancer patients using volunteers who are cancer survivors. This program is not site specific like Reach to Recovery.

EDUCATION AND INFORMATION – *I Can Cope* – An eight-session educational class providing information for survivors on their families about both medical and psychosocial adjustment to cancer.

Look Good…Feel Better – Co-sponsored by the Cosmetic, Toiletry and Fragrance Association and National Cosmetology Association, helps women deal with side effects of cancer and its treatment by providing assistance with hair and skin care.

Finding Cancer Information on the Internet

Carla Sofka, PhD, MSW
University at Albany, State University of New York

Cancer survivors often spend much time looking for information about their cancers and treatments. Some information previously available only in books, medical journals and educational pamphlets, is now available via computer. Survivors now can access a wealth of general and medical information about cancer by searching the Internet.

What is the Internet and the World Wide Web?

The Internet is an international network of computers. The World Wide Web ("WWW" or "the Web") is a system that disseminates information through the Internet so you can access the information. Thousands of cancer-related files or "sites" are available on the World Wide Web (just as thousands of books are available through a library or bookstore). Each site has a unique combination of letters and characters (a Uniform Resource Locator or "URL") that serves as an address that tells your computer how to connect to the information stored at that site.

What types of sites contain cancer information?

The World Wide Web contains many sites that provide information and support. As with any information you find about cancer and treatments, you should note the source of the information and discuss it with your doctor. For example, the National Cancer Institute is a more reliable source of information about a specific treatment than is a consumer magazine. The types of cancer-related sites available include:
- Educational sites such as those that provide descriptions of different types of stages of cancer.
- Treatment-related sites such as those that provide potential options for treatment as well as descriptions of clinical trials.
- Chat groups or discussion groups or online support groups that provide forums for communicating with other cancer survivors to share experiences and coping strategies.
- Home pages, sites created by individuals, agencies, or organizations that can contain practically anything. Some describe personal experiences through stories, poetry or artwork.

Others include referral information about resources for support, such as peer support groups and counseling services. Many sites contain an electronic mail address through which you can correspond with the individual, agency, or organization.

How can I access the World Wide Web?

You need two things to access online services: a computer with a modem and an online provider that provides a connection to the Internet. Many national commercial providers offer free trial subscriptions to try their services. You can obtain more information from:

America Online (800) 975-7700
Compuserve (800) 848-8990
Prodigy (800) 776-3449

Some providers service local geographic regions. To find local providers, look in the classified ads in your local newspaper under computer services or Internet providers. They also may be listed in your Yellow Pages. Additionally, community-based organizations known as "Freenets" provide free services. Look in the computer section of your local library or bookstore for a listing of Freenets and useful hints for choosing an Internet provider. Be sure to choose a provider with a local telephone number to avoid long distance phone charges.

If you do not own a computer, you may be able to gain access through a local public or university library. A community health resource center, medical school library, or friend with a home computer may also be able to help you. If you are not able to gain free access, some copy centers and "cyber cafes" (coffee shops that rent computers by the hour) sell Internet access time.

What should I do before I search for cancer-related information on the World Wide Web?

1. TAKE A DEEP BREATH AND BE PATIENT. At times, many people are using the Internet and you may have to wait for information. If you are not comfortable with computers, try to search with someone who is familiar with online services.

2. FAMILIARIZE YOURSELF WITH HOW YOUR COMPUTER ACCESS SITES ON THE WEB. You probably will use a searching mechanism called a "browser" that allows you to visit sites for which you have

an address or to locate sites that are relevant to a particular topic.

3. IDENTIFY AND PRIORITIZED THE TYPE OF INFORMATION YOU WANT NOW. If you are using a web browser to search for sites, define keywords as specifically as possible. For example, if you want to learn about the side effects of drugs used to treat breast cancer, "breast cancer" would yield too many files to read, while "chemotherapy and breast cancer and side effects" may give you a more narrow selection.

4. YOU CAN SPEND HOURS OR DAYS WADING THROUGH ALL OF THE AVAILABLE INFORMATION. Some sites offer automatic links to related sites. Be selective; if you do not have free access, costs can accumulate quickly.

5. REMEMBER THAT ANYONE CAN POST INFORMATION ON THE WEB. Be a wise consumer. Make sure that the information comes from an accurate and reliable source. Always discuss the information with your doctor.

WHERE SHOULD I START TO SEARCH FOR CANCER INFORMATION ON THE WORLD WIDE WEB?

Every month, many new sites are added to the Internet that provide information, resources, and support about cancer. The following sites are good places to start. They provide reliable, valuable information and have links to other relevant sites.

NAME: CANSEARCH – Type this address to access it: http://www.access.digex.net/~mkragen/cansearch.htm1.

This site, developed by a cancer survivor, helps inexperienced Internet users locate sites on the Web quickly to gain disease and treatment-specific information and identify resources for support. It has automatic links to multiple sites on the Web, including the two described below. CANSEARCH is sponsored by the National Coalition for Cancer Survivorship.

NATIONAL CANCER INSTITUTE AND CANCERNET – Type this address to access it: http://wwwicic.nci.nih.gov

This government sponsored site provides access to information statements from the National Cancer Institute's Physician Data Query (PDQ) database, fact sheets on various cancer topics, and describes services provided by the Cancer Information Service (available by telephone at (800) 4-CANCER).

ONCOLINK – Type this address to access it:
http://cancer.med.upenn.edu/

This site, developed and maintained through the University of Pennsylvania, contains links to educational, information, and supportive resource sites on the Web. Unique to this site is a gallery of artwork produced by children coping with cancer.

MEDINFO.ORG – Type this address to access it:
http://cure.medinfo.org

This site provides a list of cancer discussion groups, home pages written by cancer survivors, and links to other cancer sites.

HOW CAN I LEARN MORE ABOUT THE INTERNET AND THE WORLD WIDE WEB?

Most bookstores have numerous user guides in the computer section. Some commercial providers publish guides specific to their service that include free access for a limited number of hours. Free assistance may be available through your local public library. For a fee, some computer stores and adult education programs offer classes about the Internet.

C. Professional Medical Societies

American Association of Sex Education,
Counselors and Therapists
Box 238
Mt. Vernon, IA 52314-0238
(319) 895-8407
   Provides names of registered sex therapists in your area.

American Board of Medical Specialties
One Rotary Center, Suite 805
Evanston, IL 60201
(800) 776-2378
   The American Board of Medical Specialties is the umbrella organization for all specialty boards that certify physicians. It can tell you if your physician is board certified in his or her specialty. Board certification does not guarantee a physician's expertise, but it does signify meeting rigorous standards established by his or her peers. The organization also publishes the ABMS Compendium of Certified Medical Specialists, the only biographic directory that is authorized by all specialty boards. The Compendium, which is available in public and medical libraries, is published every even-numbered year, with an annual supplement.

American College of Radiology
1891 Preston White Drive
Reston, VA 20191
(703) 648-8900
   Provides a list of accredited mammography facilities and conducts a voluntary peer review of mammography facilities to determine if they meet accreditation standards designed to ensure that services are provided by qualified staff, and that equipment used is specially designed and properly maintained for mammography.

American College of Surgeons
Office of Public Information
55 East Erie Street
Chicago, IL 60611
(312) 664-4050
   Provides a geographic list of Fellows of the American College of

Surgeons (who are board-certified surgeons), including type of specialty. It prefers written requests.

AMERICAN SOCIETY OF CLINICAL ONCOLOGY
225 Reinekers Lane, Suite 650
Alexandria, VA 22314

AMERICAN SOCIETY OF PLASTIC AND
RECONSTRUCTIVE SURGEONS
444 East Algonquin Road
Arlington Heights, IL 60005
(847) 228-9900; (800) 635-0635 (referral message tape)

Will provide written information on reconstruction and mail a list of certified reconstructive surgeons by geographical area after callers provide details on the above (800) message tape.

ASSOCIATION OF ONCOLOGY SOCIAL WORKERS (AOSW)
1910 East Jefferson Street
Baltimore, MD 21205
(410) 614-3990

COLLEGE OF AMERICAN PATHOLOGISTS
325 Waukegan Road
Northfield, IL 60093-2750
(847) 446-8800

Surveys hospital and nonhospital laboratories to determine if they met CAP Standards for accreditation. CAP standards are voluntary, but approximately 4,000 laboratories in the United States have asked CAP to survey their facilities and received accreditation. You can call CAP to find out if a particular lab is accredited.

COMMUNITY HEALTH ACCREDITATION PROGRAM
350 Hudson Street
New York, NY 10014
(800) 669-1656

Accredits home-care organizations for minimum standards of safety and care. It will provide callers with a list of accredited and nonaccredited agencies in your community.

JOINT COMMISSION ON ACCREDITATION
OF HEALTHCARE ORGANIZATIONS
Public Information Coordinator
Department of Corporate Relations
One Renaissance Boulevard

Oakbrook Terrace, IL 60181
(708) 916-5632

This joint commission of the American Hospital Association, the American Medical Association, the American College of Physicians, the American College of Surgeons, and the American Dental Association establishes standards for hospital care. The commission accredits hospitals that meet its standards. The Public Information Coordinator can tell you if a particular hospital is accredited.

ONCOLOGY NURSING SOCIETY
501 Holiday Drive
Pittsburgh, PA 15220
(412) 921-7373

Professional organization of oncology nurses who receive regular updates on the latest issues in oncology nursing.

SOCIETY OF GYNECOLOGIC ONCOLOGISTS
401 North Michigan Avenue
Chicago, IL 60611
(312) 644-6610, (800) 444-4441

Resource information on cancers of the female reproductive tract and referral services for oncologists in your area.

VISITING NURSE ASSOCIATIONS OF AMERICA
3801 East Florida Ave., Suite 900
Denver, CO 80210
(888) 866-8773

Provides callers with names of visiting-nurse associations in their community. More than 500 non-profit visiting-nurse associations in the United States provide community-based home care services including skilled nurses, therapists, and home health care aides.

II. COMMUNITY RESOURCES FOR CANCER SURVIVORS AND CONSUMERS

A. NATIONAL AGENCIES THAT PROVIDE INFORMATION AND SERVICES TO CANCER SURVIVORS

AMERICAN ASSOCIATION OF RETIRED PEOPLE (AARP)
601 E Street, NW
Washington, DC 20049
(800) 424-3410, (202) 434-2277
AARP on line: (800)827-9948, Prodigy: (800)776-3449, ext.147

Compuserve: (800) 621-1258

Provides a wide range of services to the elderly. Services include information, counseling groups, advocacy, benefits and entitlement, community activities, employment opportunities, teaching opportunities, training, and assistance to the homebound. A biweekly magazine available.

AMERICAN BRAIN TUMOR ASSOCIATION (ABTA)
2720 River Road, Suite 146
Des Plaines, IL 60018
(800) 886-2282, (847) 827-9910
E-mail: ABTA@aol.com
Web Page: http://neurosurgery.mgh.harvard.edu/abta/
http://pubweb.acns.nwu.edu/~lberko/abta_html/abtal.htm

A national organization providing patients and family members with written information about brain tumors and treatment. Services include patient education materials, listing of support groups, referrals to support organizations, a pen-pal program, information on treatment facilities, and funding for research. The ABTA also publishes a newsletter and provides publications for the public.

AMERICAN FOUNDATION FOR UROLOGIC DISEASE
300 W. Pratt Street, Suite 401
Baltimore, MD 21201
(800) 828-7866

Provides information on support groups for prostate cancer survivors and their families, as well as information on prostate cancer and other urologic disorders. A national information/referral service including a phone line is available.

AMERICAN HAIR LOSS COUNCIL
P.O. Box 809313
Chicago, IL 60606-9313
(800) 274-8717

Provides information and resources on hair loss.

AMERICAN SELF-HELP CLEARINGHOUSE
St. Clares-Riverside Medical Center
25 Pocono Road
Denville, NJ 07834
(201) 625-7101, (201) 625-9565, TDD (201) 625-9053

The Self-Help Clearinghouse maintains a database of 4,000 local self help meetings throughout New Jersey, as well as 650 national self help headquarters and one of a kind groups. Publishes a national directory and a network newsletter containing articles of interest to the self help and professional community. Assistance for persons interested in starting support groups is provided by telephone consultation and with resource materials by mail.

BONE MARROW TRANSPLANT FAMILY SUPPORT NETWORK
P.O. Box 845
Avon, CT 06001
(800) 826-9376

National person to person support network. Enables families to feel "connected" when coping with the decision, daily routines prior to and following transplants, and with the follow up care after transplant.

BREAST IMPLANT INFORMATION NETWORK
(800) 887-6828

Provides medical and legal information for women with or considering breast implants.

CANCER CARE, INC.
1180 Avenue of the Americas
New York, NY 10036
(212) 302-2400 (national office)

20 Crossway Park North
Suite 304
Woodbury, NY 11797
(800) 813-HOPE (813-4673)
E-mail: cancercare@aol.com

Cancer Care is a nonprofit organization whose mission is to help people with cancer and their families. Through professional one-to-one counseling, support groups, educational programs, and telephone contact, Cancer Care provides guidance, information, and referrals to cancer patients and families, all free of charge. Cancer Care also offers limited financial assistance for treatment related costs on a restricted basis in New York City, Long Island, New Jersey, and Connecticut. Cancer Care provides direct services through offices in New York, New Jersey, and Connecticut and nationally through their toll-free number.

CANCERVIVE
6500 Wilshire Blvd.
Suite 500
Los Angeles, CA 90048
(310) 203-9232

Assists cancer survivors to face and overcome the challenges of life after cancer.

CANDLELIGHTERS CHILDHOOD CANCER FOUNDATION
7910 Woodmont Avenue, Suite 460
Bethesda, MD 20814
(800) 366-2223, (301) 657-8401
E-mail: 75717.3513@compuserve.com

Parents of children and adolescents will want to contact The Candlelighters Childhood Cancer Foundation for support, information, and advocacy regarding childhood cancer and referral to local self help groups. CCCF has a network of peer support groups for parents; publishes a quarterly *Newsletter,* youth *Newsletter,* bibliography, and other materials; answers information requests; and maintains an Ombudsman Program on insurance concerns and long-term survivor's network. Other services include bereavement counseling, pain management, speaker's bureau, and a phone line.

CAN ACT (CANCER PATIENT'S ACTION ALLIANCE)
26 College Place
Brooklyn, NY 11201
(718) 522-4607

Addresses problems of access to advanced cancer treatments, barriers created by FDA drug approval process, and restrictive insurance reimbursement policies.

CHEMOCARE
231 North Ave., West
Westfield, NJ 07090
(800) 55-CHEMO (552-4366), (908) 233-1103 (NJ Residents)

A program of personal support and encouragement offered to people undergoing chemotherapy and/or radiation therapy by people who have experienced the treatment themselves. Other services include a newsletter, volunteer training programs, cancer counseling self-help/peer support groups, family and individual groups, cancer information, patient advocacy, speaker's bureau, information/referrals for community resources, and a phone line.

CORPORATE ANGEL NETWORK
Westchester County Airport Building 1
White Plains, NY 10604
(914) 328-1313, FAX (914) 328-3938

Helps alleviate costs for cancer patients receiving specialized treatment in NCI-approved treatment centers by arranging transportation aboard corporate aircraft on routine flights when seats are available.

CURE FOR LYMPHOMA FOUNDATION
215 Lexington Avenue
New York, NY 10016
(212) 319-5857

The CFL Foundation is a nonprofit organization established to raise money for lymphoma research and to provide support and education for those whose lives have been touched by lymphoma.

DES ACTION U.S.A. (WEST COAST OFFICE)
1615 Broadway, Suite 510
Oakland, CA 94612
(800) 337-9288

This national organization with over 30 chapters in the United States and affiliates in Canada, Australia, the Netherlands, and France offers counseling, educational materials, and a newsletter about diethylstilbestrol (DES), a synthetic hormone that was once given to women during pregnancy to prevent miscarriages. DES increases the risk of certain types of cancer in those women and their daughters who were exposed to the drug in the womb.

ENCORE PLUS
YWCA of the U.S.A.
Office of Women's Health Initiatives
624 9th Street NW 3rd Floor
Washington, DC 20001-5394
(202) 628-3636

Targets medically underserved women over 50 in need of early detection education, breast and cervical cancer screening, and support services. Provides women under treatment and recovering from breast cancer with a unique combined peer support and exercise program.

GILDA RADNER OVARIAN CANCER REGISTRY
Roswell Park Cancer Institute
Elm and Carlton Streets
Buffalo, NY 14263
(800) 682-7426

National registry providing information on screening and detection for ovarian cancer.

THE HUMOR PROJECT
110 Spring Street
Saratoga Springs, NY 12866

(518) 587-8770

Provides free catalog and resources on humorous material; holds conferences on the use of humor in coping with illness.

INTERNATIONAL ASSOCIATION OF LARYNGECTOMEES
1599 Clifton Road N.E.
Atlanta, GA 30329
(404) 329-7651

Voluntary organization composed of member clubs. Assists people who have lost their voice as a result of cancer. Call to get information on meetings held monthly at local chapters. Pre and postoperative education is available. Other services include a resource list, professional education, literature and publications for the public.

SUSAN G. KOMEN BREAST CANCER FOUNDATION
5005 LBJ Freeway, Suite 370
Dallas, TX 75244
(800) IM-AWARE, (800) 462-9273

National volunteer organization working through local chapters and Race for the Cure events across the country fighting to eradicate breast cancer by advancing research, education, screening and treatment. Helpline answered by trained volunteers who provide information on breast health or answer breast cancer questions.

LET'S FACE IT
P.O. Box 29972
Bellingham, WA 98228-1972
(360) 676-7325

Mutual help network for persons with facial disfigurements..

LEUKEMIA SOCIETY OF AMERICA
600 Third Avenue
New York, NY 10016
(800) 955-4LSA, (212) 573-8484

National voluntary health agency dedicated to seeking the cause and cure of leukemia, lymphomas (including Hodgkin's disease) and multiple myeloma. All counseling groups are free of charge and open to patients and families. Other services available are financial assistance, funding grants, professional education, speaker bureau, publications, literature, and information/referrals to different resources.

LOOK GOOD... FEEL BETTER
(See information under American Cancer Society or call (800)ACS-2345).

LYMPHOMA RESEARCH FOUNDATION OF AMERICA, INC.
8800 Venice Blvd., Suite 207
Los Angeles, CA 90034
(310) 204-7040
E-mail: lrfa@aol.com

A research organization that also provides information, education and support for lymphoma patients and their families. Sponsors support groups at no charge which meet on a regular basis in Los Angeles. Currently involved in developing nationwide support groups. Literature and publications available upon request.

MAKE TODAY COUNT
c/o Connie Zimmerman
Mid-America Cancer Center
1235 E. Cherokee
Springfield, MO 65804-2263
(800) 432-2273, FAX (417) 888-7426

Mutual support organization that brings together persons affected by a life-threatening illness so they may help each other. More than 200 chapters in the United States provide formal programs, group discussions, chapter newsletters, social activities, workshops, and seminars and education activities.

THE MAUTNER PROJECT
1707 L Street NW, Suite 1060
Washington, D.C. 20036
(202) 332-5536

Provides information, support, and advocacy to lesbians with cancer and their families.

MY IMAGE AFTER BREAST CANCER
6000 Stevenson Avenue, Suite 203
Alexandria, VA 22304
(703) 461-9616

Provides a 24-hour "HOPEline" staffed by breast cancer survivors to give information and counseling.

NATIONAL ALLIANCE OF BREAST CANCER
ORGANIZATIONS (NABCO)
9 East 37th Street, 10th Floor
New York, NY 10016
(212) 719-0154, (800) 719-9154 (outside NYC), (212) 889-0606
E-mail: nabcoinfo@aol.com
Web page: http://www.nabco.org

Non-profit central information resource on breast cancer; network of 300 organizations; advocates for beneficial legislative and regulatory change. Fixed fee for membership but information is given free of charge. Physician referrals are available. Other services include job discrimination related issues, professional education, speaker's bureau and literature/publications for the public.

NATIONAL ASSOCIATION FOR HOME CARE
228 7th Street, SE
Washington, DC 20003
(202) 547-7424

Trade association that represents the nation's home care agencies, hospices, and home care aide organizations. Services include professional education, information, and referrals on a national and local level, and publications.

NATIONAL BRAIN TUMOR FOUNDATION (NBTF)
785 Market Street, Suite 1600
San Francisco, CA 94103
(800) 934-CURE, (415) 284-0208
E-mail: sstf39f@prodigy.com

Raises funds for research and provides information on local and national levels, and counseling/support services to brain tumor patients, survivors and their families. Issues a quarterly newsletter. A telephone support line is available for patient-to-patient contact. An excellent publication, *Brain Tumors: The Resource Guide,* is available free of charge.

NATIONAL BREAST CANCER COALITION
1707 L Street NW, Suite 1060
Washington, DC 20036
(202) 296-7477, FAX (202) 265-6854

Grassroots advocacy movement of more than 300 member organizations and thousands of individuals working through a National Action Network, dedicated to the eradication of breast cancer through action, policy and advocacy.

NATIONAL COALITION FOR CANCER SURVIVORSHIP (NCCS)
1010 Wayne Avenue, 5th Floor
Silver Spring, MD 20910
(301) 650-8868, FAX (301) 565-9670

A network of independent groups and individuals concerned with survivorship and support of cancer survivors and their loved ones. The primary goal is to promote a national awareness of issues affecting cancer survivors. The NCCS serves as a clearinghouse for information on services and materials on survivorship; encourages the study of survivorship; and promotes the development of cancer support activities.

NATIONAL FAMILY CAREGIVERS ASSOCIATION
9621 East Bexhill Drive
Kensington, MD 20895
(800) 896-3650, (301) 942-6430

Helps improve lives of American's 18 million caregivers by providing information and support.

NATIONAL HOSPICE ORGANIZATION
1901 N. Moore Street, Suite 901
Arlington, VA 22209
(800) 658-8898

Non-profit membership association dedicated to promoting and maintaining quality care of terminally ill people and their families, providing education, technical assistance, publications and advocacy and referral services.

NATIONAL INFERTILITY NETWORK EXCHANGE
P.O. Box 204
East Meadow, NY 11554
(516) 794-5772

Peer support groups for infertile couples, education programs, and referral service.

NATIONAL KIDNEY CANCER ASSOCIATION
1234 Sherman Avenue, #203
Evanston, IL 60202
(847) 332-1051

The Association works to improve care and increase survival of kidney cancer patients through information, research, and patient advocacy with employers, government and insurance companies.

NATIONAL LYMPHEDEMA NETWORK
2211 Post Street, Suite 404
San Francisco, CA 94115
(800) 541-3259

Nonprofit resource center that provides information about prevention and treatment of lymphedema, swelling that is a common complication of lymph node surgery. Helps organize local support groups focusing on the treatment and impact of lymphedema. Publishes a newsletter with personal stories as well as network news.

NATIONAL SELF-HELP CLEARINGHOUSE
CUNY, Graduate School and University Center
25 W. 43rd Street, Room 620
New York, NY 10036
(212) 354-8525, FAX (212) 642-1956

Provides information and referral to self-help groups and regional self-help clearinghouses. Encourages and conducts training of professionals about self help; carries out research activities. Publishes manuals, training materials and newsletter.

NATIONAL WOMEN'S HEALTH NETWORK
1325 G Street NW
Washington, DC 20005

Provides preventative diet information focused specifically on breast cancer.

NORTH AMERICAN BRAIN TUMOR COALITION
595 Second Street
Brooklyn, NY 11215-2601

PATIENT ADVOCATES FOR ADVANCED
CANCER TREATMENTS (PAACT)
1143 Parmelee NW
Grand Rapids, MI 49504
(616) 453-1477, FAX (616) 453-1846

Association for both patients and physicians for diagnostic and therapeutic treatments of prostate cancer.

PROSTATE CANCER SUPPORT GROUP NETWORK
300 West Pratt Street
Suite 401
Baltimore, MD 21201
(410) 727-2908

A national network of over 400 prostate cancer survivor support and self-help groups that promotes awareness, education, support and research. Addresses the collective needs of all the groups through increasing public awareness and advocacy, and provides current information through leadership meetings and educational seminars.

SUPPORT FOR PEOPLE WITH ORAL AND
HEAD AND NECK CANCER, INC. (SPAHNC)
PO Box 53
Locust Valley, NY 11560-0053
(516) 759-5333 (phone and FAX)

Addresses the broad emotional, psychological and humanistic needs of these cancer survivors, empowering each to take an active role in his or her recovery.

SHARE (SELF HELP FOR WOMEN
WITH BREAST OR OVARIAN CANCER)
1501 Broadway, Suite 1720
New York, NY 10036
(212) 719-0364

Provides information and support for women with breast and ovarian cancer to help them help themselves.

UNITED OSTOMY ASSOCIATION, INC.
36 Executive Park, Suite 120
Irvine, CA 92614
(800) 826-0826, (714) 660-8624, FAX (714) 660-9262

Association of ostomy chapters dedicated to complete rehabilitation of all ostomates.

US TOO INTERNATIONAL, INC.
930 North York Road, Suite 50
Hinsdale, IL 60521-2993
(800) 808-7866, (708) 323-1002, FAX (708) 323-1003

Provides prostate cancer survivors and their families emotional and educational support through an international network of chapters.

WELLNESS COMMUNITY
2716 Ocean Park Boulevard
Suite 1040
Santa Monica, CA 90405-5211
(310) 314-2555

The largest cancer support organization devoted solely to psychological and emotional support for cancer survivors and their families and serves as an adjunct to medical treatment. All services are free, including support groups, workshops, lectures, and other social events.

WELL SPOUSE FOUNDATION
17456 Drayton Hall Way
San Diego, CA 92128

Network of support and advocacy groups for families of a person with a chronic illness.

Y-ME NATIONAL ORGANIZATION FOR
BREAST CANCER INFORMATION AND SUPPORT
212 West Van Buren, 4th Floor
Chicago, IL 60607-3908
(800) 221-2141, (312) 986-8338

Provides peer-support groups, volunteer matching, educational materials, and referrals to community resources. Provides training and technical assistance to hotline staffs of other cancer support groups and a detailed self-help manual for starting support groups. Maintains a prosthesis bank for women with financial need.

B. NEWSLETTERS ABOUT CANCER SURVIVORSHIP

AMERICAN BRAIN TUMOR ASSOCIATION
2720 River Rd., Suite 146
Des Plaines, IL 60018
(847) 827-9910

AMERICAN FOUNDATION FOR UROLOGIC DISEASE
300 W. Pratt Street, Suite 401
Baltimore, MD 21201
(800) 828-7866

AMERICAN PROSTATE SOCIETY
1340F Charwood Road
Hanover, MD 21076
(410) 859-3735

BONE MARROW TRANSPLANT (BMT) NEWSLETTER
1985 Spruce Avenue
Highland Park, IL 60035
(847) 831-1913

CANCER COMMUNICATION NEWSLETTER
1143 Parmelee NW
Grand Rapids, MI 49504
(616) 453-1477
  Newsletter for men with prostate cancer

CANDLELIGHTERS
Childhood Cancer Foundation, Inc.
7910 Woodmont Ave., Suite 460
Bethesda, MD 20814
(800) 366-2223
  Publishes three different newsletters—one for parents, one for children, and one for young adult survivors of childhood cancer

CONVERSATIONS!
c/o Cindy H. Melancon
P.O. Box 7948
Amarillo, TX 79114-7948
(806) 355-2565
  The newsletter for women who are fighting ovarian cancer.

COPING MAGAZINE
Media America, Inc.
2019 North Carothers
Franklin, TN 37064
(615) 790-2400
  Magazine about living with and beyond a cancer diagnosis; published six times a year.

THE FUNLETTER
P.O. Box 4545
Santa Barbara, CA 93140
  A fun-filled newsletter for kids and families battling cancer.

INTERNATIONAL MYELOMA FOUNDATION
2120 Stanley Hills Drive
Los Angeles, CA 90046

LIVING THROUGH CANCER JOURNAL
Living Through Cancer Survivorship Center
323 Eighth Street SW
Albuquerque, NM 87102
(505) 242-3263
  Written by and for survivors and their families and includes per-

sonal stories, poetry, book reviews, articles on survivorship, and resource lists.

NCCS Networker
National Coalition for Cancer Survivorship
1010 Wayne Avenue, 5th Floor
Silver Spring, MD 20910

SEARCH
National Brain Tumor Foundation
323 Geary Street, Suite 510
San Francisco, CA 94102
(415) 296-0404

Quarterly publication reports stories of people who have been diagnosed with brain tumors and their families, as well as organizational news.

Surviving! A Patient Newsletter
Stanford University Medical Center
Patient Resource Center, Room H0108
Division of Radiation Oncology
300 Pasteur Drive
Stanford, CA 94305
(415) 723-6171

Created by Stanford University Medical Center patients primarily for survivors of Hodgkins disease, this newsletter contains original personal stories, essays, and artwork by cancer survivors as well as medical news.

Take Care!
National Family Cardgivers Association
9223 Longbranch Parkway
Silver Springs, MD 20901
(800)296-3650

Provides caregivers with "can-do" information, resources, answers to their questions, and more.

Y-ME
212 West Van Buren St.
Fourth Floor
Chicato, IL 60607-3908
(800) 221-2141

Newsletter for breast cancer survivors.

III. INSURANCE RESOURCES

LIST OF STATE INSURANCE DEPARTMENTS

For information and assistance on insurance laws, rights, and companies, contact the office listed for your state. Note: this information, current as of, January, 1995, is subject to change.

ALABAMA
Commissioner, Insurance Department
135 South Union St., Rm. 200
Montgomery, AL 36104
(334) 269-3550

ALASKA
Director, Commerce and Economic Development Department
P.O. Box 110805
Juneau, AK 99811-0805
(907) 465-2515

ARIZONA
Director, Department of Insurance
2910 N. 44th St., Ste. 210
Phoenix, AZ 85018
(602) 912-8444

ARKANSAS
Commissioner, Insurance Department
1200 West 3rd Street
Little Rock, AR 72201
(501) 371-2600

CALIFORNIA
Department of Insurance
300 South Spring St.
Los Angeles, CA 90013
(213) 897-8921

COLORADO
Acting Commissioner, Division of Insurance
Dept. of Regulatory Agencies
1560 Broadway, Ste. 1550
Denver, CO 80202
(303) 894-7855

CONNECTICUT
Commissioner, Department of Insurance
153 Market St., 11th Fl.
Hartford, CT 06103
(203) 297-3800

DELAWARE
Commissioner, Department of Insurance
841 Silver Lake Blvd.
P.O. Box 7007
Dover, DE 19903
(302) 739-4251

DISTRICT OF COLUMBIA
Administrator, Insurance Administration
Consumer & Regulatory Affairs Department
P.O. Box 37378
Washington, DC 20013
(202) 727-8000

FLORIDA
Department of Insurance
Bureau of Consumer Assistance
200 E. Gaines St.
Tallahassee, FL 32399-0322
(904) 922-3100

GEORGIA
Comptroller General & Insurance Commissioner
Office of Insurance
West Tower, 7th Fl.
2 Martin Luther King, Jr. Dr.
Atlanta, GA 30334
(404) 656-2056

HAWAII
Insurance Commissioner, Division of Insurance
Commerce & Consumer Affairs Department
250 South King St.
Honolulu, HI 96813
(808) 586-2790

ILLINOIS
Acting Director, Department of Insurance
320 W. Washington, 4th Fl.
Springfield, IL 62767-0001
(217) 782-4515

INDIANA
Director, Department of Insurance
311 W. Washington St., Ste. 300
Indianapolis, IN 46204
(317) 232-2385

IOWA
Commissioner, Insurance Division
Department of Commerce
Lucas State Office Bldg.
Des Moines, IA 50319
(515) 281-5705

KANSAS
Commissioner, Insurance Department
420 S.W. Ninth St.
Topeka, KS 66612-1678
(913) 296-3071

KENTUCKY
Commissioner, Department of Insurance
Public Protection & Regulation Cabinet
215 W. Main St.
Frankfort, KY 40601
(502) 564-6027

LOUISIANA
Commissioner, Department of Insurance
P.O. Box 94214
Baton Rouge, LA 70804-9214
(504) 342-5900
(800) 259-5300 in state

MAINE
Superintendent, Bureau of Insurance
Professional & Financial Regulations Department
46 State House Station
Augusta, ME 04333-0046
(207) 287-3461

MARYLAND
Commissioner, Division of Insurance
Licensing & Regulation Department
501 St. Paul Pl.
Baltimore, MD 21202-2272
(410) 333-2521

MASSACHUSETTS
Commissioner, Division of Insurance
Executive Office of Consumer Affairs
470 Atlantic Avenue
Boston, MA 02210
(617) 521-7794

MICHIGAN
Commissioner of Insurance
Licensing & Regulation Dept.
611 W. Ottawa
P.O. Box 30220
Lansing, MI 48909
(517) 373-9273

MINNESOTA
Commissioner, Department of Commerce
133 East 7th St.
St. Paul, MN 55101
(612) 296-6848

MISSISSIPPI
Commissioner, Department of Insurance
1804 Sillers Bldg.
Jackson, MS 39201
(601) 359-3569

RESOURCES

MISSOURI
Director, Division of Insurance
Department of Economic Development
Truman Bldg., Box 690
Jefferson City, MO 65102
(800) 726-7390

MONTANA
Chief Deputy Commissioner,
Office of State Insurance Division Auditor
Mitchell Bldg., Room 130
Helena, MT 59620
(406) 444-3871

NEBRASKA
Director, Department of Insurance
The Terminal Bldg.
941 O St., Ste. 400
Lincoln, NE 68508
(402) 471-2200

NEVADA
Commissioner, Insurance Division
Department of Commerce
3406 Centennial Park Dr.
Carson City, NV 89706
(702) 687-4270

NEW HAMPSHIRE
New Hampshire Insurance Department
169 Manchester St.
Concord, NH 03301-5151
(603) 271-2261

NEW JERSEY
Commissioner, Department of Insurance
20 W. State St., CN325
Trenton, NJ 08625
(609) 292-5360

NEW MEXICO
Superintendent, State Insurance Division
State Corporation Commission
500 Old Santa Fe Trail
Rm. 428, PERA Bldg.
Santa Fe, NM 87504
(505) 827-4297

NEW YORK
Superintendent of Insurance
Insurance Department
Empire State Plaza, Bldg. #1
Albany, NY 12257
(518) 474-4550

NORTH CAROLINA
Commissioner
430 N. Salisbury St.
Raleigh, NC 27603-5908
(919) 733-7343
(800) 662-7777

NORTH DAKOTA
Commissioner, Insurance Department
State Capitol
600 E. Blvd., 5th Fl.
Bismarck, ND 58505-0320

OHIO
Director, Department of Insurance
2100 Stella Ct.
Columbus, OH 43215-1067
(614) 644-2658

OKLAHOMA
Commissioner, Insurance Department
3814 North Santa Fe
Oklahoma City, OK 73118
(405) 521-2828

OREGON
Director, Department of Consumer & Business Services
350 Winter Street NE
Salem, OR 97310
(503) 378-4120

PENNSYLVANIA
Commissioner, Insurance Department
1321 Strawberry Sq.
Harrisburg, PA 17120
(717) 787-2317

RHODE ISLAND
Department of Business Regulation
233 Richmond St.
Providence, RI 02903
(401) 277-2246

SOUTH CAROLINA
Chief Insurance Commissioner
Department of Insurance
120 East Alpine Road
Columbia, SC 29219
(803) 788-0500

SOUTH DAKOTA
Secretary, Division of Insurance
Commerce & Regulations Dept.
500 East Capitol
Pierre, SD 57501
(605) 773-3563

TENNESSEE
Commissioner, Department of Commerce & Insurance
Volunteer Plaza
500 James Robertson Pkwy.
Nashville, TN 37243
(615) 741-2241

TEXAS
Commissioner, Board of Insurance
111-A P.O. Box 149091
Austin, TX 78714-9091
(512) 463-6464

UTAH
Commissioner, Department of Insurance
State Office Bldg., Rm. 3110
Salt Lake City, UT 84114
(801) 538-3800

VERMONT
Commissioner, Department of Banking & Insurance
89 Main St., Drawer 20
Montpelier, VT 05620-3101
(802) 828-3301

VIRGINIA
Chairman, State Corporation Commission
1300 East Main St.
Richmond, VA 23219
(804) 371-9694

WASHINGTON
Insurance Commissioner
Office of the Insurance Commissioner
P.O. Box 40256
Olympia, WA 98504-0256
(360) 753-3613

WASHINGTON, DC.
See District of Columbia

WEST VIRGINIA
Commissioner, Division of Insurance
P.O. Box 50540
Charleston, WV 25305-0540
(304) 558-3394

WISCONSIN
Commissioner, Office of Commissioner of Insurance
123 W. Washington Avenue
P.O. Box 7873
Madison, WI 53707
(608) 267-2305

WYOMING
Commissioner, Insurance Department
Herschler Building, 3 Floor East
122 W. 25th St.
Cheyenne, WY 82002
(307) 777-7401

ADDITIONAL SOURCES FOR INSURANCE INFORMATION

AIDS BENEFITS HANDBOOK (mail order only)
P.O. Box 209040
Yale University Press
New Haven, CT 06520-9040
(203) 432-0940

Provides valuable information on social security, welfare, medicaid, medicare, food stamps, housing, drugs and other benefits for AIDS survivors and cancer survivors as well.

CONSUMER FEDERATION OF AMERICAS GROUP
(Formerly, National Insurance Consumer Organization)
414 A Street, SE
Washington, DC 20003
(202) 547-6426

Offers tips on topics such as how to select an insurance agent and what coverage to avoid. For list of publications, send a self-addressed stamped envelope.

MEDICAL INFORMATION BUREAU, INC.
P.O. Box 105, Essex Station
Boston, MA 02112
(617) 426-3660

Keeps data about your health on file for insurance companies. You can verify that any information they have about you is correct by writing for a form requesting disclosure of the information the bureau has. The records must be sent to a "licensed medical professional" whom you designate.

MEDICARE RIGHTS CENTER
1460 Broadway, 8th Floor
New York, NY 10036-7393
(212) 869-3850 or (800) 333-4114 (northeastern states only)

Dedicated to ensuring the rights of seniors and people with disabilities to quality, affordable health care through direct services, public education and public policy.

NATIONAL ASSOCIATION OF PERSONAL FINANCIAL ADVISORS
1130 Lake Cook Rd. #150
Buffalo Grove, Il
(847) 537-7722

Professional association of fee-based personal financial advisors who can refer individuals to financial planners who concentrate their practices on the needs of people with serious illness.

NATIONAL INSURANCE CONSUMER HELPLINE (NIAA)
(800) 942-4242

Provides free information and publications on insurance, including health and disability insurance.

IV. LEGAL AND FINANCIAL RESOURCES

STATE EMPLOYMENT DISCRIMINATION LAWS AND ENFORCING AGENCIES (AS OF FEBRUARY, 1996)

Every state has a law that prohibits employment discrimination based on disability. State laws that cover employers who have fewer than 15 employees may protect cancer survivors whose employers are not covered by the Americans with Disabilities Act.

Most states have an agency that enforces the employment discrimination law. Some states require you to file a complaint with the state agency before or instead of filing a complaint in state court. If you live and work in different states, contact the agency where you work. If your state has no enforcing agency, contact an attorney or the Equal Employment Opportunity Commission at (800) 669-4000 for how to file a complaint directly in state court or for further information.

STATE	EMPLOYERS COVERED	ENFORCING AGENCY
ALABAMA	public employers	none
ALASKA	min. 1 employee	Human Rights Commission 800 A Street, Suite 204 Anchorage, AL 99501 (907) 274-4692

ARIZONA
min. 15 employees

Civil Rights Division
1275 West Washington Street
Phoenix, AZ 85007
(602) 542-5263

ARKANSAS
min. 9 employees

none

CALIFORNIA
min. 5 employees

Department of Fair Employment
   and Housing
2014 T Street, Suite 210
Sacramento, CA 95814
(916) 445-9918

COLORADO
min. 1 employee

Civil Rights Commission
1560 Broadway, Suite 1050
Denver, CO 80202-5143
(303) 894-2997

CONNECTICUT
min. 3 employees

Commission on Human Rights
   and Opportunities
21 Grand Street
Hartford, CT 06106
(860) 541-3400

DELAWARE
min. 20 employees

Department of Labor
Labor Law Enforcement Section
State Office Building,
   6th Floor
820 North French Street
Wilmington, DE 19801
(302) 577-2011

DISTRICT OF COLUMBIA
min. 1 employee

Human Rights Commission
441 4th Street NW,
Room 970 North
Washington, DC 20001
(202) 724-1385

FLORIDA
    min. 15 employees   Commission on Human
                                Relations
                             325 John Knox Road,
                             Bldg. F, Suite 240
                             Tallahassee, FL 32303-4149
                             (904) 488-7082

GEORGIA
    min. 15 employees   Public employment only:
                             Georgia Office of Fair
                                Employment Practices
                             156 Trinity Avenue, S.W.
                             Suite 208
                             Atlanta, GA 30303
                             (404) 656-1736

HAWAII
    min. 1 employee   Hawaii Civil Rights Commission
                             888 Mililani Street, 2nd Floor
                             Honolulu, HI 96813
                             (808) 586-8640

IDAHO
    min. 5 employees   Commission on Human Rights
                             1109 Main Street, #400
                             Boise, ID 83720-0040
                             (208) 334-2873

ILLINOIS
    min. 1 employee   Department of Human Rights
                             James R. Thompson Center
                             100 West Randolph Street,
                                10th Floor
                             Chicago, IL 60601
                             (312) 814-6245

INDIANA
    min. 15 employees   Civil Rights Commission
                             103 N. Senate Avenue,
                                Room N
                             Indianapolis, IN 46204
                             (317) 232-2600

IOWA
 min. 4 employees Civil Rights Commission
211 East Maple Street,
 2nd Floor
Des Moines, IA 50319
(515) 281-4121

KANSAS
 min. 4 employees Civil Rights Commission
Landon State Office Building
900 SW Jackson St.,
 Suite 851 South
Topeka, KS 66612-1258
(913) 296-3206

KENTUCKY
 min. 8 employees Human Rights Commission
332 West Broadway, 7th Floor
Louisville, KY 40202
(502) 595-4024

LOUISIANA
 min. 15 employees none

MAINE
 min. 1 employee Human Rights Commission
Statehouse, Station 51
Augusta, ME 04333
(207) 624-6050

MARYLAND
 min. 15 employees Commission on Human
 Relations
William Donald Shafer Tower,
 #900
6 St. Paul Street
Baltimore, MD 21202
(410) 767-8600

MASSACHUSETTS
    min. 6 employees   Commission Against
                                       Discrimination
                                  One Ashburton Place
                                  Boston, MA 02108
                                  (617) 727-3990

MICHIGAN
    min. 1 employee   Department of Civil Rights
                                  1200 6th Street,
                                      5th Floor North Tower
                                  Detroit Ml 48226
                                  (313) 256-2615

MINNESOTA
    min. 1 employee   Department of Human Rights
                                  Bremer Tower
                                  7th Place and Minnesota Street
                                  St. Paul, MN 55101
                                  (612) 296-5663

MISSISSIPPI
    public and private   none
    employers that receive
    public funds

MISSOURI
    min. 6 employees   Commission on Human Rights
                                      3315 West Truman Boulevard
                                  Jefferson City, MO
                                  65102-1129
                                  (573) 751-3325

MONTANA
    min. 1 employee   Human Rights Commission
                                  PO Box 1728
                                  616 Helena Avenue
                                  Helena MT 59624
                                  (406)444-2884

NEBRASKA
min. 15 employees
Equal Opportunity Commission
301 Centennial Mall South
PO Box 94934
Lincoln, NE 68509-4934
(402) 471-2024

NEVADA
min. 15 employees
Equal Rights Commission
2450 Wrondel Way, Suite C
Reno, NV 89502
(702) 688-1288

NEW HAMPSHIRE
min. 6 employees
Human Rights Commission
163 Loudon Road
Concord, NH 03301
(603) 271-2767

NEW JERSEY
min. 1 employee
Division of Civil Rights
31 Clinton Street, 3rd Floor
Newark, NJ 07102
(201) 648-2700

NEW MEXICO
min. 4 employees
Human Rights Commission
1596 Pacheco Street
Aspen Plaza
Santa Fe, NM 87505
(505) 827-6838

NEW YORK
min. 4 employees
Division of Human Rights
55 West 125th Street
New York, NY 10027
(212) 961-8400

NORTH CAROLINA
min. 15 employees
Human Relations Commission
217 West Jones Street
Raleigh, NC 27603
(919) 733-7996

Office of Administrative Hearings
424 North Blount
Raleigh, NC 27601
(919) 733-2691

NORTH DAKOTA
    min. 1 employee   none

OHIO
    min. 4 employees   Civil Rights Commission
220 Parsons Avenue
Columbus, OH 43215-5385
(614) 466-5928

OKLAHOMA
    min. 15 employees   Human Rights Commission
2101 North Lincoln Boulevard,
    Room 480
Oklahoma City, OK 73105
(405) 521-2360

OREGON
    min. 6 employees   Civil Rights Division
Bureau of Labor & Industry
800 NE Oregon Street, #1070
Box #32
Portland, OR 97232
(503) 731-4075

PENNSYLVANIA
    min. 4 employees   Human Relations Commission
1001 South 2nd Street, #300
Harrisburg, PA 17105
(717) 783-8266

RHODE ISLAND
    min. 4 employees   Commission for Human Rights
10 Abbott Park Place
Providence, RI 02903-3768
(401) 277-2661

SOUTH CAROLINA
min. 15 employees

Human Affairs Commission
2611 Forest Drive, Suite 200
Columbia, SC 29204
(803) 253-6336

SOUTH DAKOTA
min. 1 employee

Commission on Human
    Relations
224 West 9th Street
Sioux Falls, SD 57104-6407
(605) 367-7039

TENNESSEE
min. 8 employees

Human Rights Commission
531 Henley Street, Suite 701
Knoxville, TN 37902
(423) 594-6500

TEXAS
min. 15 employees

Commission on Human
    Rights
Box 13493
Austin, TX 78711
(512) 437-3450

UTAH
min. 15 employees

Anti-Discrimination Division
    of the Industrial Commission
160 East Third S, 3rd floor
Salt Lake City, UT 84111
(801) 530-6801

VERMONT
min. 1 employee

Attorney General's Office
Civil Rights Division
109 Slate Street
Montpelier, VT 05609
(802) 828-3657

VIRGINIA
    min. 6 employees   Council on Human Rights
                                   1100 Bank Street
                                   Richmond, VA 23219
                                   (804) 225-2292

WASHINGTON
    min. 8 employees   Human Rights Commission
                                   1511 Third Avenue, Suite 921
                                   Seattle, WA 98101
                                   (206) 464-6500

WEST VIRGINIA
    min. 12 employees   West Virginia Human Rights
                                      Commission
                                   1321 Plaza East, Room 108A
                                   Charleston, WV 25301-1400
                                   (304) 558-2616

WISCONSIN
    min. 1 employee   Equal Rights Division
                                   201 East Washington Avenue,
                                       Room 117
                                   PO Box 8928
                                   Madison, WI 53708
                                   (608) 266-6860

WYOMING
    min. 2 employees   Fair Employment Commission
                                   6101 Yellowstone,
                                       Room 259C
                                   Cheyenne, WY 82002
                                   (307) 777-7262

FEDERAL GOVERNMENT AGENCIES

EQUAL EMPLOYMENT OPPORTUNITIES COMMISSION
1801 L Street NW, Room 9405
Washington, DC 20507
(800) 669-3362
   Provides information in English and Spanish on how to enforce your rights under the Americans with Disabilities Act

JOB ACCOMMODATION NETWORK (JAN)
President's Committee on Employment of the Handicapped
918 Chestnut Ridge Road, #1
PO Box 6080
Morgantown, WV 26505
(800) JAN-PCEH (526-7234)

   JAN provides information to employers on how to accommodate a handicapped worker.

NATIONAL REHABILITATION INFORMATION CENTER
8455 Colesville Road, Suite 935
Silver Spring, MD 20910
(800) 346-2742

   Government-funded information service that provides access to comprehensive information on disability-related products, research, and resources. Provides publications and referrals to support groups.

REHABILITATION SERVICES ADMINISTRATION
United States Department of Education
Office of the Commissioner
330 C Street, S.W.
Washington, DC 20202
(202) 205-5482

   Responsible for ensuring that your state rehabilitation services agency complies with federal law.

PUBLIC INTEREST RESOURCES

AMERICAN CIVIL LIBERTIES UNION (ACLU)
132 West 43rd Street
New York, NY 10036
(212) 944-9800 (or call local listings)

   Provides legal assistance for victims of discrimination.

BONE MARROW TREATMENT NEWSLETTER
1985 Spruce Ave.
Highland Park, IL 60035
(847) 831-1913

   Provides a list of attorneys who handle legal issues arising from bone marrow transplant.

CHOICE IN DYING
200 Varick Street, Room 1001
New York, NY 10014

(212) 366-5540

This not-for-profit organization working for recognition of an individual's right to die with dignity provides information about living wills.

NATIONAL ACADEMY OF ELDER LAW ATTORNEYS
1604 North Country Club Road
Tucson, AZ 85716
(602) 881-4005

Provides information about how to identify and select an attorney experienced in dealing with elderly clients and their families as well as the special areas of law that affect the elderly. Prefers written inquiries with a stamped, self-addressed envelope for replies.

NATIONAL ASSOCIATION OF MEAL PROGRAMS
204 E Street, N.W.
Washington, D.C. 20002
(202) 547-6157

Provides information about meal programs (Meals on Wheels, etc.) in your community. Such programs, which provide at least one hot meal a day to individuals who are housebound, may be run by private agencies; local departments of health, public welfare, or aging; church groups; or community volunteer organizations. Other Meals-on-Wheels programs may be listed in your telephone directory under "Meals on Wheels."

NATIONAL EMPLOYMENT LAWYER'S ASSOCIATION
600 Harrison Street, Suite 535
San Francisco, CA 94107
nelahq@igc.apc.org

The NELA is a nonprofit, professional membership organization of more than 2,600 lawyers from around the country who represent employees in employment matters. To request a state listing of employment lawyers, please send a written request and a self-addressed envelope to NELA and allow four to six weeks for delivery.

Index

abdominoperineal resection, 22
ADA. See Americans with Disabilities Act
adjuvant therapy, 10, 15, 26
adopting a child, 255–56
advance health directives, 245.
   See also refusing treatment
advocating for cancer survivors. See advocacy
advocacy,
   advocating for cancer survivors 275–80
   definition of, 276
   self-advocacy, 276–280.
   See also empowerment
affirmations, 101
Agency for Health Care Policy and Research (AHCPR), 14
alcohol and cancer, 28
alternative systems of medical practice, 77.
   See also unconventional treatment
American Academy of Allergy Asthma and Immunology (AAAI), 39
American Cancer Society, 68, 285
"American Cancer Society's Survivor's Bill of Rights," 38
American Hospital Association Guide to the Health Care Field, 45
American Medical Directory, 36
Americans with Disabilities Act, 57, 184, 210–13, 254–55
anxiety, 98
appetite, loss of, 15
aspirin, in clinical trials, 29
assertiveness. See empowerment
attitudes toward cancer, of friends and relatives of survivors, 104, 105
autogenic exercise, 106–7
autogenics, 110

basic credentials, of medical practitioners, 36
Benjamin, Harold, 81
bereaved, rights of, 135
beta-carotene, 76
bioelectromagnetic applications, 77.
   See also unconventional treatment
biologic treatments, 77.
   See also unconventional treatment
biopsy, definition of, 7
bleomycin, 24
blood and immune system problems, 25

blood cell counts. See low blood counts
Blum, Diane, 62
board certification, 36
bone marrow and blood cell production, 18.
   See also growth factor
bone marrow transplantation, 10
   allogeneic, 10
   autologous, 10
Bone Marrow Transplant Newsletter, 195
breast, radiation to, 22
breast cancer, 26
breathing. See respiratory problems

calcium, 29
Calder, Kimberley, 168
CAnCare, 157
cancer,
   cells, growth of, 6
   definition, 5
   detection, 27
   emotions and, 95
   long-term control of, 7
   metastasis, 8
   myths about, 263–64
   screening, goals of, 5
   stages of. (See survivorship, stages of)
   subclinical form, 7
   symptom relief, 7
   symptoms, 12
   treatment, definition of, 6. (See also treatment plan.)
   See also under specific headings
cancer and personal attitude, 93, 94
Cancer Care, Inc., 68
cancer centers, 44
cancer experience, benefits of, 111
CancerFax, 284
Cancer Information Service, 283
cancer insurance. See health insurance
CancerNet, 284
Cancer Pain Guideline, 14
"Cancer Survivors' Bill of Rights," 59–60
Candlelighters Childhood Cancer Foundation, 68
Candlelighters Quarterly, 140
Candlelighters Youth Newsletter, 140
CanSurmount, 140
Card, Irene, 168
caregivers. See health-care providers
Cassileth, Barrie, MD, 78, 82, 84
Catholic Charities, 70
centering, 110, 111
certification, of a doctor, 36

Chapman, Christoper, 84
Chasen, Nancy, 32
chemoprevention trials, 29
chemotherapy, 9
   and fetal development, 21
   and nausea and vomiting, 17
   and sexual problems 22.
   See also treatment types
childhood cancer survivors, 25
children,
   and coping with cancer in the family, 122
   and informed consent, 52
Choices in Healing, 80
choosing a doctor, 33, 35–39
choosing a hospital, 43–47
City of Hope research project, 77
Clark, Elizabeth Johns, 116
Claudet, Ann, 251
clergy, 70
clinical trials, 8, 11–12, 29.
   See also unconventional treatment
COBRA. See Comprehensive Omnibus Budget Reconciliation Act
colon cancer, 29
communication,
   patient-doctor, 39–43, 85
   among family members, 118–19, 121–24, 130
Communication: It's Good for Your Health, 39
communication skills, developing, 278
community resources for cancer survivors and consumers, 292
Comprehensive Omnibus Budget Reconciliation Act, 185–86
consent. See informed consent
concentration, loss of, 19–20
conception and sterility, 21
confidentiality, 50, 52–54, 58
   challenges to, 56
   and support groups, 57
conization of cervix, 22
consultations with a caregiver, 40–43
Consumers' Guide to Health Plans, 199
coping styles, 42
   I Can Cope, 125, 140
   children and, 122
coronary artery disease, 24
costs of cancer treatment. See financial impact of cancer
Council of Churches, 70
counseling. (See social workers)
   different from peer support groups, 144
Cousins, Norman, 82

A CANCER *survivor's* ALMANAC

crisis of cancer, 118
Cruzan, Nancy, 247
curative intent, definition of, 6
cure, medical definition of, 6
cystectomy, radical, 22

Department of Veterans Affairs, 243
Dependent Equity Fiscal Responsibility Act (DEFRA), 178
depression, 100, 102
detection of cancer, early, 27
diagnosis,
 negative reactions to, 97
 the initial crisis of, 117
dialogue. See communication, patient-doctor
diet, and cancer prevention, 28. See also nutrition
dietary problems, 15
dietary services, 68
dietitians, 69
disability insurance, 172
discrimination in employment. See employment discrimination
DNA-based testing, 57
dry mouth, 16
durable power of attorney for health care, 245, 246
Dying at Home, 131
dysfunction, 27

Eating Hints for Cancer Patients, 68
emotions,
 coping with, 97
 expressing, 95
Employee Retirement and Income Security Act. See ERISA
employment,
 avoiding discrimination, 222
 and cancer survivors, 207
 discrimination, 207–31
  and federal agencies, 323
  and state employment discrimination laws, 315
 employment rights, 207–31
  enforcing 225–30.
 See also Americans with Disabilities Act
empowerment, 5, 34, 277
 in the hospital, 49, 50, 94
endocrine problems, 26
Engel, Renee, 217
ERISA, 184, 186–88, 216
Essiac, 78
expenses. See financial impact of cancer
experimental treatment. See clinical trials; unconventional treatment

Family and Medical Leave Act, 215
family members,
 coping styles, 121
 children, 122
 family burnout, 12
 reactions to cancer patients,
Fawzy, Fawzy I, MD, 80
Federal Rehabilitation Act, 213–15
Federation of Jewish Philanthropy, 70
Federation of Protestant Welfare Agencies, 70
female sexual problems. See sexual problems
fiber in diet, 29
finasteride, 29
fertility 21, 23, 26
fetal development, 21
financial impact of cancer, 239–45
 credit, 254
 financial information resources, 315
 financial planning, 244, 248–49
  trusts and estates, 249
 financial support, 240
  private, 240
  public, 241. (See also Social Security)
 power of attorney, 250
 taxes, deducting medical expenses from, 243–44
 wills, traditional, 248
Fiore, Neil, 92
Food and Drug Administration Cancer Liaison Office, 84
Freedom of Information Act, 56
From Victim to Victor, 81

Ganz, Patricia, MD, 4
G-CSF. See growth factor
gender differences in coping, 120
genetic information, 56
GM-CSF. See growth factor
Goldsmith, Lisa, MD, 219–220
gonadal failure, 27
grief. See loss and grief
growth factor, 18–19
Guide to Health Insurance for People with Medicare, 178
guilt, 81, 95–96, 120

hair loss, 17, 68
 minimizing, 18
 preparation for, 18
halitosis, 16
healing strategies, 94

health-care providers. See clergy, dietary services, hospice care, nurses, psychologists and psychiatrists, rehabilitation specialists, social workers
health insurance, 169–195, 199
 collecting benefits, 192–94
 obtaining, 182
 purchasing, 189–91
 reasonable and customary charges, 170
 regulation of, 188
 and rights of individuals, 189
 right to, 185
 Social Security benefits, 241–42
 strictures regarding hospital stays, 47
 types of, 170
  cancer insurance, 171
  catastrophic insurance, 170
  fee-for-service, 170
  hospital indemnity policy, 175
  lifetime maximum benefits, 170
  long-term care insurance, 175
  Medicaid, 181
  medical savings accounts, 171
  Medicare, 176–77, 178–81
  Medicare HMOs, 180–81
  Medigap 178, 179
 and unconventional treatment, 195
 veteran's benefits, 243
Health Insurance Portability and Accountability Act of 1996, 184
health maintenance organization, 173
healthy imagining, 110, 111, 112–13
heart muscle injury, 24
Henning, Margherita, 252
herbal medicine, 78. See also unconventional treatment
HMO. See health maintenance organization; managed care plans
Hodgkin's disease, 26
Hoffman, Barbara, 206
Holland, Jimmie, 80, 100
hope, 125–26
hormone treatment for prostrate cancer, 22
hospice care, 69–70, 131
Hospital and Community Psychiatry, 57
hospital experience, 47–49
 admission, 47–48
 leaving, 50
 preadmission, 47
hospital indemnity policy, 175
hospitals,
 evaluating, 4
 types of, 44
 accreditation, 45
hospital stays, 47

How to Select a Home Care Agency, 67
Human Dimensions of Cancer Care: Principles and Guidelines for Action, The, 71
hyperthermia treatment, 1
hysterectomy. See radical hysterectomy

I Can Cope, 140
ice turban, 18
identifying feelings and beliefs, 98
imagery, 109
  autogenics, 106–7, 110
  centering, 110, 111
  healthy imagining, 110, 111, 112–13
immune system problems. See blood and immune system problems
indemnity insurance. See disability insurance
infertility. See fertility
information,
  about medical procedures, 50
  and children, 52
  Freedom of Information Act, 56
  genetic, 56
information seeking skills, developing, 278
information sources.
  See American Cancer Society, Cancer Care, Inc., Candlelighters Childhood Cancer Foundation, community resources, insurance resources, legal information resources, Leukemia Society, National Alliance of Breast Cancer Organizations, National Cancer Institute, National Coalition for Cancer Survivorship, newsletters, UsToo, Y-Me.
  See also resources; Internet
informed consent, 12, 50–51
insurance. See disability insurance, health insurance, life insurance, Social Security benefits, veteran's benefits
insurance resources, 306
insurance terms, 201–4
interferon, 11
interleukin–2, 11
Internet, cancer information on the, 286–89
IRS. See financial impact of cancer, deducting medical expenses from taxes

Job Accommodation Network, 232, 234
job accommodation, 233
job discrimination. See employment and cancer survivors

Joint Commission on Accreditation of Healthcare Organizations (JCAHO), 45
Joshua's Tent, 131
Journal of the National Cancer Institute, 82

Karuschkat, Jane, 217–218
Keeling, Wayne, 103
kidney damage, 25
Klein, Carol, 218
Kushner, Rabbi Harold, 96

laetrile, 79
late effects, 23–24, 26
legal concerns, 244–54
legal information resources, 315–23
Lehman, Betsy, 48
Leigh, Susan, 262
Lerner, Michael, 80, 81
leukemia,
  acute myelogenous, 25
  treatment related, 25–26
Leukemia Society, 68
Levy, Sandra, MD, 94
liability, doctor's, 51
life insurance, 196–98
  and living benefits, 198
    viaticating, 198
    accelerating, 198
living benefits. See life insurance
Living Through Cancer Journal, 80
living will, 246
Logan-Carrillo, Catherine, 138
long-term effects, 23–24
long-term survivors, and medical problems, 23
loss and grief, 130
  grieving behaviors, 133
  hiding grief, 133
  managing grief, 132
Love, Medicine, and Miracles, 81
low blood counts, 18–19, 25
lung tissue injury, 24

macrobiotic diet, 76. See also nutrition
ma huang. See treatments, herbal medicine
Make Today Count, 140
Making the Most of Your Next Doctor Visit, 39
male sexual problems. See sexual problems
malpractice, 250–54
managed care plans, 173
manual healing, 77.

See also therapeutic touch; unconventional treatment
massage, 77
mastectomy, 22
Medicaid, and home health aides, 67
Medicaid, 181
  eligibility, 182
medical information. See resources
Medical Information Bureau, 191
medical records,
  confidentiality of, 52
  access to, 53, 55, 56
Medical Records: Getting Yours, 56
medical savings account, 171
Medicare, 176–77, 178–81
  eligibility, 182
Medicare, and home health aides, 67
Medicare HMOs, 180–81
Medigap, 178, 179
menopause, 21, 26
menstrual period, 20–21
metastasis, definition of, 8
mind/body control, 76, 81
Modern Healthcare, 45
modification of the immunologic system, 11
MSA. See medical savings account
Mullan, Fitzhugh, xvi
myths about cancer, 263–64

National Alliance of Breast Cancer Organizations, 68
National Association for Home Care, 67
National Cancer Institute, 44, 68, 283
National Cancer Institute's Cancer Information Service, 12
  publications of, 283.
  See also CancerFax, CancerNet
National Coalition for Cancer Survivorship (NCCS), 68, 141
  Eighth Annual Assembly of, 57
  founding of 265–66
National Committee for Quality Assurance (NCQA), 175, 199
National Hospice Organization, 70
National Institute of Health Office of Alternative Medicine.
  See Office of Alternative Medicine
nausea and vomiting, 7, 15–17
  antinausea medications, 7
negotiation skills, 279
nervous system injury, 24
neurotoxicity, 19
neutropenia. See low blood counts
new approaches, 9, 10.
  See also adjuvant therapy, bone mar-

row transplantation, modification of
   the immunologic system, hyperthermia treatment
New England Journal of Medicine, 82
newsletters about cancer survivorship,
   303
nurses, private duty, 66
nutrition, 15–16, 28, 76
nutritional services, 68

O'Connor, Sandra Day, 117
Office of Alternative Medicine (OAM),
   76
Office of Consumer Protection, 55
Official Directory of Medical Specialists
oncologist, selecting an, 35
oncology social workers. See social
   workers
oophorectomy, 22
Operation Uplift, 160
orchiectomy, 22
ostomy, 67
   intercourse after, 67

pain, 12
   acute pain, 12
   chronic pain, 13
   controlling pain,
      medication, 13
   pain clinic, 14
   relaxation techniques, 14
   treatment of, 12
palliation, 7
palliative care, 69
partial penectomy, 22
patient's rights, 51
PDQ, 12, 284
peer support, 141–62
   145, 146, 147
   established organizations, 155.
      See also peer-support groups
peer-support groups, 139, 141–43,
   145–62
   confidentiality and, 57
   multicultural, 155
   organizing, 151–53
   resources for, 153–55
pelvic radiation therapy, 22
penectomy. See partial penectomy; total
   penectomy
People Living Through Cancer, 141,
   158–59
Persons With Cancer Speak Out, 267
pharmacologic treatments, 77.
   See also unconventional treatment
phases of treatment, 7

initial diagnostic and treatment phase,
   7
Phoenix, The, 140
physician, choosing, 33, 35
   See also oncologist; primary care
      physician
Physician Data Query. See PDQ
platelets, 18
point-of-service, 44, 173
posttreatment care, 50
power of attorney, 250
prevention of cancer, 27
primary care physician, selecting a, 35
privacy. See confidentiality
Privacy Act of 1974, 54, 55
privilege, doctor-patient.
   See confidentiality
problem solving skills, developing, 279
professional medical societies, 290
prostate cancer,
   and finasteride, 29
   hormone treatment for, 22
prostatectomy. See radical prostatectomy
pruritus. See skin changes
psychiatrists, 65
psychologists, 65
Public Citizen's Health Research
   Group, 56

quality of life concerns, 71
Questionable Methods of Cancer
   Treatment Management, 85
QT alumni, 156

radiation,
   and fetal development, 21
   avoiding excess, 28.
   See also treatment types
radiation to breast, 22
radical cystectomy, 22
radical hysterectomy, 22
radical prostatectomy, 22
radical vulvectomy, 22
radon, and cancer, 28–29
Reach for Recovery, 140–141
Ready to Live, Prepared to Die, 131
records, patient's medical, 50
rectal cancer, 29
recurrence, monitoring for, 25
red blood cells. See low blood counts
refusing treatment, 50, 52, 247
rehabilitation
   activities, 104
   resources,
      federal vocational, 234
      state vocational, 233

zxspecialists, 67
resources, 283–325.
   See also information sources
respiratory problems, 20
retroperitoneal lymph node dissection,
   22
Ritchie, Walter, 215
Rieger, Regina, 251
rights of bereaved, 135
rights of patients, 50, 51, 52, 54–55, 56

screening, cancer, goals of, 5
selenium, 76
self-blame. See guilt
self-esteem, 106
self-image, 101, 102
self-worth, 106
sexual desire. See sexual functioning
sexual functioning, 20–22
sexual problems associated with cancer,
   20–22
sexually transmitted diseases and cancer,
   29
shortness of breath, with lung tissue
   injury, 24.
   See also respiratory problems
side effects, 12
Siegel, Bernie, MD, 81
Siegel, David, MD, 80, 82
skin changes, 19
social impact of cancer, 102.
   See also attitudes toward cancer; social
      stigma of cancer
Social Security benefits, 241
social stigma of cancer, 104
social workers, 63–64
solid tumors, 26
Spingarn, Natalie Davis, 32
Stanford Health Services, 160
sterility. See conception and sterility
stomatitis, 16
Stovall, Ellen, 274
stress and cancer, 81,
   coping with, 108–10
support groups. See peer-support
   groups
surgery. See also treatment types
Surviving!, 161
survivor, definitions of, 276
survivor organizations, 162.
   See also peer-support groups
survivors,
   advocating for. (See advocacy)
   childhood, 25
survivorship, 63, 162
   movement, 265

A CANCER *survivor's* ALMANAC

stages of, 267–71
    acute stage, 268
    extended stage, 268
    permanent stage, 269.
    See also empowerment
symptoms of cancer, 12

T cells, 76, 109
taste, 16
Tax Equity Fiscal Responsibility Act (TEFRA), 178
terminal illness, 130
Texas Cancer Council, 71
therapeutic touch, 78.
    See also unconventional treatment
therapy, 99
    enterostomal, 67
    occupational, 67
    physical, 67
    sexual, 67
    speech, 67
tobacco, cancer and, 27
total pelvic extenteration with vaginal reconstruction, 22
total penectomy, 22
transplantation. See bone marrow transplantation
treatment,
    cancer recurrence, 8
    follow-up care, 8, 64
    initial diagnostic and treatment phase, 7
    maintenance phase, 8
        nurses and, 66
    phases of, 7, 8
    refusing, 50, 52
    side effects of, 12
treatment plan, 6, 7, 34, 43
treatments
    alternative. (See unconventional treatments; clinical trials)
    biologic, 77
    experimental. (See unconventional treatment; clinical trials)
    unconventional, 75. (See also clinical trials)
        biooelectromagnetic, 77
        biologic treatment, 77
        herbal medicine, 78
        laetrile, 79
        manual healing, 77
        pharmacologic treatment, 77
        therapeutic touch, 78
treatment side effects, 12
treatment types,
    surgery, 9

radiation, 9
chemotherapy, 9
tumor necrosis factor, 11
turban, ice, 18

unconventional treatment, 75–85
    alternative systems of medical practice, 77
    bioelectromagnetic application, 77
    biologic treatment, 77
    cost of, 82
    herbal medicine, 77
    issues involved in, 79–80
    manual healing, 77
    pharmacologic treatment, 77
    therapeutic touch, 78.
    See also clinical trials
Unconventional Drug Treatments, 85
unemployment disability laws, 232
United Jewish Appeal, 70
United Ostomy Association, 139
Us Too, 68, 155–57

VA. See the Department of Veterans Affairs
veteran's benefits, 243
Visiting Nurses Association, 70
visiting your doctor. See consultations with a caregiver
vitamin C, 76
vitamin E, 76
vocational rehabilitation, 232–34
vomiting, 15–17
vulvectomy. See radical vulvectomy

warning signs of cancer, 30
weight gain, 15
weight maintenance, 15
Weyrich, Dr. Raymond, 251
When Bad Things Happen to Good People, 70, 96
white cell counts. See low blood counts
white cell growth factor. See growth factor
wigs, 18
Words That Heal, Words That Harm, 40
worker's compensation, 231–32
World Wide Web. See Internet

Y-Me, 68, 155–56

About the NCCS

The National Coalition for Cancer Survivorship (NCCS) is a nonprofit organization that informs, serves, and advocates on behalf of its members and in support of the more than 8 million cancer survivors in the United States. Founded in 1986, NCCS is a national consumer network of individuals, organizations, and institutions serving tens of thousands of cancer survivors and those who care for them.

Join/Support NCCS ■ Annual Membership Options:

- ❏ Individual Membership—$35
- ❏ Individual Sustaining—$65
- ❏ Individual Patron—$500
- ❏ Physician-Friend—$100
- ❏ Organizations (budgets < $150,000)—$65
- ❏ Organizations (budgets $150,000–$1 million)—$125
- ❏ Organizations (budgets > $1 million)—$250
- ❏ Institutions (budgets < $1 million)—$200
- ❏ Institutions (budgets > $1 million)—$350

Donations

❏ $500   ❏ $250   ❏ $100   ❏ $50   ❏ Other $_____

This donation is:

- ❏ In memory of _____
- ❏ In honor of the (specify milestone) of _____
- ❏ Send acknowledgement to _____

Please indicate whether you are contributing as an individual or an organization.

Name _____   Phone _____
Organization (if any) _____
Institution (if any) _____   Department _____
Address _____
City _____   State _____   Zip _____

NCCS is a 501(c)3, tax-exempt organization. Send checks payable to the NCCS to:

NCCS
1010 Wayne Avenue, 5th Floor
Silver Spring, MD 20910
301-650-8868